AESTHETIC DERMATOLOGY

NOTICE

AESTHETIC DERMATOLOGY

Lawrence Charles Parish, M.D.

Gary P. Lask, M.D.

McGRAW-HILL, INC.
Health Professions Division

*New York • St. Louis • San Francisco • Colorado Springs • Auckland • Bogotá
Caracas • Hamburg • Lisbon • London • Madrid • Mexico • Milan • Montreal
New Delhi • Paris • San Juan • São • Paulo • Singapore • Sydney • Tokyo • Toronto*

AESTHETIC DERMATOLOGY

The editors were Ellen Datloff and Gail Gavert.
The production supervisor was Annette Mayeski.
The cover was designed by York Graphic Services, Inc.
who set this book in Trump Medieval.
Kingsport/Arcata was printer and binder.

1 2 3 4 5 6 7 8 9 KGSKGS 9 7 6 5 4 3 2 1

ISBN 0-07-048476-7

Library of Congress Cataloging-in-Publication Data
Aesthetic dermatology/[edited by] Lawrence Charles Parish, Gary P. Lask.
p. cm.
Includes bibliographical references.
ISBN 0-07-048476-7:
1. Skin—Diseases—Treatment. 2. Beauty, Personal. I. Parish, Lawrence Charles.
[DNLM: 1. Dermatology—methods. 2. Esthetics. WR 100 A254]
RL110.A33 1991
616.5—dc20
DNLM/DLC
for Library of Congress 89-13810
CIP

To Sheila and Karen

Contents

PART II

GENERAL CONSIDERATIONS

31

CHAPTER

PART IV

SKIN STRUCTURES

PART V

TISSUE INCREASES AND DECREASES

Contributors

Mohamed Amer, M.D. [20]
Professor and Chairman of Dermatology and Venereology, Zagazig University Faculty of Medicine, Zagazig, Egypt; Visiting Professor of Dermatology, Jefferson Medical College, Thomas Jefferson University, Philadelphia, Pennsylvania.

Robert N. Axelrod, M.D. [19]
Associate Clinical Professor of Ophthalmology, University of California at Los Angeles School of Medicine, Los Angeles, California.

Robert Baran, M.D. [25]
Head of the Division of Dermatology, Centre Hospitalier, Cannes, France.

Daniel Beniamini-Loker, M.D. [5]
Dermatologist, Instituto de Biomedicina, Vargas School of Medicine, Central University of Venezuela, Caracas, Venezuela.

Earle W. Brauer, M.D. [3]
Associate Professor of Clinical Dermatology, New York University School of Medicine, New York, New York.

William P. Coleman III, M.D. [29]
Clinical Associate Professor of Dermatology, Tulane University School of Medicine, New Orleans, Louisiana.

Gustavo Colon, M.D. [29]
Clinical Associate Professor of Plastic Surgery, Tulane University School of Medicine, New Orleans, Louisiana.

Laurence M. David, M.D. [7]
Director, Institute of Laser and Cosmetic Surgery, Hermosa Beach, California.

David M. Duffy, M.D. [27]
Assistant Clinical Professor of Medicine (Dermatology), University of California at Los Angeles School of Medicine, Los Angeles, California.

Pierre F. Fournier, M.D. [28, 30]
President, the French Society of Aesthetic Surgery, Paris, France.

Robert P. Friedman, M.D. [2]
Assistant Clinical Lecturer in Internal Medicine (Dermatology), University of Arizona College of Medicine, Tucson, Arizona.

Edward Glassberg, M.D. [7]
Resident in Dermatology, Thomas Jefferson University Hospital, Philadelphia, Pennsylvania

Mauricio Goihman-Yahr, M.D., Ph.D. [5]
Professor of Dermatology and Head of Section of Immunology I, Instituto de Biomedicina, Vargas School of Medicine, Central University of Venezuela, Caracas, Venezuela.

Norman Goldstein, M.D. [13]
Clinical Professor of Dermatology, John A. Burns School of Medicine, University of Hawaii, Manoa, Hawaii.

Charles H. Greenbaum, M.D. [4]
Clinical Professor of Dermatology, Jefferson Medical College, Thomas Jefferson University, Philadelphia, Pennsylvania.

Steven S. Greenbaum, M.D. [4, 16, 20]
Assistant Professor of Dermatology, Jefferson Medical College, Thomas Jefferson University, Philadelphia, Pennsylvania.

Eckart Haneke, M.D. [25]
Professor and Chairman of Dermatology, Ferdinand Sauerbruch Klinikum, Wuppertal, Federal Republic of Germany.

Elliot M. Heiman, M.D. [2]
Clinical Professor of Psychiatry, University of Arizona College of Medicine, Tucson, Arizona.

Harry M. Humeniuk, M.D. [6]
Resident in Dermatology, Thomas Jefferson University Hospital, Philadelphia, Pennsylvania.

Robert W. Hutcherson, M.D. [18]
Clinical Professor of Surgery (Head and Neck), University of California at Los Angeles School of Medicine, Los Angeles, California.

Waine C. Johnson, M.D. [14]
Clinical Professor of Dermatology, University of Pennsylvania School of Medicine, Philadelphia, Pennsylvania.

A. Paul Kelly, M.D. [8]
Professor of Internal Medicine (Dermatology) and Chairman of Dermatology, Charles R. Drew University of Science, Los Angeles, California, Clinical Associate Professor of Medicine (Dermatology), University of California at Los Angeles School of Medicine, Los Angeles, California.

Francisco Kerdel-Vegas, M.D. [Introduction]
Ambassador to the Court of Saint James from the Republic of Venezuela, London, England; Visiting Professor of Dermatology, Jefferson Medical College, Thomas Jefferson University, Philadelphia, Pennsylvania.

Robert Kotler, M.D. [15]
Associate Clinical Professor of Surgery (Head and Neck), University of California at Los Angeles School of Medicine, Los Angeles, California.

Gary P. Lask, M.D. [6, 7, 16, 20]
Associate Clinical Professor of Medicine (Dermatology), University of California at Los Angeles School of Medicine, Los Angeles, California.

Giovanni Micali, M.D. [11]
Professor of Plastic Surgery, University of Catania Faculty of Medicine, Catania, Italy.

Larry E. Millikan, M.D. [22, 26]
Professor and Chairman of Dermatology, Tulane University School of Medicine, New Orleans, Louisiana.

Frederic E. Mohs, M.D. [9]
Emeritus Clinical Professor of Surgery, University of Wisconsin School of Medicine, Madison, Wisconsin.

Ronald L. Moy, M.D. [17]
Associate Clinical Professor of Medicine (Dermatology), University of California at Los Angeles School of Medicine, Los Angeles, California.

Jean-Paul Ortonne, M.D. [10]
Professor and Chairman of Dermatology, Nice Medical School, Hôpital Pasteur, University of Sophia-Antipolis, Nice, France.

Emiliano Panconesi, M.D. [1]
Professor and Chairman of Dermatology I, University of Florence Faculty of Medicine, Florence, Italy.

Lawrence Charles Parish, M.D. [12, 20]
Clinical Professor of Dermatology and Director, Jefferson Center for International Dermatology, Jefferson Medical College, Thomas Jefferson University, Philadelphia, Pennsylvania; Visiting Professor of Dermatology, Yonsei University College of Medicine, Seoul, South Korea; Visiting Professor of Dermatology and Venereology, Zagazig University Faculty of Medicine, Zagazig, Egypt.

Umberto M. Reali, M.D. [11]
Associate Professor of Plastic Surgery, Department of Dermatology I, University of Florence Faculty of Medicine, Florence, Italy.

Terence J. Ryan, D.M., F.R.C.P. (U.K.) [21]
Consultant Dermatologist, Oxford University, Oxford, England; Visiting Professor of Dermatology, Jefferson Medical College, Thomas Jefferson University, Philadelphia, Pennsylvania.

Richard K. Scher, M.D. [24]
Professor of Clinical Dermatology, Columbia University College of Physicians and Surgeons, New York, New York.

Stephen N. Snow, M.D. [9]
Assistant Professor of Surgery, University of Wisconsin School of Medicine, Madison, Wisconsin.

Susan C. Taylor, M.D. [24]
Clinical Associate in Dermatology, University of Pennsylvania School of Medicine, Philadelphia, Pennsylvania.

Walter P. Unger, M.D. [23]
Assistant Professor of Medicine (Dermatology), University of Toronto Faculty of Medicine, Toronto, Ontario, Canada.

Joseph A. Witkowski, M.D. [12]
Clinical Professor of Dermatology, University of Pennsylvania School of Medicine, Philadelphia, Pennsylvania.

John M. Yarborough, M.D. [26]
Clinical Professor of Dermatology, Tulane University School of Medicine, New Orleans, Louisiana.

Preface

The concept of aesthetic or cosmetic dermatology is not a revolutionary, new discovery. About a century ago, Edmund Saalfield of Berlin prepared a small manual, translated into English as *Lectures on Cosmetic Treatment.* He told his readers:

> Only a short time has elapsed since the Art of Cosmetics has obtained recognition in medical circles. This special branch of Dermatology has indeed been left too long in the hands of quacks, and even to-day in many newspapers one is able to see how much mischief is done in this department.[1]

Physicians such as John Woodbury of New York, who wrote *What Dermatology Has to Do with Beauty: How to Relieve All Imperfections of the Skin,*[2] illustrated this concept and discouraged ethical dermatologists from the area. Fortunately, books like *Personal Beauty: How to Cultivate and Preserve it in Accordance with the Laws of Health*[3] and *The Care of the Skin*[4] by C.J. White, professor of dermatology at Harvard University, indicate that some in the medical community, nevertheless, had a little interest in helping people improve their appearance.

Dermatology once shunned any therapeutic modality that focused solely on the patient's emotional well-being as opposed to disease alteration. Cutaneous medicine and surgery now accept the challenge of correcting and improving the patient's appearance. Pigmentary changes that cause social ostracism can be remedied with photo-activated chemicals. Devastating birthmarks can be eliminated through the use of lasers. Disfiguring scars can be repaired. Even the ravages of aging can be reduced. Cosmetics can be used to advantage to diminish dermatologic abnormalities or to make one more attractive.

This text concentrates on those aspects of dermatology for which therapeutic intervention may be needed. Diagnosis and clinical description are included only when they may assist the practitioner in choosing the most appropriate therapy.

Details of medical and surgical therapy will be given in a straightforward fashion. In some instances, the treatment or procedure can be carried out after studying the particular chapter. In other situations, additional training or reading is needed; it is hoped that in these cases enough information is presented for the practitioner to be able to make an appropriate choice.

The inspiration for this project came from the late Jerry Stone, an outstanding medical editor. We are most appreciative of the secretarial skills of Carmela Ciferni. Lastly, Ellen Datloff, Editorial Director; Gail Gavert, Development Editor; and the staff at McGraw-Hill deserve a special vote of thanks for their support and encouragement.

Lawrence Charles Parish, M.D.
Gary P. Lask, M.D.

References

1. Saalfield E. Lectures on Cosmetic Treatment. New York: Paul B. Hoeber, 1910:1.
2. Woodbury JH. What Dermatology Has to Do with Beauty: How to remove all imperfections of the Skin. New York; private printing, ?1888.
3. Brinton DG, Napheys GH. Personal Beauty: How to Cultivate and Preserve it in Accordance with the Laws of Health. Springfield, MA: WJ Holland, 1890.
4. White CJ. The Care of the Skin. Cambridge, MA: Harvard University Press, 1914.

Introduction

FRANCISCO KERDEL-VEGAS

Aesthesis is the perception of the senses, or, more specifically, of the beautiful. In relation to the skin, it can be limited to the physical appearance: shape, color, texture, and suppleness. The odor emanating from the skin has its own characteristics. The descriptive term aesthetic can be said to be "the science of the conditions of sensuous perception."[1] When we couple it with the word for the study of the skin, we arrive at the term *aesthetic dermatology*.

The skin, the largest organ of the body, has many functions, including sensation, temperature control, fluid balance, immunological recognition, and ultraviolet protection. The functions are not unique to this organ, but they are significant. Racial and sexual characteristics are also demonstrated by the ectoderm and its appendages.

FIRST IMPRESSIONS

The skin, to paraphrase Argentinian author Marcial Quiroga, is the organ of introduction. The first visual impression we receive on meeting another person consists of the characteristics of the skin, especially that of the face. Special importance has been given to the aesthetics of the skin from the

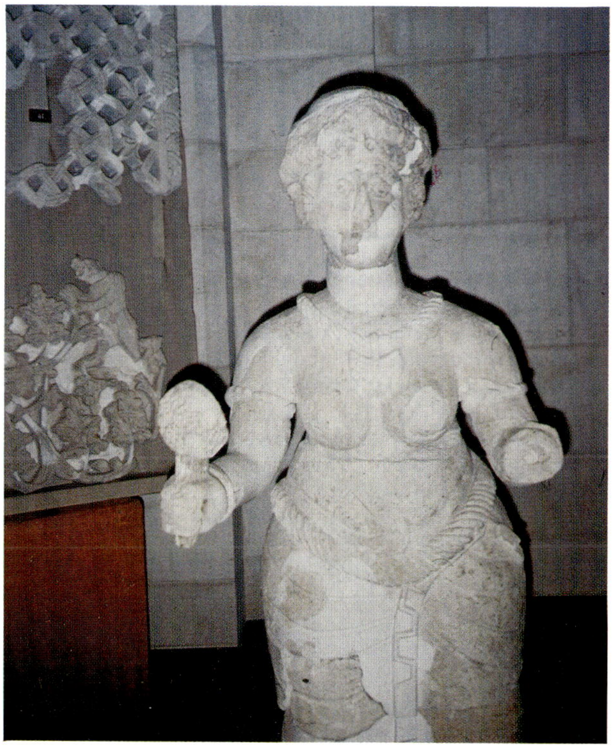

FIGURE 1
Dancer's statue, eighth century. *(Courtesy of the Israel Department of Antiquities and Museums.)*

PART I

BACKGROUND

CHAPTER

1

Cultural and Psychological Aspects of Aesthetic Dermatology

EMILIANO PANCONESI

In terms of aesthetic dermatology, the appearance of the skin is everything. It may only be a symptom of the underlying dermatologic *disease* or a manifestation of other disease, but these symptoms represent all, or almost all, of the problem of cosmetic *alterations* of the skin. Thus, it is often difficult to determine just where the boundary lies between disease and aesthetically disturbing symptoms. For one patient a "minor" cutaneous disease may have disproportionately severe psychological consequences, whereas another patient with a serious disease is apparently able to underestimate or ignore even obvious disfigurement. Every dermatologist is familiar with the obsessively insistent pleas of the acne patient to "get rid of the horror," contrasting starkly with the stoic endurance of so many patients with facial cancer.

Even before birth, when the central nervous system develops out of the ectoderm, the mind and the skin of the individual are intimately related. The appearance of the skin so conditions an individual's self-image that any pathological alteration can have psychological consequences.

HISTORICAL BACKGROUND

As far as we know, only human beings take an aesthetic interest in their appearance. They defend it from the attacks of time and climate, trying whenever possible to modify it, usually to better it. They even try to falsify their appearances. Attempts are sometimes made to construct a different identity in the process of falsifying the appearance.

This obsession with appearance is not entirely the product of the modern mass media. It is a very old and voluminously discussed aspect of human nature. What is new, perhaps, is the way in which the mass media promote rapid change in terms of detail, custom, and overall trends. The basic idea of cosmetics, the artificial creation of "order," in Greek *cosmos*, can be traced to the oldest of recorded civilizations. In 2200 BCE, it is reported that King Meri of Egypt spent a patrimony, all his earnings from fishing in a great lake, on unguents and perfumes for his wife.

For the ancient Greeks and Romans, the problem of cosmetics was one of morality, or truth and the appearance of truth. Xenophon reports the story of Iscomac who told Socrates that he had succeeded in convincing his wife to choose "true beauty," the virtues of the good housewife, rather than the "appearance of beauty," the product of cosmetics and Oriental frivolities.

Galen, one of the great physicians of ancient times, took a moderate position: he distinguished between good cosmetic, *kosmetiké techne,* which preserved and protected beauty, and bad cosmetic, *kommotiké techne,* which was artificially constructed and could be "bought." Despite this distinction, Galen shared the prevailing view that cosmetics were somehow "immoral," a frequently unfair attitude that appears elsewhere both in classical sources on the subject of beauty and cosmetics and in even more pronounced examples found in other cultures and historical periods.

This prejudice and moralizing is still with us. Girls with a "soap and water" look are presumed virtuous, whereas those who use heavy makeup are presumed immoral. Despite this residual moralizing, most women wear some makeup, and some try at any cost to be more attractive by eliminating or covering up defects and trying to look younger. Youth, closely related to the ideal of beauty, is a *leit motiv* of cosmetics.

THE PSYCHOLOGICAL SIGNIFICANCE OF THE SKIN

Because of its critical role in an individual's self-image, the skin has always attracted the attention of psychologists. The connection between the skin and self-image begins very early in our ontogenesis.[1] In fact, as Anna Freud tells us, at the beginning of life, being hugged, caressed, and blandished make the various parts of the child's body sensitive. It helps the child construct a healthy body image and makes his narcissistic libido grow and simultaneously promotes the love object by consolidating the bond between mother and child.

The skin is important in relation to the development of the body-self and the mental-self because of (and together with) its fundamental tactile function. Among its many other functions is a "dermo-optical" function, so defined by the well-known psychoanalyst Didier Anzieu.[2] This function presumes that the skin has some visional capacity (!) as well as and perhaps because of its "visibility." It is to this latter function, the visibility of the skin, that cosmetology is related above all. Another function or capacity of the skin is thought to be that it inscribes "sensorial traces," a sort of *pictogram.*[3] Dermato-cosmetologists are reminded immediately of the painting of faces and bodies (including the application of makeup, pomades, or medications) in various cultural-anthropological settings from prehistoric times on, as if the skin were a mirror or like Perseus' shield,[5] which reflects the picture of reality.

The skin constitutes what René Thom calls an *interface,* serving as an envelope which simultaneously limits or contains the body, conditions exchanges between inside and outside, and most important of all for the aesthetic dermatologist, presents its visible self.

Because it is visible, the skin is the site where conflicts regarding exhibitionism find expression.[4] A study of the amount of exhibitionism contained in cosmetological rituals and requests for cosmetic procedures might be an important reference in the psychological study of an individual and would be relevant to the general problem of psychological motivations in patients seeking professional aesthetic dermatological help.

CUTANEOUS FOCAL POINTS FOR AESTHETIC ATTENTION

The aesthetic cosmetological skin ego (an extension of Didier Anzieu's idea of Moi-Peau?[2]) is part of an *aesthetic ego,* which is expressed in and by a body ego that observes the skin and itself, with attention being focused on particular features and portions of the skin. Perhaps each distinct portion of the puzzle that forms our cutaneous covering merits consideration in terms of psychological significance, but for our purposes we can say that our patients give particular attention to the face (mouth, hair, eyes) and perhaps to the body itself taken as a whole. The latter belongs to the field of aesthetic medicine as opposed to cosmetic dermatology and does not enter into this discussion.

THE FACE

The face, and the mouth or eyes alone, is known for its profound psychological resonance. St. Jerome (letter 54) said, "The face is the mirror of the mind. . . and eyes without speaking confess the secrets of the heart." In terms of individual identity, these are the most important of all body parts. They are the features that make the strongest impression on other people, a basic component of sexual attraction and the changing ideal of beauty.

Because of the importance of the face, the use of makeup is a common practice, although opinions have long been divided on the proper use of makeup. Ovid wrote that cosmetics on the face should not be noticeable.[5] This contrasts with Baudelaire's opinion in his "Eloge du Maquillage," when he talks about makeup as preparing a mask or disguise.

> The painting of one's face should not be done with the vulgar, inadmissible aim of imitating beautiful nature and trying to rival youth. . . . Who would dare assign to art the sterile function of imitating nature? Makeup must not be hidden to avoid being noticed, it must, on the contrary, be displayed, if not with affection, at least with some sort of candor.[6]

In either manner makeup on the face plays a large part in the restoration of one's body image; for example, eliminating impressions of oily, dirty, or dull skin, or trying to harmonize colors, making them blend with that of the hair, which can also change color to match even one's clothes! An error in the choice of lipstick or mascara can "ruin" a face or give it a grotesque aspect, as in the case of bright red lipstick on the pale skin of an elderly woman. The right shade of makeup can favor the look of light skin, classically favored for women, or dark, once preferred for men but much appreciated also in women now that the tanned sporty look is in favor (despite the risk of skin cancer posed by excessive exposure to sunlight).

We also know how sweet and romantic the blush of an adolescent can be, but blushing can become a torment if it happens too often and, above all, when it leads to erythrophobia. In the latter case, the ultrasensitive subject can find help in makeup that makes the flushing less evident and partially interrupts the vicious circle which is often the base of the disturbance.

THE MOUTH

The lips "talk," even psychologically and without opening. According to Knapp[10], often nonverbal communication depends very much on the lips: if their characteristics are able to tell us something about personality, in particular, as far as we know, about sensuality (a woman with thick or fleshy lips is considered sensuous) and temperament, their makeup (like that of the cheeks) has for centuries (the *polderos* of the ancient Greeks, the *focus* of the ancient Romans!) tried to deceive, suggesting variations on the theme of attractiveness. Unfortunately, the makeup chosen follows the dictates of fashion more often than one's desires regarding self-representation: just think of the variations in the shades of lipsticks during our lifetime, over 10-year periods, from bright red to pale pink to almost white, and then bright red again.

THE HAIR

The "crowning glory" is of such great importance, symbolic and real, that it has always been bought by those who did not have or like their own. The particular position which hair held in the past is valid still today; the hair is important and it is perfectly acceptable to buy and wear wigs of other people's hair. Hair loss is a threat, and causes great suffering, even to men who are often the subjects of such loss, and particularly to young men (who may suffer premature androgenetic defluvium). It may be psychogenic (as in telogen effluvium) and have important somatopsychic implications with various, well-known psychological and symbolic motivations.

Over the centuries many different cultures* have paid special attention to the hair which has represented power and force (including sexual prowess), beauty, physical strength (the Biblical Samson!), and social position (in relation to the quantity and quality of one's hair and the perfec-

* *ietroi kefalés:* According to Herodotus, these were the "doctors of the head." He also wrote of an unguent made of "kiki" that made the hair beautiful.

tion of the hair-do). It can be a status symbol or an indication of one's conservatism or liberalism, a sign of liberty or transgression (as in the 1960s) or disorder. Short hair can call to mind the idea of order (as in the case of soldiers) and it has been used as a punishment or sign of condemnation (during World War II, women's heads were shaved if they were considered too friendly with Nazi soldiers, as were the heads of Irish women who made friends with British soldiers in other times).

Hair has always been used in witchcraft and black magic. Sorceresses could purportedly tell a lot about a person from a lock of hair and even use it to influence the person's destiny. In Greek mythology, Persephone cut hair from her victims to consecrate them to the powers of the underworld. Myths, rites, and written history have all supplied us with explanations as to why problems of appearance related to the hair are among those most suffered, and therefore most instrumentalized. Promises of miracles on the part of charlatans as well as honest attempts to realize difficult cures on the part of honest cosmetologists have all been heeded at one time or another. Some dermatologists, besieged by patients who want their hair to grow back, let it be known that they do not treat hair problems. Others try to alleviate the patient's suffering from thinning hair or onset of baldness by prescribing topical minoxidil.

One thing is certain: "The hair or hair-do is halfway between nature and culture, between skin and clothes, an ornament which delimits something visible and something hidden."[7] It is a fundamental, natural covering that extends the body past its very cephalic extreme with "offshoots" that are particularly evident to all. The hair is clothing that is considered tragically unchangeable because it is alive. In fact, it can be modified, cut, modelled, and dyed time after time, unlike any other part of the body.

In agreement with some psychiatrists there is no reason to marvel, after all, if the hair is a "source of intense ideological and emotional, affective conditioning" and "a means of nonverbal communication, an instrument for relating, a part of the body that is objectified as if it were something out of context and invested with special social, religious, magico-mystical meanings" (A. Cossidente, personal communication, 1989).

The result is the special position of the hair, that of an object which influences the mind and is at the same time the terrain on which the mind externalizes its fantasies. The bidirectional psychological interaction between the mind and hair creates a complex situation with intricate dynamics in cases of alterations to the hair leading to very diverse behavioral and emotional-affective modifications, depending on individual personality characteristics.[7]

CONCLUSIONS

Knowledge of the cultural, historical, and psychological aspects of appearance and cosmetics should be part of the cultural background of every aesthetic dermatologist. These principles should be the pillars of medical practice, and will allow the realization of empathy between doctor and patient, always important but particularly necessary in aesthetic dermatology.

An aesthetic *disorder,* a disturbance of a patient's *cosmos,* whether real or imaginary, serious or minor, causes suffering and upsets the patient. A patient's self-image is different from the doctor's objective evaluation. A doctor who minimizes or refuses to consider the patient's perspective will not be successful.

One must always remember that a patient has special expectations when the reasons for visiting the doctor have aesthetic implications. For such a patient, the office visit is a magical moment, and the doctor must be aware of this and use the moment to satisfy these expectations and help the patient.

The Visit

A visit to the doctor is an important ritual, one of a lifetime of rituals of coming close, being close, experiencing gratifying contact. It is an extension of the first formative magic contact with the mother through the skin. The visit to the aesthetic dermatologist is particularly significant because it involves the surface on which individual's self-image is based. It might be said that the patient is like a child asking for help to correct some disorder, to restore the *cosmos.* The doctor, like a mother, must understand, reassure, and cure, providing alternative forms of the original comforting and caressing.

Thus, at the outset, in the womb of the office,

the aesthetic dermatologist must make a special effort to reassure the patient. As an example, the doctor might inquire of the patient—who may be noticeably disfigured—why he or she has come to the doctor or who is the patient—the parent or the child? Such an approach can reassure the patient, if done with ease, without exaggeration, and in a credible manner. Touch the patient. Patients who have dermatologic disorders often feel like lepers, untouchable and unclean. Offer words of encouragement.

Physicians should develop their own rituals to follow in reassuring their patients with *love* in the very broadest sense. The doctor in this way helps and cures patients, helping them to accept and thus helping to cure themselves.[7,8,9]

REFERENCES

1. Cossidente A. Il significato psicologico della pelle, in Panconesi E. (ed) Lo stress, le emozioni e la pelle. Milan: Masson, 1989.
2. Anzieu D. Le Moi-peau. Paris: Borda, 1985.
3. Castoriadis-Aulaguier P. La violence de l'interpretation. Paris: P.U.F., 1975.
4. Shilder P. The image and appearance of the human body, London: P. Regan, 1985.
5. Ovidio. I cosmetici delle donne, a cura di Rosati G. Venice: Marsilio Ed, 1985.
6. Baudelaire C. Curiosités esthétiques. Paris: Editions Garnier Freres, 1962.
7. Pomey-Rey D. Capelli e psicologia, in Zviak C. (ed) Scienza della cura dei capelli. Milan: Masson, 1987.
8. Moravia S. La cattura dell'invisible, in Panconesi E. (ed). Lo stress, le emozioni e la pelle. Milan: Masson, 1989.
9. Panconesi E. Stress and skin diseases: Psychosomatic dermatology. Clin Dermatol. 1984; 2(4):1–282.

CHAPTER

2

Psychiatric Screening of Patients for Aesthetic Procedures

ROBERT P. FRIEDMAN
ELLIOTT M. HEIMAN

Although dermatologists have long recognized the dynamic interplay between the psyche and the skin, the burgeoning field of aesthetic dermatology demands new skills that reflect a heightened awareness of mind/body interactions. Aesthetic surgeons are faced with the difficult task of evaluating the psychological suitability of patients for a wide variety of major and minor cosmetic procedures.

Reaching an understanding of the prospective cosmetic surgery patient's motivation, expectations, and underlying psychological makeup is a vital step in achieving a satisfactory result. Elective cosmetic surgery is designed to produce a happy patient[1]; however, in cosmetic surgery the surgeon's appraisal of the result is less important than the patient's level of satisfaction. For this reason, an astute presurgical psychological evaluation is essential and at times may be more important than a proficient technical procedure.[2]

PSYCHOLOGICAL PROBLEMS

Psychiatrists have found a high incidence of psychological problems and neurotic traits in persons who wish to have aesthetic surgery, including an increased frequency of emotional lability, depression, latent aggressiveness, high sensitivity, low self-confidence, introversion, and frequent somatic signs of anxiety manifested by cardiac, respiratory, and gastrointestinal disturbances.[3] In spite of the fact that many candidates for cosmetic surgery have psychological problems, there is a high success rate for cosmetic surgery, and many patients experience an enhanced feeling of well-being after such surgery.[4] This is probably because physical attractiveness is perceived as being an extremely important aspect of an individual's life. A person who is thought of as "attractive" is also considered to be "sensitive, kind, interesting, strong, poised, modest, sociable, outgoing, exciting, and sexually warm."[5] In addition, a person who considers herself or himself to be unattractive may act in a self-defeating manner. When such a person believes that the cosmetic problem has been corrected, that person is able to act in a much more positive manner, thereby eliciting more positive responses from others. Cosmetic surgery is therefore well justified in such cases.

MOTIVATION AND EXPECTATION

Effective psychological screening of cosmetic surgery candidates must include two fundamental issues: *motivation* and *expectation*.[4] In assessing a patient's reason for seeking surgery (motivation), the physician must be able to discover the true reason for the request.[6] Motivations are classified as being *internal* or *external*. It is generally believed that surgical candidates with internal motives—e.g., "I want to feel more attractive"—are more likely to be pleased with the surgical result than are those with external motives—e.g., "My mother wants me to have this done."[7] In practice, however, most patients exhibit a mixture of internal and external motivation, making this portion of the assessment difficult.

In examining the second fundamental issue—patient expectations—*body image* is an important concept. Body image may be defined as the mental representation of one's body at any moment. When the perception of one's body image is unrealistic, a distortion of body image exists.[2] Any gross distortion will persist postoperatively and can be expected to result in a very dissatisfied patient. Even among individuals with an essentially correct body image, unrealistic expectations often lead to unhappiness, because such patients expect the impossible and are never satisfied with reasonable results. An example would be a patient who expects surgery to save a marriage.

PATIENT CATEGORIES

Although various categories of problem patients are encountered in screening, a few patient types are clear-cut good candidates for aesthetic surgery. The first category includes patients with an obvious disfigurement in whom the need is great and the chances are good that appearance will be improved.[8] Psychological issues are usually minimal, and these patients are the most acceptable candidates for surgery. A second group includes patients whose occupations—entertainers, artists, and business persons—reward them for being more attractive. A third group includes patients who do not like their aging appearance or changes caused by weight loss. A fourth group includes patients with minor cosmetic problems who have long planned to have them corrected.[9]

At the other end of the spectrum are patients whom the surgeon should absolutely exclude from surgery by preoperative screening, for example, those who have serious mental illness, such as schizophrenia with delusions of disfigurement. A physician cannot correct a delusion by means of surgery. Although some individuals with a history of severe mental illness may be reasonable candidates for surgery, it is wise to first obtain a psychiatric consultation.[4]

The second group to be avoided consists of patients who have a history of repeated surgeries or repeated physician visits with chronic dissatisfaction. These patients may make a strong emotional appeal to the surgeon with such phrases as "just a little here" or "the last doctor did it wrong" that may seduce the unwary physician into accepting the case as a challenge. Surgeons should be aware of their own fantasies of omnipotence, because they have no better likelihood of succeeding than did their predecessors.[6]

Another problem group consists of patients who seek surgery in the middle of a life crisis, e.g., a middle-aged woman with recent losses, perhaps a widow or divorcee, who wishes to regain confidence by looking more attractive. Such a goal can be realistic if the individual has the necessary psychological stability and does not view the surgery as solving all of life's problems. If there is uncertainty concerning the suitability or timing of such surgery, a psychiatric evaluation should be requested or a final decision delayed.

A final group of problem patients are those with a distorted body image, as discussed earlier. Individuals having bizarre distortions of body image of delusional proportions should be avoided without exception. On the other hand, a certain degree of distortion is quite common. For instance, people frequently have trouble recognizing themselves on a recording or in a photograph. Often, prospective patients fall somewhere between the delusional and the normal, having a mild degree of distortion of body image. An example of this might be an attractive person who exaggerates the degree of imperfection caused by a few scars and wants a major procedure when a minor procedure would suffice.

For most problem patients, cosmetic surgery is clearly not contraindicated if the surgeon recognizes the need for careful handling and is willing to exert the required effort to meet the patients' emotional demands. In this group are patients who have purely external motivations and unrealistic expectations not associated with a grossly distorted body image.

Certain personality styles may cause problems for the surgeon and therefore should be recognized. Some of these personality types include the following.

1. The *rude* patient is hypercritical and demanding and can be a problem for both the physician and the office staff.[1]
2. The *schizoid* or *isolated* patient may have flat affect, poor eye contact, and a blank stare and be generally vague. As a result, the physician may have difficulty establishing rapport and/or even knowing what the patient expects from the aesthetic procedure.[6]
3. The *obsessive* or *perfectionistic* patient, as well as the *paranoid* patient, pays extreme attention to detail and must have an excessive amount of control over all decisions. Such a patient should be given a detailed plan and must know precisely what is going to happen before, during, and after surgery.[9]
4. The *dependent* patient is often childlike. Such a patient may not ask even the most appropriate questions about the procedure, takes little responsibility for personal care, and may not comply with follow-up.[2]
5. The *hysterical* patient is dramatic and theatrical as well as flirtatious and preoccupied with personal attractiveness. Such a patient may not pay sufficient attention to detail and may be very emotional.[6]

PATIENT SCREENING

The initial patient interview must be done by the aesthetic surgeon, not relegated to other staff members, audiovisual devices, or questionnaires. A relaxed atmosphere, free of interruption, and an adequate time allowance are essential.[2] The surgeon should be prepared to have a second meeting if a final decision cannot be reached.

The screening begins with the initial telephone call and includes interaction with the office staff. Therefore, the staff members must communicate their observations and impressions of the patient to the physician. For instance, a demanding or rude patient should be identified immediately. On first encountering the prospective patient face to face, the surgeon should observe the patient's appearance and behavior, noting the quality of dress (slovenly or meticulous), the quality of eye contact, the ability of the patient to express himself or herself in an organized fashion, the degree of assertiveness or obsequiousness, the attention or inattention to detail, and the quality of affect (depressed or overly expansive).

The physician should then determine the motivation for the individual's request for treatment. Is the motivation primarily internal, such as the improvement of self-esteem, or is it external, such as the urging of a significant person in the patient's life? Is there an obvious reason for surgery, such as a clear disfigurement, or a "payoff," such as career improvement? Establishing how long the person has been considering surgery is also very important, because a patient who is acting on a whim is a poor surgical candidate, whereas an individual who has been considering surgery for a long time has a good prognosis. This information can be easily elicited by asking such questions as, "How long have you wanted this surgery?" and "To what extent have you investigated this procedure?" If the patient seems to be acting on a whim, the best strategy is to temporize and encourage the patient to think more carefully about the decision.

Next, the surgeon must obtain a clear history of past cosmetic procedures, with an eye toward identifying insatiable surgical candidates and patients who express repeated dissatisfaction with preceding physicians.

The presence of unrealistic expectations must be recognized. A question such as "In what way do you expect your life to be different?" will illicit revealing responses regarding expectations. A more open-ended question such as "Why do you want the surgery?" will clarify both motivation and expectations.[10]

The physician should assess the patient's general

psychological strengths and weaknesses by obtaining a careful history, including psychological problems and past treatment, the quality of interpersonal relationships (e.g., marital status and significant others), and life accomplishments (employment, interests, and hobbies). The physician should also directly question the patient about the use of alcohol and other mind-altering substances, as these could impair the patient's judgment concerning the procedure.

Most important, the physician must discuss plainly and fully the risk/benefit ratio of the procedure, making certain that the patient understands both the expected positive results and the possible adverse effects.[11] In cosmetic surgery it is especially important for patients to give informed consent for the procedure. Patients must clearly comprehend the changes that can be expected from the procedure. Any risks, including those attributable to the anesthetic, must be carefully discussed. It is also essential that the physician be sure of having rapport with a prospective cosmetic surgery patient. Does the patient understand what the surgeon is saying, and is there a reasonable doctor-patient relationship so that effective interaction is possible? Although this determination may not be rational and scientific, the surgeon must have a good sense that the patient has the capacity to work with the surgeon before proceeding to surgery.

RECOMMENDATIONS

The dermatologic surgeon must recognize the need to invest a large amount of time and energy in the psychological evaluation of patients. The surgeon must be aware of the psychological issues involved in screening out patients who may not be suitable candidates for surgery as well as identifying patients who, while they are reasonable candidates for surgery, require special attention. The interview must be conducted in an atmosphere that is relaxed and unrushed. The surgeon must also be aware of his or her own personality and recognize those types of patients with whom he or she can and cannot deal. If the surgeon gives psychological issues this kind of attention and approaches the interview with a clear understanding of what information is required, greater patient satisfaction and a sense of increased control over the surgeon's practice will result.

REFERENCES

1. Rees TD. Selection of patients, in Rees TD, Wood-Smith D, Cosmetic Facial Surgery, Philadelphia: WB Saunders, 1973, 17–26.
2. Goin JM, Goin MK. Psychological understanding and management of the plastic surgery patient, in Georgiade NG, Georgiade GS, Riefkohl R, et al. Essentials of Plastic, Maxillofacial, and Reconstructive Surgery. Baltimore: Williams and Wilkins, 1986, 1127–1143.
3. Meyer L, Jacobsson S. Psychiatric and psychosocial characteristics of patients accepted for rhinoplasty. Ann Plastic Surg. 1987; 19:117–130.
4. Thomson JA, Knorr NJ, Edgerton MT. Cosmetic surgery: The psychiatric perspective. Psychosomatics. 1978; 19:7–15.
5. Berscheid E, Gangestad S. The social psychological implications of facial physical attractiveness. Clin Plast Surg. 1982; 9: 289–296.
6. Shulman BH. Psychiatric assessment of the candidate for cosmetic surgery. Otolaryngol Clin North Am. 1980; 13:383–389.
7. Mohl PC. Psychiatric consultation in plastic surgery: The psychiatrist's perspective. Psychosomatics. 1984; 25:474–476.
8. Stegman SJ, Tromovitch TA. Cosmetic Dermatologic Surgery. Chicago: Year Book, 1984, 61–65.
9. Reich J. The interface of plastic surgery and psychiatry. Clin Plast Surg. 1982; 9:367–377.
10. Lavell S, Lewis CM. Safe: A practical guide to psychological factors in selecting patients for facial cosmetic surgery. Ann Plast Surg. 1984; 12:256–259.
11. Schweitzer I. The psychiatric assessment of the patient requesting facial surgery. Austral NZ J Psych. 1989; 23:249–254.

CHAPTER

3

Cosmetics

EARLE W. BRAUER

DEFINITION

In this chapter the term *cosmetics* refers to those substances applied topically to the skin, hair, and nails which influence the appreciation of light and shadow emanating from these structures. These products consist of pigments, dyes, and lakes in a variety of vehicles such as solids and solutions as well as thick and thin emulsion systems. Their skillful application can augment or conceal natural or acquired personal physical attributes to achieve a visual and sensual effect that is considered pleasing, desirable, and advantageous by a particular society and a cultural level within that society. The products considered are standard, conventional stock items: foundation, lipstick, eye makeup, blusher, highlighter, concealer, nail enamel, hair coloring, and perfume. These products are readily available under commonly recognizable brand names everywhere in the world. Package components and product formulation are designed to foster easy application and removal.

INTRODUCTION

Through the ages, almost all societies have tampered to some extent with natural body appearance. Social, economic, and political station are announced and measured through the trappings of personal adornment, e.g., physiognomy, costume, and jewels, as well as life-style, e.g., real property, livestock, and sportscars. Currently, the demographics of population reveal a distinct shift to older age groups at a time when there is a premium on the appearance of youthfulness, which is interpreted as *attractiveness*. The success of a wage earner in maintaining or advacing in a job, the ability of a homemaker to weather the mental depression of the "empty nest syndrome" as children leave the home and menopause begins, the pressure to gain acceptance by one's peer group when a trick of nature or the end result of disease or an accident sets one apart, and the desire to look good because it feels good are only a few of the cogent reasons for seeking the noninvasive, quick, simple, reversible benefits of cosmetics. While the wearing of applied skin color is now widely accepted among women, this practice is for the most part shunned by men, with the exception of hair coloring.

PRINCIPLES OF COSMETIC USE

The observing eye registers form and pattern by the reflected light and shadow an object creates. A teacup is differentiated from its saucer in this manner; similarly, a rough surface can be distinguished from one that is smooth. Alteration in the direction and intensity of the light source also changes one's appreciation of these relationships. The strategic placement of particular colors can mimic this effect when the light source cannot be altered or has been predetermined, for example, the achievement of a three-dimensional effect by an artist working in a two-dimensional medium. This positioning of color, along with its extent, spectrum, and intensity, attracts the eye and "toys" with that which is registered by the brain. This is easy to accept in an actor wearing stage makeup. It can also be achieved with modern cosmetics by anyone with a modicum of dexterity and a genuine desire to improve personal appearance. The face, less so the hair and nails, can be considered an artist's canvas, while cosmetic products with their array of colors constitute the artist's palette. The fundamentals of utilizing these tools are simple; however, just as with a portrait artist, the quality of the end result depends on the skill and technique that can be acquired only through practice.

Acquisition of the cosmetics is only the first step. Familiarity with the products, including how they are applied, how much time one has during the process of application before the product dries or resists further spread, what products can be applied on top of one another, what shades are necessary to achieve the desired results, how shades are blended, and when fingers are the best applicator instruments compared to brushes, are but a few of the technical skills that can be learned only by trial and error.

The desire to improve one's appearance is often stimulated by an important social function such as an anniversary or wedding. A person in this situation will purchase a few "interesting" makeup products, usually without an overall plan. A scant hour or two before the social event, an attempt is made to create an aesthetic miracle. What is achieved, if anything, may be ignoble. The moment is filled with anxiety, time is short, the tools are often strange, and their selection is limited. In desperation, everything is wiped off and the individual returns to the usual products and tired routine, vowing never to fall victim to another urge to improve self-image. The older the individual—older women are the ones likely to benefit most from an attractive make-over—the more likely she is to lack the confidence to use cosmetics to project a more attractive appearance.

PROGRAM FOR SUCCESS

Motivation

An individual frequently possesses the self-motivation to improve his or her appearance.* She may correctly judge that some of her facial features—e.g., roundness of face, width of nose, size of eyes, and prominence of chin—detract from her appearance. The assessment may not be correct, but that does not matter. The woman has an image of the appearance she would like to project, one that will make her feel comfortable or satisfied. Perhaps the drive is economic: Obvious gray hair may hinder the opportunity for a promotion in job status or the chance of success in gaining employment. Often the desire is just to "look more fashionable." Only rarely does a physician—the person whose opinions are the most respected and the one who may provide the greatest influence—include in a treatment program for anxiety, depression, or a psychosomatic illness the simple suggestion: "Sometimes looking better on the outside can help your internal process as well. Have you considered having a facial or splurging on some new eye makeup?" Motivation is necessary regardless of its genesis; the physician can be its most powerful source.

Goal

Most people want to be as attractive as others in their (age) group. But an otherwise level-headed 45-year-old woman should not expect that cosmetics, no matter how skillfully applied, will make her appear to be 25. What cosmetics can do is modify

* For the sake of brevity, pronouns in this chapter will reflect the feminine only.

her appearance so that she feels she is the best and perhaps the youngest-looking in her age group. Women, especially mature ones, must be cautioned not to overapply makeup or emphasize color brightness. Subtlety should be the rule.

Preparation

A woman can regard herself as if she were a portrait artist. She requires a comfortable chair and table (the artist's easel), as large a mirror as convenient with a magnifying lens on the reverse side (the reflection is the canvas), and good light of average intensity. A palette of several colors is necessary for each type of cosmetic: foundation, eye makeup, highlighter, lipstick, etc. It is not necessary at this stage to purchase costly products, but unless enough shades are at hand with which to work and experiment, the end product will be of limited quality. Finally, she may wish to purchase or borrow from the local library a simple makeup manual.* Helpful diagrams and sketches showing what can be achieved with colors, shading, and highlighting can be a shortcut to the acquisition of skill and technique.

Practice and Performance

Once equipped, the motivated woman should set aside a period of time, free from outside disturbances, exclusively for experimentation. There should be no urgency to accomplish anything, merely a desire to gain familiarity with all the tools of the trade and their application and removal. With guidance and support from an experienced friend or reference to a "how-to" manual and a measure of patience, satisfying rewards can be registered at each practice session. These sessions should be limited to about 20 or 30 min in the beginning, since the friction of repeated removal and cleansing may cause contact irritation. As skill is acquired, the original natural timidity is replaced by a spirit of adventure.

* An abundance of these books can be found in the health section of any bookstore. I was associated with *Revlon Art of Beauty*, Dolphin Books, Doubleday, New York, 1982. It is written in a simple, lively style with a multitude of sketches, diagrams, and color swatches to teach skills that lead to confidence in one's personal appearance and fitness.

BASIC SYSTEM

Although they cannot serve as a substitute for a good manual, selected basic principles of cosmetic application deserve mention.

Topographic Survey

Identification of the anatomic features (personal physical attributes) with which one must work is essential. This is an honest, nondisparaging itemization of normal characteristics. (Congenital or acquired defects are similarly evaluated but require greater skill and experimentation in management.) The survey should include the following elements.

Face: round, ovoid, square, rectangular, triangular, pronounced mentum or malar eminences
Lips: average, full, thin, long horizontally
Eyes: small, prominent, round, almond-shaped, deep-set, hooded, closely set, widely spaced
Nails: plate length, shape, integrity (ridged, ragged, etc.)
Hair: color, length, amplitude of wave or curl

Materials and Techniques

Also essential is a descriptive inventory of topically applied, readily removable agents—especially color, simple prosthetics, and fragrance—and the basic principles of their use.

Foundation Foundations are available in *lotion*, *cream*, or *solid cake* forms in all normal skin tones. Foundation is applied broadly with the fingers or a sponge to the cleansed and moisturized forehead, face, and neck to project symmetry of the skin surface. Pigmentations and other minor surface "flaws" are camouflaged because the light striking the skin is reflected more uniformly. Moisturizer applied before the foundation acts as a priming coat to permit easier skin acceptance and longer wear. In most instances the foundation color should closely match skin coloration. The goal is to achieve a balanced canvas upon which a portrait will be painted.

Lip Makeup Lip makeup is most commonly seen in the *stick* or *swivel tube* form but is also available in a *vial* with its own *sponge-tip applicator wand*, a *pencil* to lay down a fine line at the edge of the vermilion, or a *pot* for application with a fingertip. Lip makeup is the most frequently used of all these products, often the only makeup used. It is produced in all colors, including white and black. A young woman can experiment with any shade, while a more mature woman should select shades that are less bright. Each lip product is also produced as a *cream* to create a creamy, moist look (having nothing to do with its viscosity), a *frost* for a glazed or shimmering effect, a *gloss* to apply over and emphasize the shine of a previously applied product, and a *transparent* for inducing a gloss or shine to one's natural lip color. To deemphasize full lips, one can extend the application of foundation over the lip area; then, using a well-pointed lip pencil, one can lay down a line of color inside the vermilion border including the lateral angles of the mouth. The final step involves the careful filling in of this outlined area. To overcome thin lips using a well-pointed lip pencil, one can lay down a line of color outside the vermilion border and then add color to the lips within the new outline. To minimize long, horizontal lips, one extends the application of foundation into the corners of the mouth and avoids the placement of lip color to the angles of the vermilion.

Eye Makeup Four forms of eye makeup are commonly used. "Dressing" the eye plays an important role in changing one's appearance, for, like the lips, the eyes are extremely expressive and readily capture the attention of an observer. As with the lips, color selection can complement one's costume to create additional emphasis. *Eye shadow* comes in a multiplicity of matte (flat) and frosted colors in *cake, powder*, and *liquid* forms. It is applied to the skin surface encompassing the eyebrow superiorly, the upper eyelid margin inferiorly, the bridge of the nose medially, and the most lateral edge of the orbital ridge. Several colors may be used simultaneously to achieve the desired effect. Small eyes will appear larger if a dark shade is applied to the lower segment of this area while the upper portion is highlighted with a lighter, frosted shade. Eyes will appear less prominent if flat dark shades are used. Extending color beyond the outer canthus makes the eyes appear less round. These principles can be practiced to achieve a change in the appearance of any eye configuration. *Eyeliner* is used to draw a line of emphasis about the open eye. Liners are available in many colors and are packaged in *vials* with an *applicator wand*, as *pencils*, and even as *solid cakes* or *liquids* for application with a brush. The product should be deposited on the true skin lid margin at the base of the cilia, usually the upper or both the upper and lower for greater emphasis. Younger individuals often abuse the product by applying it to the mucosal margin of the lid to provide additional emphasis. This practice should be discouraged, as it may lead to asymptomatic tattooing in the conjunctival sac as a result of product debris entering this area. Eyes that are set widely apart should have eyeliner extended to encroach upon the inner canthus while neglecting the outer canthus. The reverse should be done for eyes that are closely set. *Mascara* is a product that comes in *cream, cake*, and *liquid* forms for application to the cilia. The mass and color create lash prominence to further increase an observer's attention. The most popular packaging at present is a vial with its own brush that not only dispenses the product but can also curl the lash. *Brow makeup* in *cake* or *pencil* form adds emphasis and color uniformity to attractively shaped eyebrows. However, the brow shape can be changed by means of physical interference, such as plucking with a tweezer. For reducing the effect of closely set eyes, the medial edge of the brow should begin laterally to an imaginary line drawn vertically through the inner canthus. It should also extend significantly lateral to the outer canthus. Hair should be plucked to give the brow a tapered shape with an arch, or high point, lateral to the center of the eye. Exactly the opposite should be done to minimize the effect of widely spaced eyes. The shape, color, and size of eyeglass frames exert powerful effects on all aspects of the face; *tinted contact lenses* are available to alter the color of eyes. For individuals with little or no lashes and others who wish to create a dramatic effect, *false eyelashes* in a wide variety of shapes, sizes, configurations, and colors can be easily affixed with adhesive.

Blusher These products are usually *loose* or *cake powders* in shades from dark red to brown for application in broad strokes with a soft, long-bristle brush. Blusher is applied in the form of an arc extending from above and lateral to the eyebrow down to cover the malar prominence. The width of the arc over the temporal area should be narrow and should widen gradually as it terminates over the cheekbone. For a *round* face, an additional touch of blusher over the mentum promotes the illusion of facial length. For a *triangular* face, blusher should not be applied to the chin, while for a *square* face, additional blusher should be applied to both the forehead and the mentum. Experimenting with the placement and configuration of blusher color as well as the color itself will *sculpt* the face to achieve a variety of illusions. Blusher in cream form for application with the fingertip is also available. This is the rouge of ancient origin, but it is no longer limited to bright reds. However, its application requires considerable skill and should be avoided by the novice.

Concealer or Highlighter Flesh-toned *creams* packaged in *stick form* or *pots* for finger application have an important but limited function. They are applied before the foundation to conceal or emphasize an attribute. For example, patting on concealer in a shade lighter than the normal skin tone to the commonly observed areas of increased pigmentation below the lower eyelids (familiarly known as *circles*) will camouflage this cosmetic deficit more efficiently than will the use of foundation alone. Likewise, application to the tip of the nose in a dark shade will reduce its appearance or highlight it if a lighter shade is used.

Nail Enamel Nail enamel consists of a *lacquer* in a glass bottle with its own *applicator brush*. It is available in hundreds of shades to match lip makeup. Well-cared-for hands are important eye-catchers. Nail colors that blend with the lips and costume create a pleasing effect which is considerably enhanced if the nail plates are long enough to extend beyond the fingertip and well shaped. The impression created is one of long and graceful fingers. For most individuals, occupation permitting, this can be accomplished through a regular program of nail care that encourages the conversion of the proximal cuticular border of the nail plate from an almost horizontal band to a narrow arc that exposes more of the proximal lunula. Nail plate awareness is essential to minimize its use as a manipulative tool subject to injury, fracture, and general wear and tear. Artificial *preformed nails* can be affixed to the true nail plate or just to the tip, or an entire prosthetic plate can be fabricated (sculptured) on the true nail surface using plastic monomers and polymers. These procedures require the attention of a professional manicurist.

Hair Grooming and Coloring Hair should be considered as a frame for a picture—the face. Its color, shape, bulk, and contour have a great influence on facial appearance. Hair is subject to and has the same influence as style and fashion. This can be seen by thumbing through a family album, in which some relatives are hardly recognizable because of the hairstyles of a previous generation. Comb, brush, shampoo, conditioner, setting lotion, spray fixative, hair waver, and hair straightener (relaxer) easily and conveniently permit conformance to fashion and the achievement of an attractive appearance. Hair *coloring* is available in temporary and permanent forms so that any color can be created not only to cover gray but to change the appearance of an individual. Not so long ago, women depended on milliners to provide hats to change mood and affect. Hair coloring is a substitute for that procedure. Its influence is of paramount importance in aesthetic dermatology.

Fragrance All the tools itemized above have visible impact only; however, aesthetic benefit via the olfactory route should not be overlooked. One's appetite for food can be made or destroyed by odor. In a similar manner, compatible fragrance—since body chemistry differs—can enhance a person's overall presence and linger long after the wearer has left.

AN EXAMPLE

A mature woman has expressed the desire to improve her personal appearance. In the accompanying photographs one can observe a few simple and extensive modifications.

Figure 1 represents the woman's normal appearance. She has a rather small, round head, small eyes, and an asymmetrical smile. The lips seem to be lost. The full head of gray hair, the jowling, and the horizontal wrinkle lines across the forehead are representative of her age group. Light reflects from the overall skin surface in a nonuniform pattern to emphasize its deficits. While the hair is neatly combed, it is "plastered" down, emphasizing the smallness and roundness of the head.

In Fig. 2 the only physical and/or cosmetic

change has been to the coiffure. The hair is the original gray; it has been set and combed to lift it away from the head and face. The head no longer appears to be small and round. This single change has done much to alter the woman's appearance.

In Fig. 3 one can observe what happens with the subtle application of color to the face. Light reflects from the face without "hot spots." The skin appears to be uniform. Shadows about the eyes, nose, and mouth have been deemphasized. The eyes look alive because of the blue shadow that has been added to the lateral aspects of both lids and the mascara that has been applied to the cilia. The brows have been given color which has made the orbital ridge more prominent. The application of reddish-brown color to the lateral aspects of the face and the cheeks (known as *highlighting* or *contouring*) has given the face a longer appearance, while the addition of a minimal amount of lipstick has provided accent and uniformity to the mouth.

Figure 4 represents only a change in coiffure. The subject is wearing no makeup. Compare it with Fig. 2. This demonstrates how appearance can be altered by changing the shape and characteristics of the frame about the face.

In Fig. 5, with the more bouffant hair style shown in Fig. 4, makeup has been applied in a manner similar to that shown in Fig. 3.

In Fig. 6 a more extensive alteration has been wrought. Most dramatic is the change in hair color. There is also a different coiffure. The facial makeup is the same.

FIGURE 1

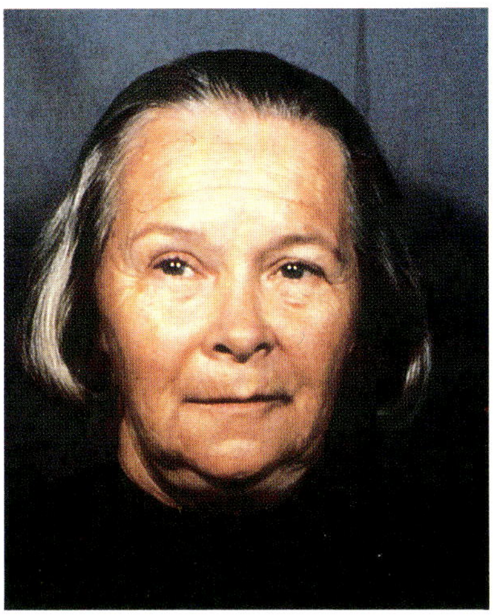

FIGURE 2

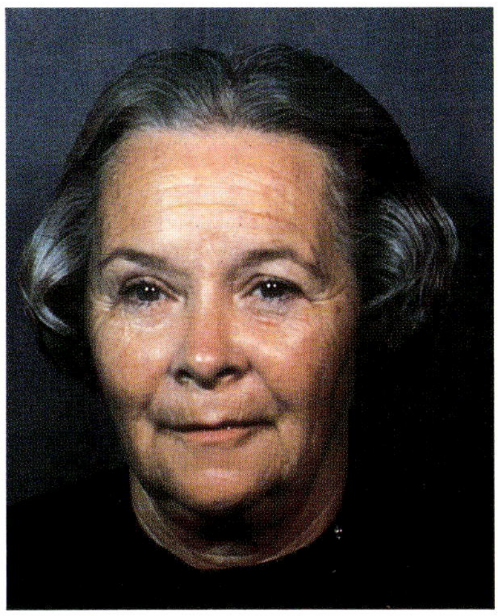

FIGURE 3

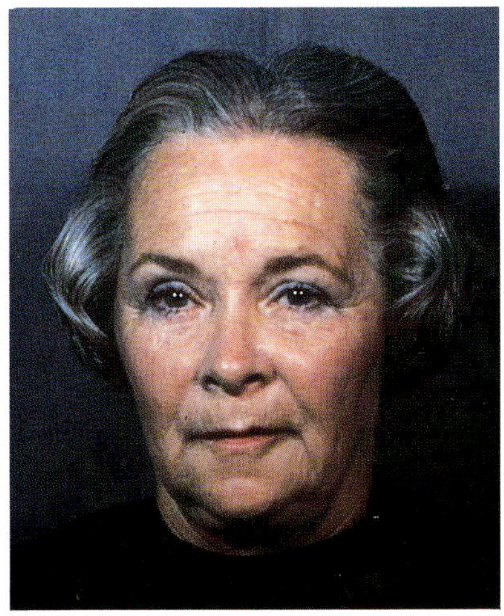

FIGURE 4

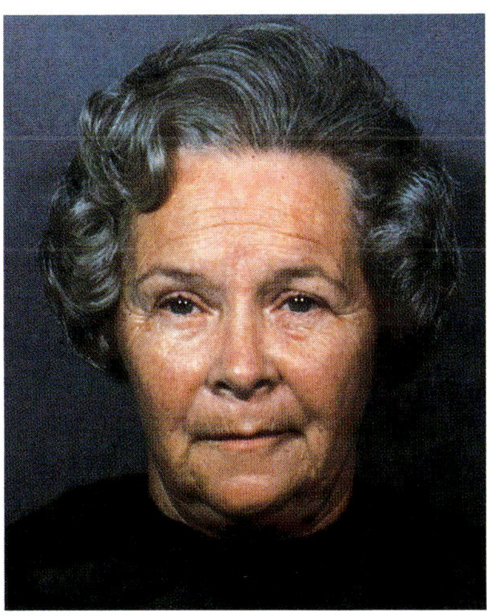

FIGURE 5

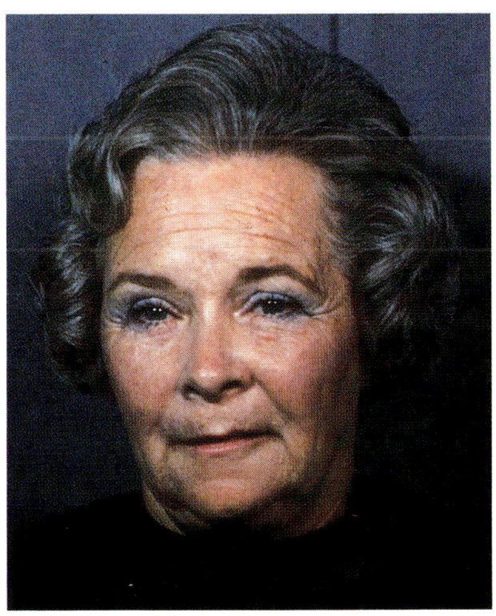

FIGURE 6

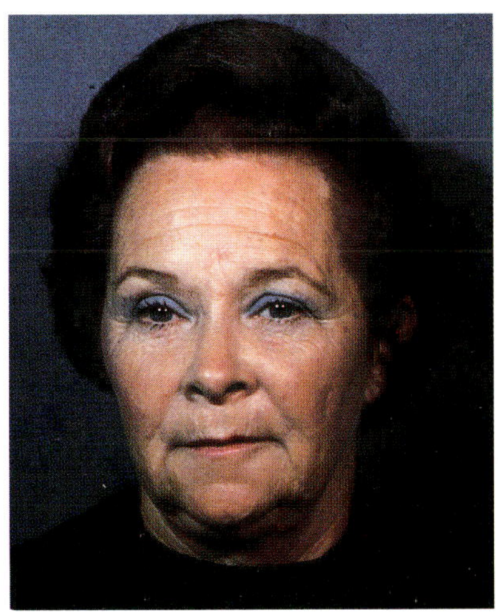

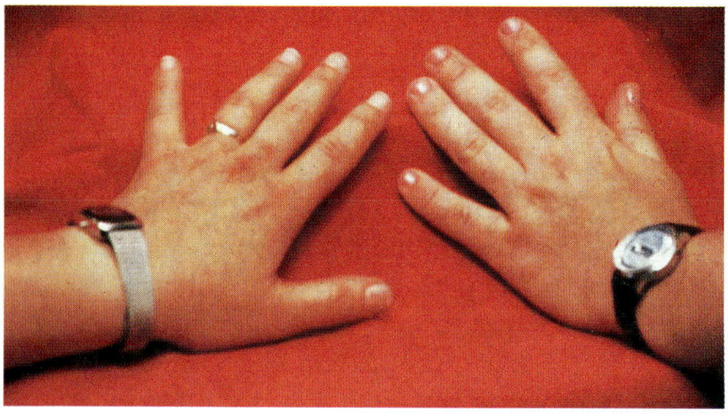

FIGURE 7

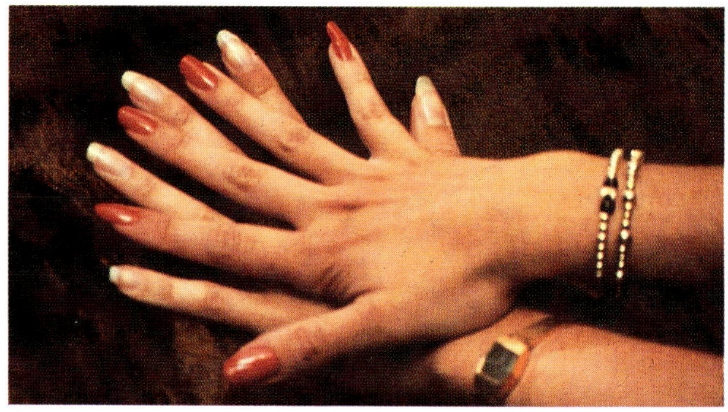

FIGURE 8

These photographs clearly demonstrate how dramatically one can alter appearance through the use of conventional cosmetic products.* It remains for the subject to select what pleases her, vary it, or start all over again.

Figures 7 and 8 illustrate how the hands play a prominent role in appearance and the projection of image. The short nails and stubby-looking fingers of the subjects in Fig. 7 are neat and clean but nothing else. In Fig. 8 the long nails convey the impression of slim, tapered, graceful fingers, and the addition of color is attractive. Much time and effort are required to possess long nails. Too frequently, genetic background, climate, season, and occupation defeat one's dedication to a manicure program. Preformed plastic nails may be affixed to natural nail plates. Also, monomer and/or polymer materials can be applied to natural fingernails to actually sculpture an attractive "nail" *in situ*. Both procedures are most successful when performed by experts. These procedures are costly, and touch-ups are necessary about every 10 days. Unfortunately, nail salons where this work is performed tend to use their own proprietary formulas composed of industrial materials mixed to achieve the desired results with little attention to biological tolerance, and adverse reactions have occurred.

* This procedure is highly successful in mitigating the cosmetic deficits caused by disease, neoplasm, genetic defects, and surgery. Color photographs have been published in Brauer EW. Cosmetics for the dermatologist, in DJ Demis (ed.) Clinical Dermatology. Philadelphia: Harper & Row, 1987; 4(38-1): 1–24, and Brauer EW: Coloring and corrective makeup procedures, *Clin Dermatol* 1988; 3:62–67.

CONCLUSION

A cosmetic make-over successfully serves aesthetic needs. This can be accomplished with conventional, readily available products at a modest cost. The procedure is noninvasive, reversible, and available to anyone at home or abroad. It lends itself to self-application with skills that can be mastered by most individuals. It is incumbent upon physicians to promote this form of aesthetic improvement in their practices.

CHAPTER

4

Local Anesthesia

STEVEN S. GREENBAUM
CHARLES H. GREENBAUM

HISTORY

Although many physicians believe anesthesia was used locally and developed in the United States, the beginning of anesthesia is actually obscure.[1] We do know that the numbing effect of cocaine was well known to the ancient Incas, who chewed coca leaves to render their saliva anesthetic when dripped into the wounds of trephination.[2]

More recently, after experimentation with cocaine in 1884 by ophthalmologist Karl Koller (1857–1944) and Sigmund Freud (1856–1939), Koller reported successful topical anesthesia of the cornea in frogs and in himself. In 1898, French and German workers utilized spinal and nerve blocks to achieve regional anesthesia. Cocaine was the first agent used, but its toxicity and potential for addiction led to a search for safer material. The isolation of epinephrine in 1897 by John Jacob Abel (1857–1938) of Johns Hopkins was a major step in this direction. Procaine hydrochloride, an ester developed by Alfred Einhorn, was the next step, but the greatest impetus to the use of regional and local anesthesia was the development of the amide group of anesthetics.

It was long known that compressed, solidified white poppy seeds produce opium, which was used by the ancients to induce artificial sleep.[3] Such material varied in strength and was unpredictable in its effects. In 1806, Friedrich Sertürner (1783–1841), an Austrian chemist, purified opium to produce morphia, or morphine. The problem was now how to administer it. Lafargue in 1836 produced local anesthesia with the subcutaneous injection of morphia paste, using a needle trocar. Other physicians selected solutions instead of pastes. By 1853, Alexander Wood and Charles-Gabriel Pravaz (1791–1853) had introduced the hypodermic syringe and hollow needle.

By 1878, Von Anrep had produced local anesthesia by subcutaneous injection, so that Koller's use of cocaine for eye surgery was a natural progression. William Halstead (1852–1927) in 1884 began to employ cocaine for nerve blocks. The following

TABLE 1
CLINICALLY IMPORTANT LOCAL ANESTHETICS

Generic Name	Trade Name	Main Use	Date of Initial Clinical Use	Maximum Dose (Approximate) Without Epinephrine Added
Esters				
Cocaine		Topical 4% solution	1884	4 ml or 3 mg/kg
Ethyl aminobenzoate	Benzocaine, Americaine	Topical 20%	1900	
		Cream or ointment 1–5%		
		Aerosol 20%		
Procaine hydrochloride	Novocain	Oral	1905	200 ml or 14 mg/kg
		Local infiltration 0.5%		1 g
		Peripheral nerve block 1–2%		1 g
2-Chloroprocaine hydrochloride	Nesacaine hydrochloride	Infiltration 0.5%	1955	1 g (200 ml)
		Peripheral nerve block 1–2%		1 g
		Epidural		1000 mg
Tetracaine hydrochloride	Amethocaine Hydrochloride, Pontocaine	Topical ointment 0.5–1%	1930	14 mg/kg
		Cream 0.5–1%		1.5 mg/kg
		Solution 0.25–1%		100 mg
		Spinal 1%		100 mg
Amides				
Dibucaine hydrochloride	Nupercaine Hydrochloride	Spinal	1929	0.667, 2.5, 5 mg/ml solutions
Prilocaine hydrochloride	Citanest	Infiltration 0.5%	1960	600 mg
		Peripheral nerve block 0.5%		10 mg/kg
		Epidural		
Lidocaine	Xylocaine	Infiltration 0.5–2%	1944	300 mg
		Topical 2–6%		
		Peripheral nerve block 0.5–2.0%		300 mg
		Epidural		
		Spinal		
Mepivacaine hydrochloride	Carbocaine hydrochloride	Infiltration 0.5–1.0%	1957	500 mg
		Peripheral nerve block 1–2%		500 mg
		Epidural		
Bupivacaine hydrochloride	Marcain	Infiltration 0.25%	1963	250 mg
		Peripheral nerve block 0.75%		250 mg
		Epidural 0.75%		
Etidocaine	Duranest	Infiltration 0.25%	1972	250 mg
		Peripheral nerve block 0.75%		
		Epidural 0.75%		

Source: Altman et al.[4] and Covino and Vassallo.[5]

year J. L. Corning (1855–1923) introduced spinal anesthesia with cocaine. Although the use of cold to dull pain had been known for some time, ether spray was not introduced until 1867. Later modifications have included the use of ethyl chloride, freon, and liquid nitrogen.

The growth of cutaneous surgery is linked to the use of appropriate local anesthesia. Many procedures would be considerably more complicated or impossible. Local anesthesia enables the patient to be awake and oriented, allowing communication between physician and patient to take place. In purely "dermal" local anesthesia, motor nerve function remains unimpaired, making it easier for the surgeon to evaluate the patient. Local anesthetics generally do not impair the sensorium of the patient, and so that phase of the recovery period is eliminated. Local anesthesia greatly facilitates the work of the physician, enabling the patient to be comfortable and making outpatient ambulatory surgery the predominant form of day-to-day dermatologic surgery practice.

HOW LOCAL ANESTHETICS WORK

Local anesthetics have traditionally been classified as esters or amides. Their structures are similar, with each being composed of an aromatic ring, an intermediate chain, and a terminal amine group.[4]

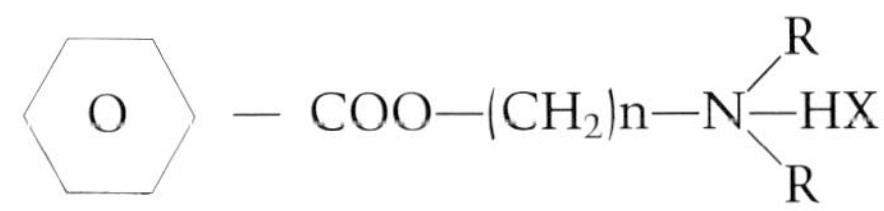

Ester

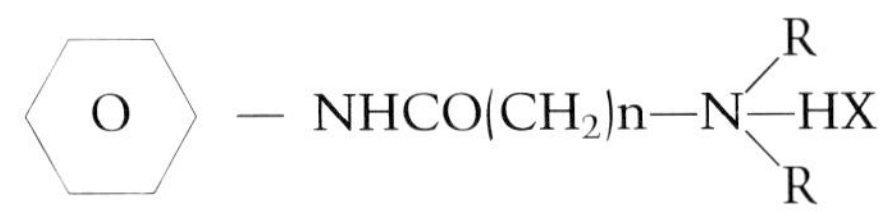

Amide

Tables 1 and 2 list clinically important local anesthetics and describe their characteristics.[4–6]

Local anesthetics can work by reversibly blocking the generation and transmission of action potentials along an excitable membrane. The formation of these action potentials requires the gating

TABLE 2
CHARACTERISTICS OF CLINICALLY IMPORTANT LOCAL ANESTHETICS

Agent	Onset	Duration	Relative Potency	Site of Metabolization
Esters				
Cocaine	Slow	Short		Liver
Ethylaminobenzoate (Benzocaine, Americaine)	Slow	Long		Plasma
Procaine hydrochloride (Novocain)	Moderate	Short	Low	Plasma
2-Chloroprocaine hydrochloride (Nesacaine Hydrochloride)	Rapid	Short	Moderate	Plasma
Tetracaine hydrochloride (Amethocaine Hydrochloride, Pontocaine)	Moderate	Long	Moderate	Plasma
Amides				
Dibucaine hydrochloride (Nupercaine Hydrochloride	Moderate to slow	Long	High	Liver
Prilocaine hydrochloride (Citanest)	Rapid	Moderate	Moderate	Liver
Lidocaine (Xylocaine)	Rapid	Moderate	Moderate	Liver
Mepivacaine hydrochloride (Carbocaine hydrochloride)	Rapid	Moderate	Moderate	Liver
Bupivacaine hydrochloride (Marcain)	Moderate	Long	High	Liver
Etidocaine (Duranest)	Moderate	Long	High	Liver

Source: Covino.[6]

of sodium and potassium ions. Local anesthetics interfere with the flow of these ions and thus block the action potentials. It is likely that the local anesthetic molecule binds to a "voltage-dependent, modulated receptor" to directly inhibit the sodium channel.[7] The blockade that ensues occurs in a defined sequence. Smaller (fine) fibers are blocked before large (coarse) ones. Hence pain and temperature sensations are lost first and motor function is lost last[8] (see Table 3).

The effect of a specific local anesthetic depends on its structure. For example, the esters are less stable chemically than are the amides and are hydrolyzed more easily in plasma by plasma pseudocholinesterase. The amide compounds are hydrolyzed in the liver at a slower rate.

Anesthetics in vivo are judged by their potency, duration of action, and speed of onset. The chemical features of an anesthetic that determine these activities are lipid solubility, protein-binding ability, and pK_a. Ultimately, the overall physical structure of the compound determines its physical activities.[7]

The *potency* of an anesthetic is directly proportional to its lipid solubility because axonal membranes constitute a lipoprotein matrix. Compounds that are lipid-soluble enter the neural membrane more easily to exert their effect. The potency of a local anesthetic is not determined solely by its lipid solubility but also by other features such as its vasodilatory effect, which can directly affect the quantity of anesthetic in an area at a given time. In addition, increased lipid solubility means that the anesthetic is more readily absorbed by the adipose tissue surrounding the injection site, and this may decrease the number of molecules available for neural blockade. For this reason accuracy of injection is critical to minimize absorption of the anesthetic by the surrounding fat.

TABLE 3
SEQUENTIAL EFFECTS OF NEURAL BLOCKADE BY LOCAL ANESTHETICS

1. Blockade of B fibers: elevation of skin temperature
2. Blockade of A (delta) and C fibers: loss of pain and temperature sensation
3. Blockade of A (gamma) fibers: loss of proprioception
4. Blockade of A (beta) fibers: loss of touch and pressure sensation
5. Blockade of A (alpha) fiber: loss of motor function

Source: Henderson JJ, Nimmo WS. Practical Regional Anaesthesia. Cambridge MA: Blackwell Scientific, 1983: 3. With permission.

The *duration of activity* of a local anesthetic depends primarily on the affinity with which it binds to the protein receptor in the sodium channel of the neural membrane. The more weakly a compound is bound to this receptor, the more rapidly and easily it is removed from the membrane and the shorter is its duration. Epinephrine in various concentrations is commonly added to lidocaine. It leads to increased hemostasis and increased duration of the anesthetic affect. Both sequelae are due to vasoconstriction. Many standard solutions contain epinephrine in a concentration of 1:100,000. It has been found that epinephrine can be considerably more dilute and still produce similar effects. In areas where compromised blood flow can be a problem, such as the distal digits, ears, and penis, it is often advisable to dilute the epinephrine at least to 1:200,000. Although actual tissue necrosis from epinephrine is extremely rare, it is sometimes advisable to use "plain" lidocaine, especially in patients with questionable cardiac stability. The vasoconstrictive effects of epinephrine require at least several minutes to take effect and so the surgeon should wait between injecting the anesthetic and performing the surgery.

The *speed of onset* of a local anesthetic is most directly related to the pK_a of that agent.[6] The pK_a is the pH at which there are equal quantities of the ionized and nonionized forms of the compound. The nonionized molecules cross the neural membrane more easily than do the ionized molecules. Therefore the greater the ratio of nonionized molecules to ionized molecules, the more rapid the onset of activity of the anesthetic. Because the percentage of nonionized molecules is inversely proportional to the pK_a of the agent, drugs with a lower pK_a have a more rapid onset of action.

Other factors that affect the speed of onset of an anesthetic are the concentration used and the relative rate of diffusion through the nonnervous tissue in the immediate vicinity of injection.

Lidocaine is the most commonly employed local anesthetic in dermatologic surgery. Table 4 lists its key features.

TOPICAL ANESTHETICS

Topical anesthetics may be effective agents when applied to surfaces such as the conjuctiva, oropharynx, anal mucosa, tympanic membrane, genitourinary tract, and tracheobronchial tree. The evaluation of topical anesthetics is difficult because of the large number of variables. The usefulness of these agents is restricted by the fact that they are unable to reach subepithelial pain receptors.[11] Topical anesthetics are often rapidly absorbed from mucosal surfaces as a result of the relatively increased surface area provide by numerous villous projections. These anesthetics allow easier passage of instrumentation including nasogastric tubes, vaginal speculums, endoscopes, and artifical airways. Topical anesthetics have been applied to the skin to treat numerous disorders, including burns, scrapes, and pruritus.[11]

Delivery methods for topical anesthetics include sprays, powders, solutions, jellies, pastes, lozenges, and suppositories. Caution must be used with all these methods to avoid serious toxicity from overzealous application and rapid absorption. In anesthetizing the oropharynx, it is especially important to be aware of the diminished or absent gag reflex and the resultant increased risk of aspiration. Any topically applied medicament can result in contact sensitivity, and a careful history must be obtained before administering a topical anesthetic.[13] EMLA (eutectic mixture of local anesthetics)[12] is a form of topical anesthesia that was introduced in Europe around 1980. The two agents employed are lidocaine and prilocaine. The mixture is applied to the skin surface and requires at least 45 min to 1 h to take effect.[11] Topical anesthetics are classified in Table 5.

TABLE 4
LIDOCAINE

Less toxic than procaine
Twice as potent as procaine
Longer duration of anesthesia than procaine
Good topical anesthetic properties
Not inactivated by cholinesterase
Causes vasoconstriction of arterioles
Mixes well with epinephrine
Metabolized by the liver, not in the bloodstream
Greater risk of adverse reactions than with anesthetics metabolized in the bloodstream
Distributed in kidneys, brain, liver, lungs, and heart
Does not cross-react with ester-derived anesthetics
Good anesthetic effect when applied topically to oral mucosa
Toxicity: cardiovascular collapse, central nervous system stimulation, tinnitus, light-headedness, nystagmus, shivering, tremors, slurred speech, drowsiness, unconsciousness, apnea, hypotension

Source: Covino and Vassallo[5] and Baker and Blackman.[10]

TABLE 5
CLASSIFICATION OF TOPICAL ANESTHETICS

Alcohols
- Benzyl alcohol: 2–10% in lotions and sprays
- Phenol: 0.5–1.5% in lotions, ointments, mouthwashes, and sprays
- Resorcinol: 3–5% in creams and ointments
- Hexylresorcinol: 0.1% in mouthwashes and lozenges
- Menthol: creams, ointments, and lozenges

Amines
- Benzoic acid esters
  - Cocaine: 4–10%
  - Hexylcaine hydrochloride (Cyclaine)
  - Piperocaine (Metycaine)
- Aminobenzoates
  - Ethyl aminobenzoate (Benzocaine): more than 5%
  - Butamben
  - Tetracaine hydrochloride: 1–2%
  - Cetacaine: 14% ethyl aminobenzoate and 2% butamben
  - Proparacaine hydrochloride (Ophthaine): 0.5%
- Amides
  - Dibucaine hydrochloride
  - Lidocaine: 2, 4, 5, and 10% viscous and fluid, 5% ointment
- Noncaine amines
  - Dyclonine hydrochloride: 1%
  - Pramoxine hydrochloride
  - Antihistamines
- Others
  - EMLA (eutectic mixture of lidocaine and prilocaine)[12]

Source: Adriani et al.[11]

Toxicity of Local Anesthetics

The local anesthetics commonly used today are "tried and true." Toxicity resulting from their use is most often due to the following factors[14]:

1. Hypersensitivity of an individual to a specific agent
2. Excessively high blood levels of the anesthetic perfusing specific organs
3. Decreased tolerance to a specific anesthetic caused by the recipient's altered physical condition
4. Allergy
5. Idiosyncratic reactions

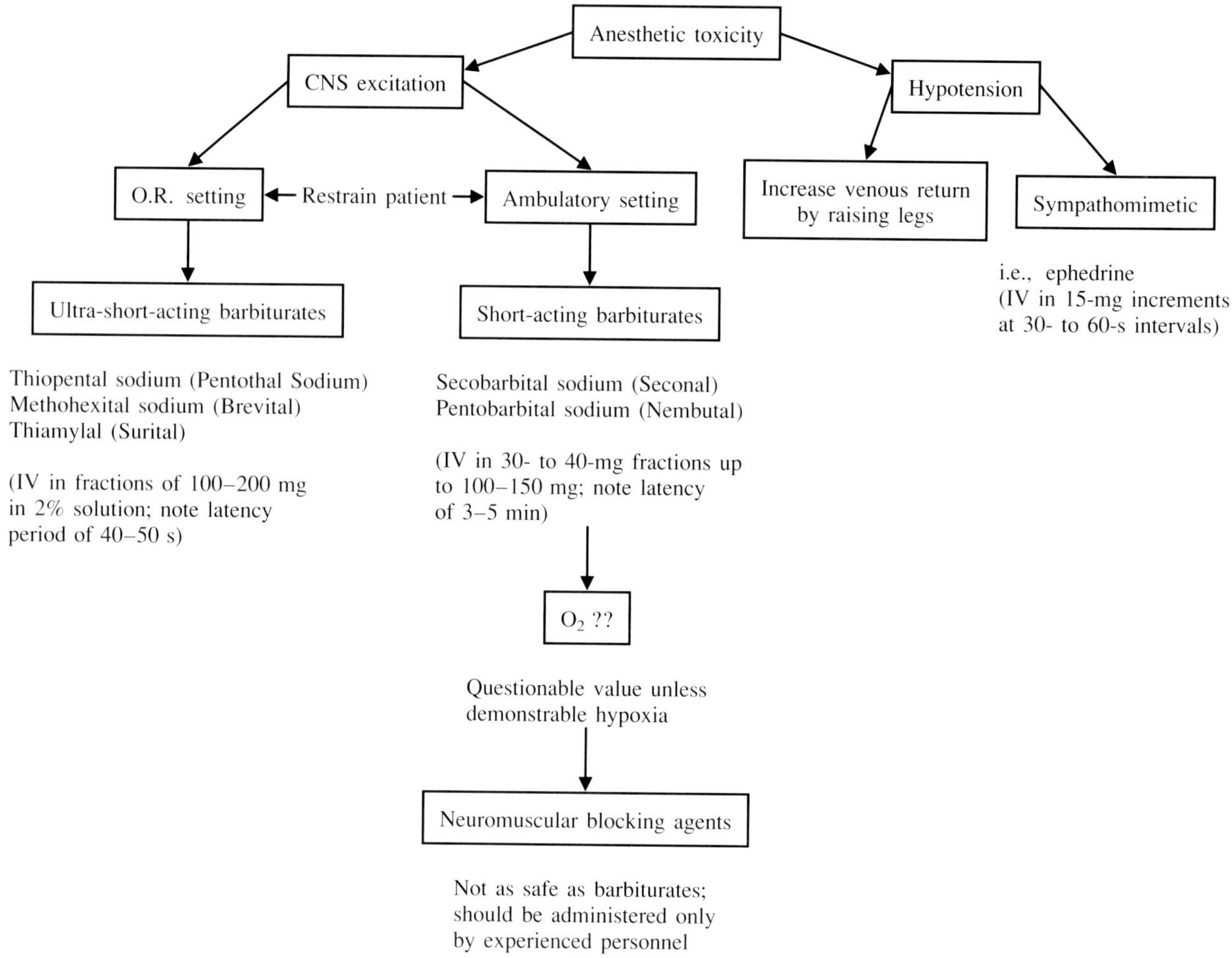

FIGURE 1
Treatment of toxicity from local anesthesia. (*From Ariani[14] and de Jong.[15]*)

Local anesthetics, when systemically absorbed, are initially distributed in the organs with the greatest blood flow, including the brain, heart, lungs, liver, spleen, adrenal glands, and kidneys. The peak plasma concentration of drug occurs 5 to 60 min after injection, after which it drops as a result of biotransformation, redistribution, and elimination.[15]

The most important organ systems affected by local anesthesia toxicity are the cardiovascular and the central nervous systems (see Table 6). Local anesthetics easily penetrate the blood-brain barrier as well as cross the placenta. Toxic reactions are more common after topical application of local anesthetic than after infiltration due to the rapid absorption of drug through mucosal membranes.[14] Figure 1 discusses the treatment of toxicity from local anesthesia.

TABLE 6
CENTRAL NERVOUS SYSTEM AND CARDIOVASCULAR SYSTEM TOXICITY FROM LOCAL ANESTHETICS

Central nervous system (in sequence as blood level increases)
- Drowsiness
- Tinnitus
- Numbness of lips and tongue with accompanying metallic taste
- Fine tremors of face and hands
- Grand mal seizures and/or apnea

Cardiovascular toxicity (in sequence as blood level increases)
- Decreased cardiac contractility
- Biphasic action on smooth muscle of blood vessel walls
  - Initial vasoconstriction
  - Later vasodilation
- Profound hypotension
- Syncope or asystole

Source: Strichartz,[7] Adriani,[14] de Jouj,[15] Privthi Raj,[16] and Sperling et al.[17]

In addition, Table 7 lists some ways to make the injection of local anesthetics more tolerable and less painful to the patient.

PERIPHERAL NERVE BLOCKS

Regional anesthesia, especially in the facial region, can be extremely useful to the dermatologic surgeon. Nerve blocks decrease the amount of anesthetic that must be used, increase the duration of the anesthesia, and often minimize anatomic distortion. Several of the major facial regional blocks are described in Table 8[8,16,19,20] and Figs. 2 through 5.

RECOMMENDATIONS

Informed consent must be obtained for any surgical procedure. Anesthesia is a part of the procedure, whether it be local or general.[21] Important risks, such as allergic reactions, need to be discussed with the patient.

TABLE 7
HOW TO EASE THE PAIN OF LOCAL ANESTHETIC INJECTION

Warn the patient about the upcoming injection.
Temperature of the injected solution does not matter.
Do not use H_2O as a local anesthetic; it is quite painful.
Stretch skin prior to injection.
Use the smallest-gauge needle possible (i.e., 30-gauge).
Inject the anesthetic through a pilosebaceous ostium if possible.
Inject the anesthetic into deep dermal subcutaneous tissue.
Inject the anesthetic as the needle is slowly withdrawn.
Inject the anesthetic slowly to avoid painful tissue distention.
Wait 5 to 6 min after deep injection for complete anesthesia.
Buffer the anesthetic with sodium bicarbonate to approach a physiologic pH of 7.4 by adding 1 ml of sodium biocarbonate (1 mEq/ml) to each 10 ml of anesthetic.

Source: Sperling et al.[17] and Arndt et al.[18]

TABLE 8
NERVE BLOCKS

Nerve Block	Technique	Field of Anesthesia
Supraorbital and supratrochlear nerves (see Figs. 2 and 3)	1. Palpate notch in supraorbital rim with finger. 2. Insert needle perpendicular to skin until paresthesias are noted or bone is felt. 3. Inject approximately 0.5–1.0 ml of anesthetic. 4. Withdraw needle slightly, then advance medially; inject 0.5–1.0 ml of anesthetic to block supratrochlear nerve.	Ipsilateral forehead and scalp as posterior as lambdoid suture.
Infraorbital nerve	Intraoral method 1. Palpate infraorbital notch and locate infraorbital foramen, which is approximately 1.0 cm below it. 2. With middle finger palpating infraorbital neurovascular bundle, elevate upper lip with thumb and index finger. 3. Insert needle into mucous membrane until tip of needle is palpated below middle finger.	Lower eyelid, lateral inferior nose, vestibule of nose, upper lip, and mucosa

(continued)

TABLE 8
NERVE BLOCKS (*CONTINUED*)

Nerve Block	Technique	Field of Anesthesia
	4. Inject approximately 2.0–3.0 ml of anesthetic. Extraoral method 1. Locate infraorbital foramen as described above. 2. Insert needle 0.5 cm inferior to and slightly medial to infraorbital bundle. 3. Advance needle to infraorbital foramen and inject 2.0–3.0 ml of anesthetic (do not inject more than 3.0 ml of anesthetic into foramen).	
Mental nerve	Intraoral method 1. Palpate from inside mouth where neurovascular bundle exits mental foramen (junction of lower lip with lower gum, posterior to first premolar). 2. Insert needle from side (medially) until tip is palpated beneath fingertip at neurovascular bundle. 3. Inject 1.0–2.0 ml of anesthetic. Extraoral method 1. Palpate neurovascular bundle exiting mental foramen from outside. 2. Insert needle in cranio-medial-posterior direction to mental foramen. 3. Inject 1.0–2.0 ml of anesthetic.	Skin and mucosa of lower lip, skin of jaw
Digital (fingers, toes)	1. Cleanse area thoroughly. 2. Inject 0.5 ml of anesthetic with 30-gauge needle at base of digit on both medial and lateral sides, making sure enough anesthetic is delivered in dorsal and ventral directions.	Sensation in fingers and toes
Ear (cranial nerves IV, VII, IX, and X and great auricular nerve) (see Fig. 4)	1. Field block around auricle anesthetizes entire ear except concha, external auditory canal, and postauricular sulcus. 2. Start field block inferiorly to anesthetize great auricular nerve first, making subsequent injections less painful.	Sensation to entire external ear

TABLE 8
NERVE BLOCKS (*CONTINUED*)

Nerve Block	Technique	Field of Anesthesia
	3. To complete anesthesia, infiltrate concha, external auditory canal, and postauricular sulcus.	
Nose (infratrochlear nerve, external branches of cranial nerve V, and infraorbital and anterior spinous branches of cranial nerve V_2) (see Fig. 5)	1. Block infraorbital nerve as described above. 2. Continue circumferentially around nose, creating field block. 3. Separately inject external nasal branch of anterior ethmoidal nerve (at columella).	Sensation to entire nose

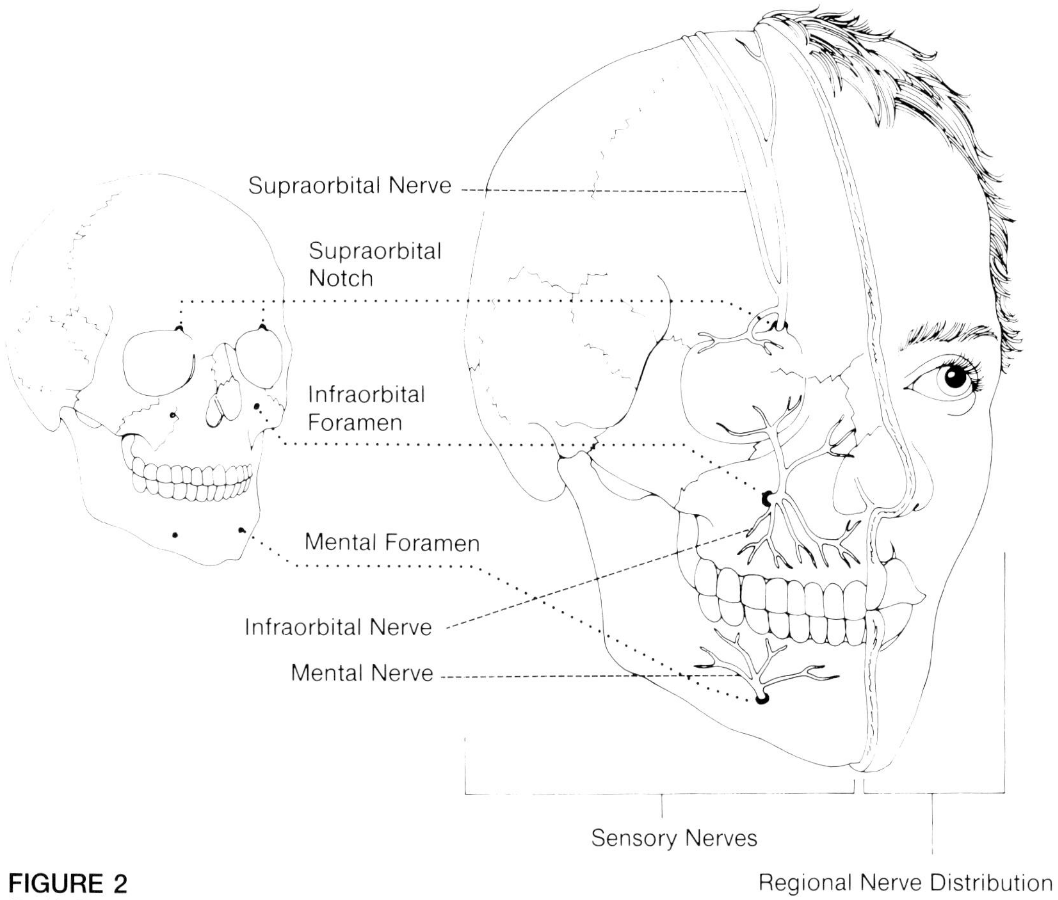

FIGURE 2
(*Left*) Skull with anatomic landmarks for supraorbital, infraorbital, and mental nerves. Note the vertical axis of the supraorbital notch, infraorbital foramen, and mental foramen. (*Right*) Supraorbital, infraorbital, and mental nerves.

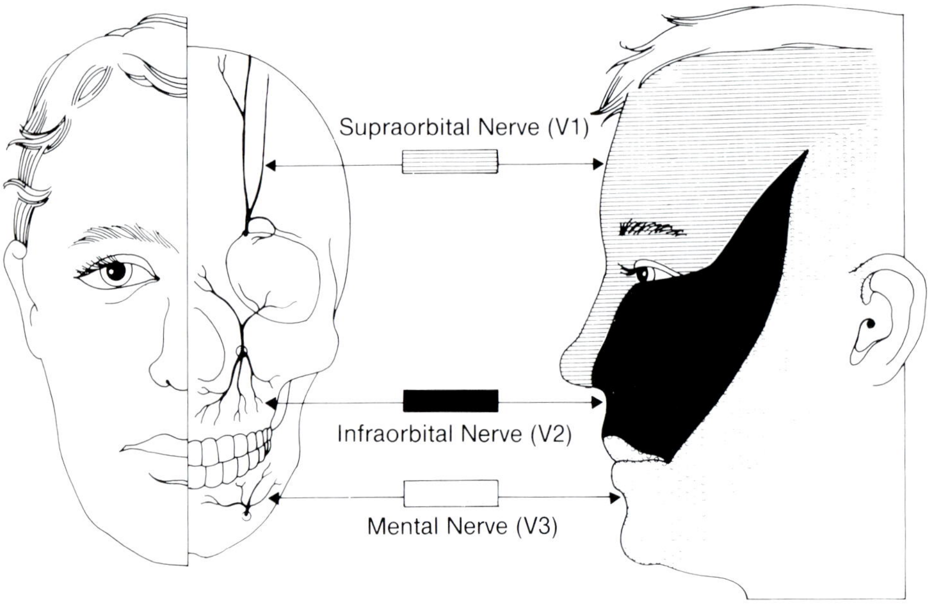

FIGURE 3
Location of the suprorbital, infraorbital, and mental nerves with their corresponding sensory distribution.

FIGURE 4
(*Left*) The lesser occipital and great auricular nerves in relation to the posterior scalp and vertebral column. (*Right*) Regional sensory nerve distribution of the lesser occipital and great auricular nerves to the external ear.

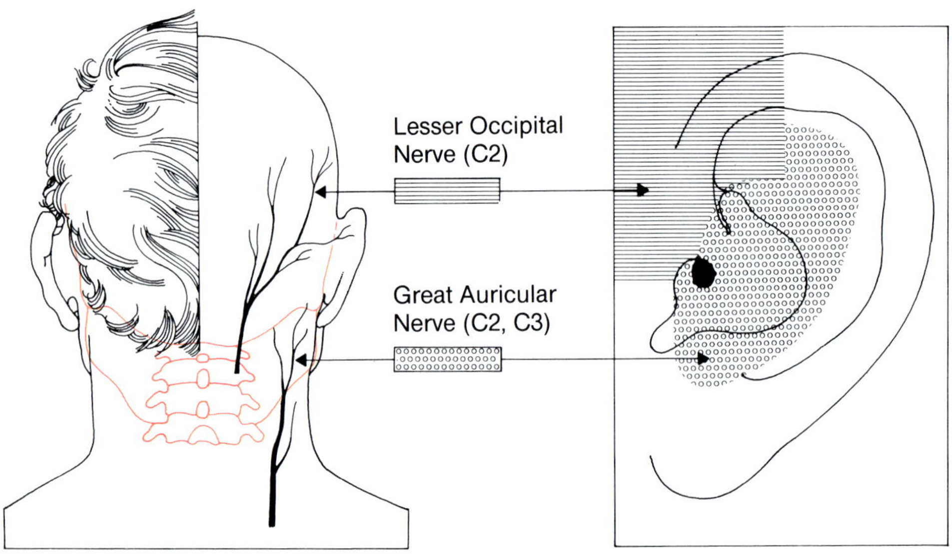

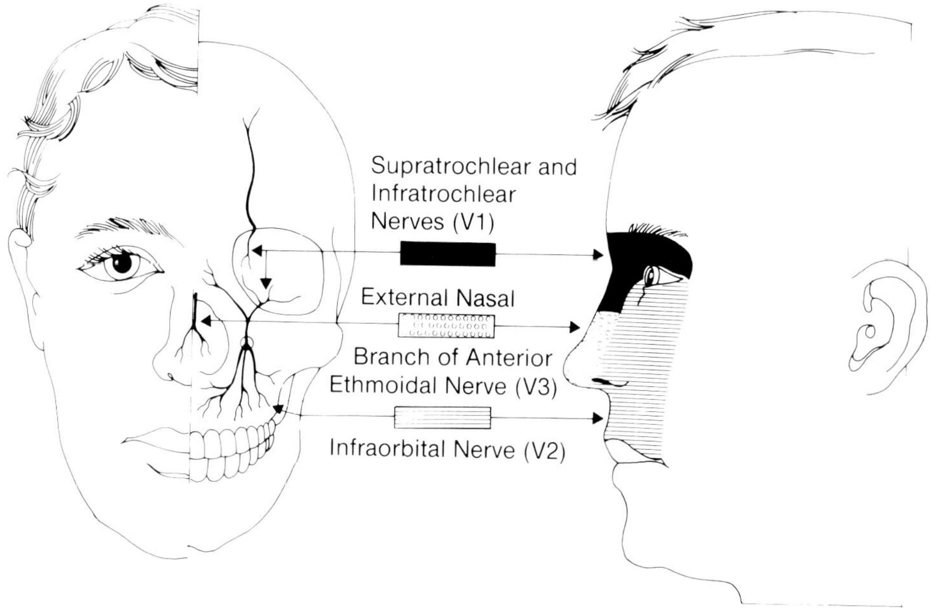

FIGURE 5
(*Left*) Major sensory nerve distribution to the nose. (*Right*) Corresponding region of sensory innervation for the supratrochlear, infratrochlear, external nasal, anterior ethmoidal, and infraorbital nerves.

REFERENCES

1. Keys TE. The development of anesthesia. Anesthesiology. 1942; 3:11–23 and 1941; 2:552–574.
2. Fink R. Leaves and needles: The introduction of surgical local anesthesia. Anesthesiology. 1985; 63:77–83.
3. Miller RD. Anesthesia, 2d ed. New York: Churchill Livingstone, 1986.
4. Altman RS, Smith-Coggins R, Ampel LL. Local anesthetics. Ann Emerg Med. 1985; 14:1207–1217.
5. Covino BG, Vassallo HG. Local Anesthetics: Mechanisms of Action and Clinical Use. New York: Grune & Stratton, 1976:3.
6. Covino BG. Pharmacology of local anesthetic agents. Br J Anaest. 1986; 58:701–716.
7. Strichartz GR. Local Anesthetics. London: Springer-Verlag, 1987:46.
8. Eriksson E. Illustrated Handbook in Local Anesthesia. Philadelphia: WB Saunders, 1980:10.
9. Henderson JJ, Nimmo WS. Practical Regional Anaesthesia. Oxford: Blackwell, 1983:9.
10. Baker JD, Blackman BB. Local Anesthesia. Clin Plast Surg. 1985; 12:25–31.
11. Adriani J, Beuttler WA, Brihmadesam L, et al. Topical anesthetics: Use and misuse. South Med J. 1985; 78:1224–1229.
12. Ehrenstrom-Reiz G, Reiz S, Stockman O. Topical anesthesia with EMLA, a new lidocaine prilocaine cream and the Cusum technique for detection of minimal application time. Acta Anaesthesiol Scand. 1983; 27:510–512.
13. Curley RK, Macfarlane AW, King CM. Contact sensitivity to the amide anesthetics lidocaine, prilocaine, and mepivacaine. Arch Dermatol. 1986; 122:924–926.
14. Adriani J. Etiology and management of adverse reactions to local anesthetics. Int Anesthesiol Clin. 1972; 10:127–130.
15. De Jong RH. Toxic effects of local anesthetics. JAMA. 1978; 239:1166–1168.
16. Prithvi Raj P. Handbook of Regional Anesthesia. New York: Churchill Livingstone, 1985:146–148.
17. Sperling LC, Weber CB, Rodman OG. Towards less painful anesthesia: Water, saline and lidocaine. J Dermatol Surg Oncol. 1981; 7:730–731.
18. Arndt KA, Burton C, Noe JM. Minimizing the pain of local anesthesia. Plast Reconstr Surg. 1983; 72:676–679.
19. Jenkner FL. Peripheral Nerve Block: Pharmacologic—By Local Anesthesia; Electric—By Transdermal Stimulation. New York: Springer-Verlag, 1977:90–93
20. Winton GB. Anesthesia for dermatologic surgery. J Dermatol Surg Oncol. 1988; 14:41–54.
21. Scarborough D, Bisaccia E, Schven W, et al. Anesthesia for the dermatologic surgeon. Int J Dermatol. 1989; 28:629–637.

PART II

GENERAL CONSIDERATIONS

CHAPTER

5

Aging and Sun Damage

MAURICIO GOIHMAN-YAHR
DANIEL BENIAMINI-LOKER

The skin is a mirror in which development and aging can be observed and monitored. Conceptually, "normal" aging should be differentiated from aging induced by light. Normal aging may be observed in areas of the skin not usually exposed to the sun. Its main features can be studied by simple inspection, magnification with a hand lens, light microscopy, electron microscopy, and a variety of physical, physiological, and biochemical techniques.[1–3]

NORMAL AGING

The salient features of aging include a lowering of the mitotic activity of keratinocytes and a decrease in the activity and number of melanocytes and Langerhans cells. There is a lowering of the number of eccrine and apocrine glands and a decrease in the total amount of collagen, which also thickens and becomes more stable. Changes occur in elastic fibers and in the elastic network. There is a reduced amount of glycosaminoglycans. In addition, there are thinning of the skin, development of canities, loss of elasticity, and a certain type of wrinkling that may be temporarily reversed by stretching. Changes occur in mechanical and functional properties, including poor adhesion between dermis and epidermis, increased bruisability and a decrease in the synthesis of vitamin D, delayed wound healing, reduced clearance of fluids and foreign materials, and diminished function of the sweat glands. Immune functions are also attenuated.[4]

PHOTOAGING

Damage induced by the sun becomes evident when sun-exposed areas are compared with otherwise equivalent regions that are protected from radia-

Supported in part by grants from CONICIT, Fundación Polar, and special funds from the Congress of Venezuela (M.G.Y.). Reina Semprúm provided secretarial assistance.

tion (e.g., the dorsal and ventral aspects of the forearms). Exposed skin shows apparent accelerated aging (dermatoheliosis, or photoaging), manifested by an increase in glycosaminoglycans and numerous hyperplastic fibroblasts. There are also changes in the elastic fibers and collagen. Pigmentary abnormalities and marked wrinkling occur. Altered dermal fibers are separated from the epidermis by a border, or "grenz," zone which has been proposed as an area of repair. Langerhans cells are damaged by photoexposure and show a diminished ability to respond to stimuli. *Photoaged skin* shows deeper wrinkling than does aged skin. The overall aspect and physiology present not only as *resting senile* structures but also as irritated and less efficient structures.[5,6] Radiation from the sun, cumulatively or by single exposure, induces changes in life span and presumably somatic mutations in cells from the diverse layers of the skin. This, plus diminished ability in antigen processing and lowered cellular immune responses, allows the development of benign and malignant neoformations. *Benign* and *malignant* are the poles of a continuous spectrum of disease.

The most common epithelial neoformations are seborrheic keratoses, actinic keratoses, Bowen's disease, basal cell epitheliomas, and squamous cell carcinomas (Figs. 1 through 4). Pigmentary changes include ephelides, lentigines, and presumably malignant melanomas. The role of the sun's rays in inducing nevi and melanocytic dysplasia is probable but has not been proved. On the other hand, ultraviolet light is considered the culprit in photoaging. Visible light may also play a role, because it is able to penetrate deeper into the skin. The exact role of infrared radiation in aging is not

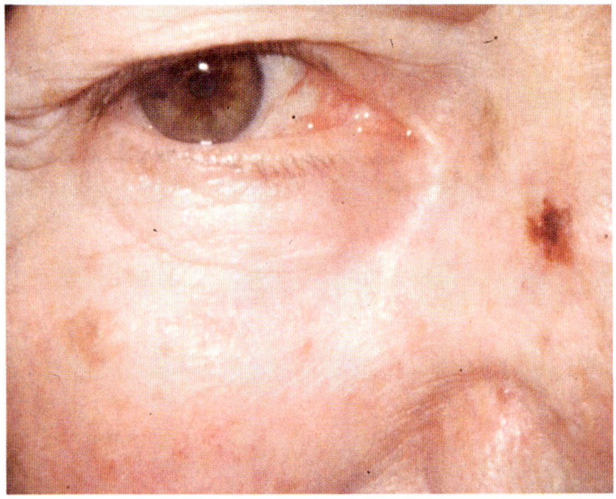

FIGURE 2
Superficial basal cell epithelioma in an old woman. Note lentigo, wrinkling, and telangiectasis.

FIGURE 1
Squamous cell carcinoma in a patient with chronic sun damage. Note wrinkling and the light color of the eyes.

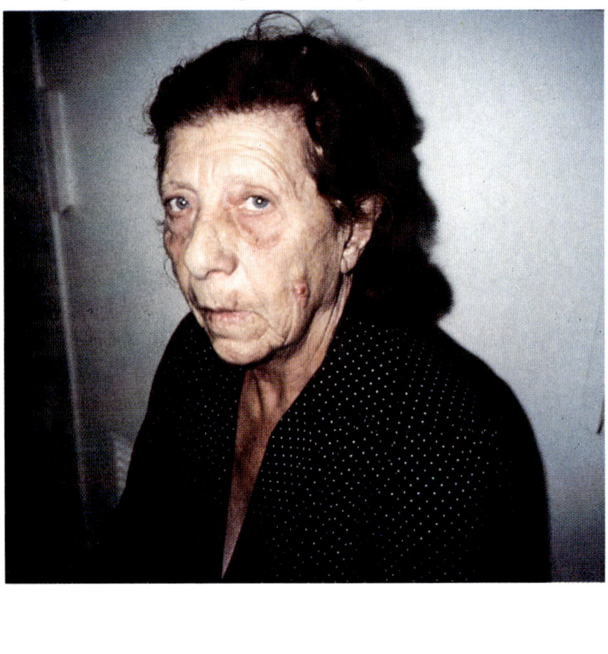

FIGURE 3
Extensive and destructive basal cell epithelioma in the earlobe. Note sun damage and "deep" wrinkles.

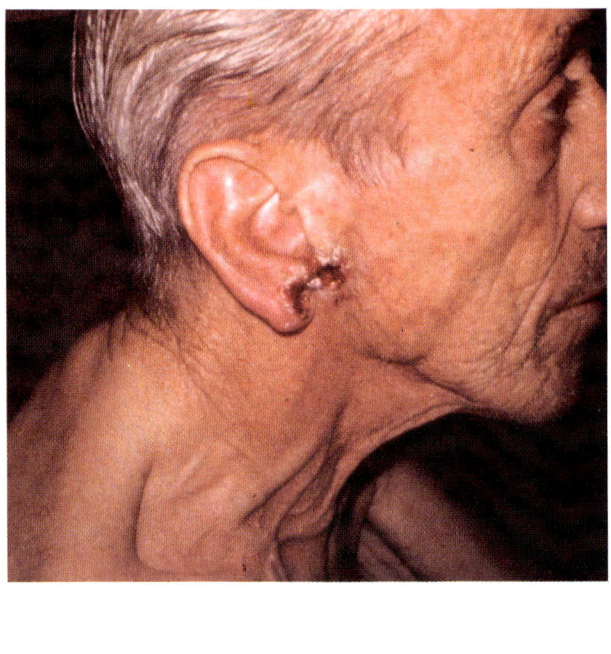

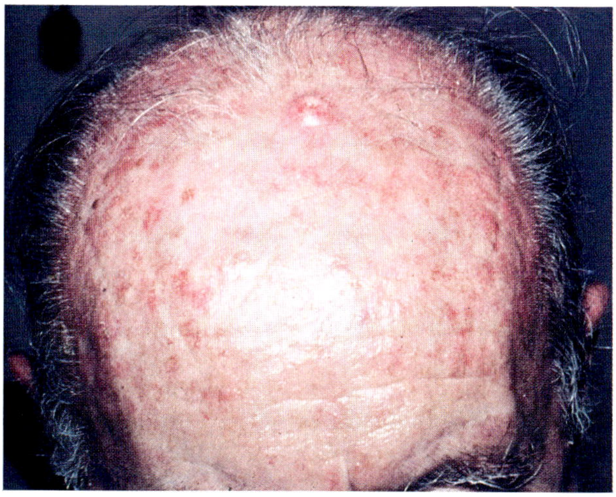

FIGURE 4
Small adenoacanthoma in exposed (bald) area of the scalp. Notice pigmentation, actinic and seborrheic keratoses, and wrinkling.

known, but this form of energy may affect the skin, as shown in erythema ab igne and other skin changes induced by chronic exposure to heat.[5–8]

Concepts of beauty change. The "milky white," almost translucent appearance that was considered so attractive in the past could be obtained in white people only by covering most of the body with vestments and strict avoidance of the sun. Neither the appearance nor the avoidance is considered desirable today.

PROTECTION

Prophylaxis includes protection from the sun and is achieved by a judicious balance of clothing and accessories, avoidance of radiation, and the use of sunscreens.[9] A commonsense knowledge of skin types (Table 1) and of the magnitude of solar radiation in the area is necessary. (Walking in the streets at noon in a tropical city constitutes significant exposure to the sun.) Physical features such as hair (or the lack of it) and anatomic prominences should be evaluated. Clothing is the single best protector, but not all textiles are equivalent in this regard. The protective potential of textiles has been quantitatively evaluated for ultraviolet light. The best protectors are cotton fibers in a brown or black color. The most important factors are the structure and weave of the material. Light may reach the skin by scattering and transmission through interstices rather than by penetrating the material.[10] A wet clinging fabric may protect less than does a dry loose garment.

Considerable effort has been spent in developing sunscreens.[9] The protective effect of sunscreens is numerically expressed as the *sun protection factor* (SPF). The SPF is the ratio between the smallest amount of radiant energy (ultraviolet B) needed to produce erythema when going through a sunscreen film applied to the skin and the amount sufficient to produce erythema in an area of skin devoid of such protection. Under standard conditions, the amount of energy is a direct function of the time of exposure. Thus, the SPF may be understood as the time needed to get erythema under a given radiant exposure. The SPF, which usually is determined in a panel of test subjects, is only a rough guide. Test conditions are not uniform, and factors such as wind, water, and radiation other than UVB are not easily quantitated.

TABLE 1
SKIN TYPES AND RELATION TO SUN EXPOSURE

Skin Type	Reaction to Sun	Appearance
I	Burns easily and severely; does not tan	Fair skin, freckles, blue eyes (e.g., Celts)
II	Burns easily and severely; tans minimally	Fair skin, hair red or blond, eyes blue, hazel, or brown (e.g., Celts)
III	Burns moderately; tans	Average white persons
IV	Burns minimally; tans readily	White or light brown skin, eyes and hair dark (e.g., Mediterraneans, Orientals)
V	Rarely burns; tans well and substantially	Brown-skinned persons, dark eyes (e.g., Amerindians, East Indians)
VI	Never burns; tans markedly	Blacks (e.g., Africans and American blacks, Australian aborigines)

TABLE 2
SELECTED SUNSCREENS

Trade Name	Main Ingredients	Appearance	Sun Protection Factor	Resistance to Water
PreSun 15	5% PABA* in ethanol	Clear lotion	15	Poor
Coppertone Super Shade 15	Octyldimethyl PABA* oxybenzone	Milky lotion	15	Good
PreSun 15 (water resistant)	Padimate O plus oxybenzone	Milky lotion	15	Good
A*-Fil	Titanium dioxide plus zinc oxide plus talc	Cream (tinted)	7	Good
RVPAQUE	Red veterinary petrolatum iron oxide	Cream (rather sticky)	10	Good

* PABA = *p*-aminobenzoic acid.

The ideal goal is to find a topical agent that protects well but is in itself invisible and undetectable. It should not be removed by sweat or water but should be easy to take off at the convenience of the user. Compromises have been found. Current sunscreens protect well against sunburn (UVB). They are cosmetically acceptable, and some are not easily removed by sweat or water. Most sunscreens do not block other forms of radiation. Opaque wide-spectrum preparations exist but are not easily adaptable to current western usage. They may nonetheless be useful in circumstances such as waterskiing, skiing in the snow, and heavy sun exposure in certain expeditions. Table 2 lists representative preparations. A comprehensive list has been published.[11] It should be noted that the ability of a given sunscreen to protect the skin from sunburn does not necessarily parallel its tumor-preventing capacity.[12]

The main purpose of a sunscreen vis à vis aging is to *protect.* Therefore, preparations with a low SPF ($\leq$8) are of little use. Arguably, screens with an SPF above 15 could be superfluous, because radiation does not exceed 15 minimal erythema doses (MED) per day[11] except under unusual conditions. Sunscreens may or may not protect against forms of radiation other than UVB. Thus, the main goal for the future will be the standardization and expansion of the measurement of protection. Oral sunscreens would be a useful alternative. Some of these sunscreens prevent light-induced damage in certain diseases such as lupus erythematosus, polymorphous light eruption, and erythropoietic protoporphyria (e.g., chloroquine, β-carotene, and canthaxanthin); however, there are no oral medications that protect from the sun and can be used by the general public for long periods of time without significant toxicity. A set of instructions to prevent sun damage is given in Table 3; it can be used as a handout for patients.

MANAGEMENT

Benign pigmentary or epithelial neoformations may be removed by mechanical, physical, or chemical means, including cold steel surgery, electrocoagulation and curettage, hot cautery, cryosurgery, and substances that have destructive properties (e.g., acids, alkalis, and biologically active compounds such as podophyllin and cantharidin). Antimetabolites such as topical 5-fluorouracil (5-FU) (Efudex, Fluroplex) may also be used for this purpose. In sunny areas, 5-FU is not well tolerated. Erythema and smarting induced by exposure of treated skin to the sun are common complaints. Side effects may be diminished by using 5-FU only at night and applying emollients and diluted topical steroids during the day. In some cases 5-FU has produced excellent improvement, but aggressive skin cancers developed later. Thus, one should exercise caution in the use of 5-FU.

Combinations are useful. For example, actinic keratoses on the arms may be destroyed by cantharidin in flexible collodion. Conspicuous keratoses near the eyes may be removed by shaving with a scalpel or razor blade and lightly cauterized (a standard hand solderer with a fine tip may be used instead of an expensive apparatus). Other lesions in the face may be treated with nightly applications of 2% or 5% 5-fluoro-uracil solution or cream. If the patient does not tolerate this therapy or if lesions recur, the lesions may be treated with cryosurgery (using liquid nitrogen or nitrous oxide) or with the old-fashioned but still useful "carbon dioxide snow pencil." (Carbon dioxide snow is made by mixing solid crushed dry ice with acetone to form a paste which is forced into a plastic syringe whose tip has been cut off. The resulting cylinder, the diameter of which varies according to the syringe used, freezes portions of a given size.) For some lesions, 50% trichloroacetic acid or pure liquified phenol may be painted on the surface. We have found cantharidin in flexible collodion (Cantharone) to be extremely useful, particularly if it is covered after application with a small square of occlusive adhesive tape for 24 to 48 h. The cosmetic results are excellent, if after the scab sloughs off the area is protected from the sun by avoidance of sunlight and the use of adequate sunscreens for several weeks.

TABLE 3
GUIDE FOR LIGHT-SKINNED INDIVIDUALS

1. Know your skin. Learn where your lesions are (if any). Look at yourself in a mirror. Ask a family member to help you analyze lesions on the back, scalp, genitals, and buttocks.
2. Have a doctor check you every year (every 6 months if you have had skin cancer).
3. Avoid damaging sun exposure:
   a. Do *not* try to get a "healthy tan." Tanning lamps or booths are as dangerous as or more dangerous than sunlight.
   b. Avoid exposure at peak hours of radiation (i.e., 10 a.m. to 3 p.m.).
4. If you must work under significant sun radiation, use a sunscreen with an SPF of 15. We recommend ________________.
5. Keep your hair loose and free-flowing. Hats or caps, long-sleeved shirts or blouses, and long trousers can help protect you from the sun. Cotton fabrics are preferable.
6. Apply these rules with common sense. Their purpose is to let you enjoy life with less danger to your skin.

The treatment of skin cancer is beyond the scope of this chapter (see Chapter 9); however, sun-damaged skin should be checked in toto at periodical intervals: every 6 months if the patient has had a skin malignancy, and yearly in other cases. Suspicious lesions should be plotted on a suitable graph. A *grid chart* on which two human figures (front and back) are plotted in a system of parallels (letters) and meridians (numbers) is very useful. Biopsies are necessary before more extensive surgical procedures are undertaken. The use of the "shave" technique is quick and safe, prevents stitching, and minimizes scarring. It is compatible with subsequent coagulation and curettage.

Xerosis cutis and pruritus are common complaints of older people. A modified Scholtz treatment is effective. This includes the following: soap should be used only once or twice weekly. Bathing may be done every 2 days or even daily in hot climates, but with water only. After bathing, the wet skin is lubricated with proprietary emollients, or with a compounded prescription of 3% lactic acid in Unibase. Dilute corticosteroids may be incorporated in this preparation at the beginning and discontinued after 1 or 2 weeks.

Peeling has been recommended to improve wrinkling and reverse the aging of collagen. Trichloracetic acid and phenol have been used for this purpose. This subject is covered in Chaps. 15 and 16. In tropical climates pigmentation is a common complication. Brunettes and individuals with pigment instability may need to avoid this treatment. Test areas should be explored first.

For a "freshening" effect and removal of superficial blemishes, the resorcinol paste treatment is effective. The paste contains 50% resorcinol, 12% zinc oxide, 6% kaolin, 14% olive oil, and equal parts of white petrolatum and lanolin. It is applied over the face with a wooden spatula. The hair is covered with a surgical cap, and the eyelids and lips are protected with petrolatum. Gowns may be used because resorcinol stains clothing. The consistency of the paste can be modified by adding small amounts of mineral oil. After application, the paste is allowed to stay on for 2 h, after which the bulk is removed with gauze impregnated with mineral oil. A thin film of paste is left. The paste is removed by the patient with soap and water at home. The number of successive daily applications determines the intensity of peeling. We usually employ three applications since four can produce a brisk reaction. When peeling starts, a sunscreen is prescribed. Beaches are avoided for several months.

Retinoids are inhibitors of tumor promotion.[13] Tretinoin (retinoic acid; Retin-A) applied topically has been proposed to prevent the development of precancerous and cancerous lesions and to enhance the repair of ultraviolet-induced dermal damage. The use of these agents has been extended recently to the treatment and prevention of wrinkling. Significant reversal of collagen changes induced by sun and time is necessary for retinoids or any other substance for that matter to annul the aging process and the resulting wrinkles. Some experimental evidence[8] has suggested that this is feasible. Only time and sober analysis will tell whether topical retinoids are able to restore youthful smoothness to aged skin. Currently, there are no grounds for systematic rejection or for euphoria.

For the prevention of cancer we have employed 0.025% retinoic acid in Unibase or in propylene glycol–alcohol–water depending upon whether the patient is old or young and has or does not have oily skin. Acceptance has not been excellent. In tropical and sunny climates there is much discomfort and itching. These symptoms may be helped to a degree by incorporating very dilute steroids and spacing the applications. This technique can be helpful when employed systematically but will probably not remain very popular. Newer retinoids will undoubtedly change the outlook.

CONCLUSIONS

The best treatment for sun-induced aging of the skin is prevention. Both attitudes about the sun and about concepts of beauty and health are acquired early. Dermatologists see teenagers with acne. Shortly thereafter, these former teenagers become parents and may bring their children to the same dermatologist. From the onset, the dermatologist should gauge the type of skin the child has and begin to warn about actinic damage: (1) Tanning booths are even more dangerous than sunlight,[14] and (2) judicious avoidance of the sun, particularly in light-skinned individuals, will prevent aging, skin cancers, and perhaps melanomas. The approach may be modified for darker complected patients and for those living in less sunny climes.

REFERENCES

1. Longas MO, Russell CS, He XY. Chemical alterations of hyaluronic acid and dermatan sulphate detected in aging human skin by infrared spectroscopy. Biochim Biophys Acta 1986; 884:265–269.
2. Chen VL, Fleischmajer R, Schwartz E, et al. Immunochemistry of elastotic material in sun-damaged skin. J Invest Dermatol. 1986; 87:334–337.
3. Plastow SR, Lovell CR, Young AR. UVB-induced collagen changes in the skin of the hairless albino mouse. J Invest Dermatol. 1987; 88:145–148.
4. Fenske NA, Lober CW. Structural and functional changes of normal aging skin. J Am Acad Dermatol. 1986; 15:571–585.
5. Kligman LH, Kligman AM. Photoaging, in Fitzpatrick TB, Eisen AZ, Wolff K, et al. (eds). Dermatology in General Medicine, 3d ed. New York: McGraw-Hill, 1987:1470–1475.
6. Pfau RG, Hood AF, Morison WL. Photoageing: The role of UVB, solar simulated UVB, visible and psoralen UVA radiation. Br J Dermatol. 1986; 114:319–327.
7. Kornhauser A, Wamer W, Giles A Jr, et al. Mechanisms of light induced dermal toxicity, in Frost P, Horwitz SN (eds). Principles of Cosmetics for the Dermatologist. St. Louis: CV Mosby, 1982:244–258.
8. Kligman LH, Kligman AM. Enhanced repair of UV: Induced dermal damage by topical retinoic acid, in Saurat JH (ed). Retinoids: New Trends in Research and Therapy. Basel: S Karger, 1985:265–271.
9. Greiter F, Bilek P, Doskoczil S. History of sun screens and the rationale for their use, in Frost P, Horwitz SN (eds). Principles of Cosmetics for the Dermatologist. St. Louis: CV Mosby, 1982:187–206.
10. Welsh C, Diffey B. Protection against solar actinic radiation afforded by common clothing fabrics. Clin Exp Dermatol. 1981; 6:577–582.
11. Pathak MA. Sunscreens: Topical and systemic approaches for the prevention of acute and chronic sun-induced skin reactions. Dermatol Clin. 1986; 6:321–334.
12. Gurish MF, Roberts LK, Krueger GG, et al. The effects of various sunscreen agents on skin damage and induction of tumor susceptibility in mice subjected to ultraviolet irradiation. J Invest Dermatol. 1981; 76:246–251.
13. Boutwell RK, Verma AK, Takigawa M, et al. Retinoids as inhibitors of tumor promotion, in Saurat JH (ed). Retinoids: New Trends in Research and Therapy. Basel: S Karger, 1985:83–96.
14. Natchwey DS, Rundel RD. Photobiologic evaluation of tanning booths. Science. 1981; 211:405–407.

CHAPTER 6

Treatment of Benign Cutaneous Lesions

HARRY M. HUMENIUK
GARY P. LASK

This chapter deals with skin lesions that are generally regarded as benign. Some of these lesions may have so-called malignant tendencies, but they generally are not destructive. Therefore, *primum non nocere* ("first, do not harm") is the rule to follow. The patient must not be left with a surgical result that is less cosmetically appealing than the lesion itself. In fact, the lesion may disappear by itself.

The most common benign lesions seen in practice are reviewed. We have included more unusual tumors when the lesion seems of importance. Concise morphologic descriptions precede outlined therapeutic modalities, but this presentation cannot replace a chapter in a general dermatology text.

ANGIOFIBROMAS

It is a histologic misnomer to refer to these lesions as adenoma sebaceum. Not infrequently, solitary angiofibromas arise and can be clinically indistinguishable from basal cell carcinoma.[1] These multiple 0.1- to 0.3-cm reddish-brown to flesh-colored smooth papules are localized to the nasolabial folds, cheeks, and chin as part of the triad of tuberous sclerosis.

Management

1. Solitary angiofibromas are best managed by simple shave excision.[2] Lidocaine 1% with or without epinephrine 1:100,000 is infiltrated into the dermis below the lesion. A 30-gauge needle may be utilized, as it causes the least discomfort for the patient. A Codman surgical marking pen may be used to delineate the lesion since a local anesthetic can blanch and obscure the margins of the lesion.

   The lesion is shaved flush with the skin, using a No. 15 blade. As the purpose is cosmetic improvement, it is better to err on the side of shaving too superficially. The procedure can be easily repeated if the initial shave is inadequate. Too deep a shave can result in a depressed depigmented area that may be more upsetting to the patient than the original lesion. The shave is

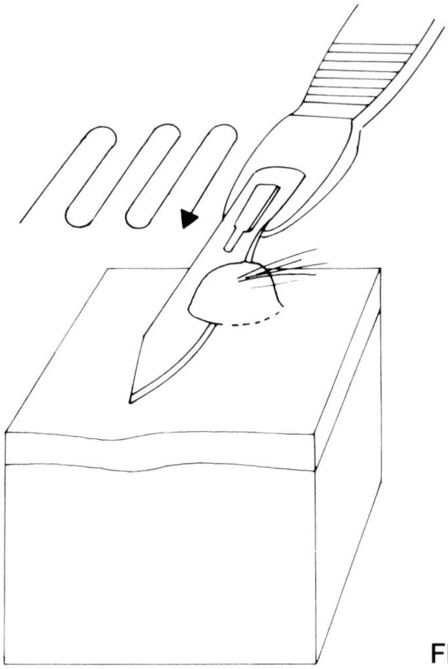

FIGURE 1

begun away from the surgeon and completed with a smooth even back and forth motion toward the operator (Fig. 1).

An alternative method is to use a Gillette Super Blue blade, which provides greater flexibility and a sharper shave.[3] Hemostasis is easily accomplished with a chemical cautery agent such as trichloroacetic acid (TCA) 20% or aluminum chloride 20% in ethyl alcohol (Drysol).

2. Dermabrasion may provide a good cosmetic result in the dominantly inherited form of multiple angiofibroma. Recurrence is to be expected, and repeat dermabrasion probably will be necessary.[4,5]
3. Ablation of multiple lesions can also be accomplished with an argon laser, CO_2 laser, or 585 pulsed dye laser.

Laser Type	Power	Spot Size, mm	Pulse Duration
Argon	0.8–1.2 W	0.2–2.0	0.2 to continuous wave
CO_2	5–10 W	1–2	Continuous wave in defocused mode
585 pulsed dye	6.25–7.25 J/cm2	5	No value applicable: standard for all pulsed dye lasers

CYSTS

Dermoid Cyst

Because they are thought to arise from sequestration of skin along lines of embryonic closure, dermoid cysts are generally present at birth; hence, these cysts are predictably localized to the face, particularly near the eyes, and the neck. Measuring 1.0 to 4.0 cm, these smooth subcutaneous nodules rarely alter the overlying epidermis. Dermoid cysts may be freely movable or can be adherent to the underlying periosteum.[6]

Midline cysts at the base of the nose must be approached with caution, as they may represent a nasal glioma.

Management See the management section for the epidermoid cyst.

Digital Mucous Cyst

These shiny, smooth, nearly translucent cystic nodules are located between the distal interphalangeal joint and the proximal nail fold. Thinned epidermis covers these 0.2- to 0.5-cm cystic lesions, which may be painful.

Management A nonsurgical initial approach is warranted since recurrence after excision is not uncommon.

1. Aspiration of the mucinous fluid followed by intralesional triamcinolone 5 to 10 mg/ml may cause resolution. Unfortunately, recurrence is common; however, repeating this procedure can lead to resolution.
2. Surgical excision: After a digital block, the overlying epidermis is incised with a No. 15 blade and retracted with skin hooks. The entire cyst and any synovial connection must be carefully dissected out. Methylene blue may be injected into the cyst to help delineate the cyst and any extensions of its synovial lining. The thinned epidermis overlying the cyst may require extension of the incisional flap to permit adequate closure.

Epidermoid Cyst

Clinically indistinguishable from pilar cysts, epidermoid cysts most commonly arise on the face, neck, shoulders, and chest. Because these cysts occur in areas where acne vulgaris is common, they used to be incorrectly termed *sebaceous cysts*. Other terms have included *keratinous cyst* and *wen*.

Clinically, a punctum usually surmounts the 0.5- to 5.0-cm freely movable firm subcutaneous protruberance. Cysts are slow in growing and become tender when inflamed. A foul-smelling cheesy substance is encountered when the cyst wall is incised and its contents are expressed.

Management

1. Inflamed cysts are best approached by intralesional injection of 2.5 to 3.3 mg/ml of triamcinolone, with each injection consisting of 0.05 to 0.25 ml.[7] Epidermoid cysts treated in this fashion may resolve completely or at least become quiescent and therefore amenable to removal, as described below.
2. Piezosurgery provides excellent cosmetic results. After appropriate anesthesia, small cysts may be removed via a small incision over the midline of the lesion. Infiltrating with lidocaine 2% without epinephrine just below the epidermis overlying the cyst is suggested. The incision is superficial and should reveal the glistening capsule of the cyst. Gentle application of pressure on both sides of the cyst generally provides adequate exposure for complete removal with curved iris scissors. The resulting defect may be closed with Steri-Strips or sutured,[8] although we prefer suturing.
3. Another approach to noninflamed cysts is to use a 2- or 3-mm punch. Larger cysts can be incised, and their contents can be expressed. The cystic sac is held with a toothed hemostat and can be easily maneuvered so that adhesions can be disrupted with small curved iris scissors. Gentle rotation of the sac in both directions can also assist in the disruption of adhesions. The entire lesion must be removed to prevent recurrence. The small defect can be closed with sutures (Fig. 2).
4. Larger lesions may be approached by making a small ellipse over the cyst. If hair is in the way, tape can be used to keep it from interfering; this precludes shaving the area.[9] This procedure pro-

FIGURE 2

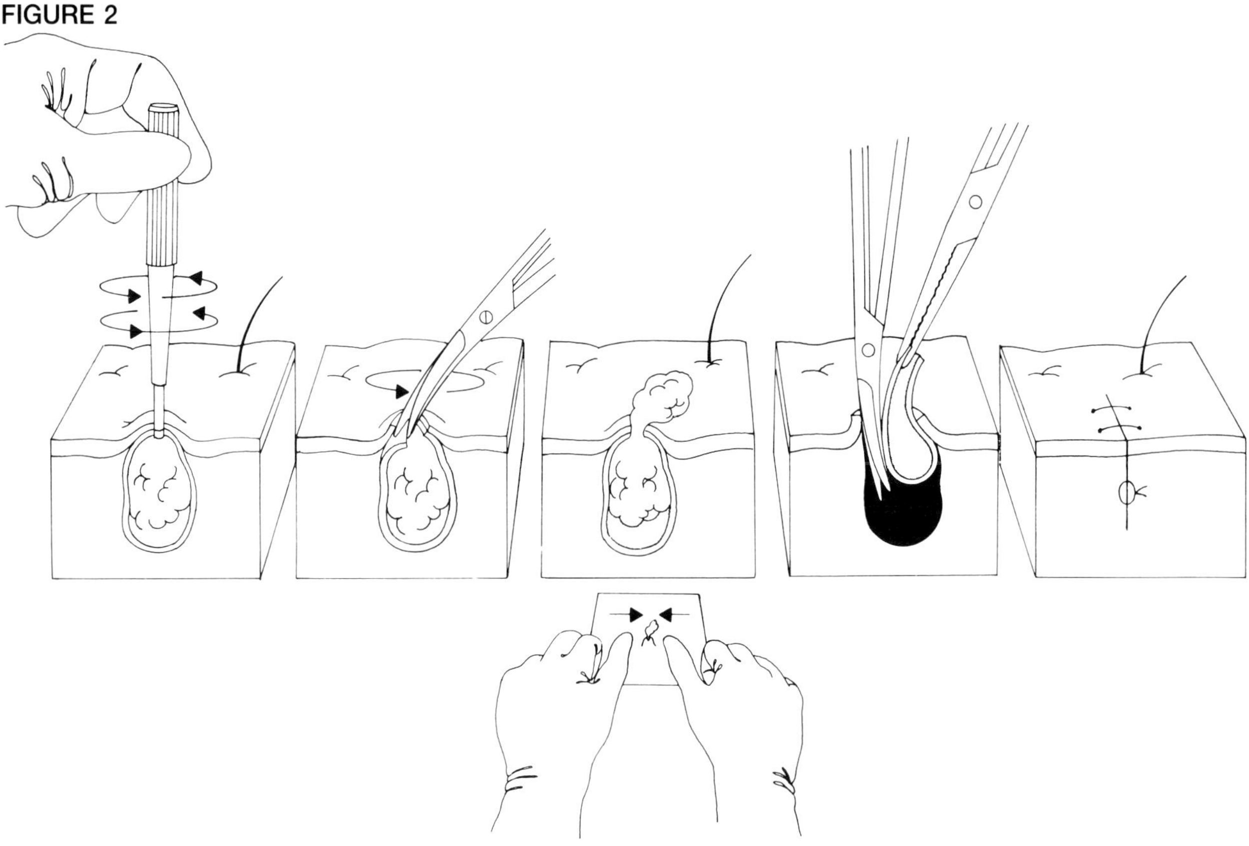

vides easy access to the underlying cyst; adhesions can be disrupted with curved iris scissors, and the lesion can be removed in toto. Primary closure smoothes out the space defect. Absorbable subcutaneous sutures may be utilized for excessively large defects. Hematoma is a rare complication requiring evacuation and consideration of drain placement.

5. Infected cysts usually require incision and drainage. An iodoform tape packing may be placed and then removed in 2 to 4 days. Antimicrobial coverage should be initiated immediately and carried out for 7 to 10 days before subsequent surgical intervention. Complete removal by one of the methods described above may be carried out 3 to 4 weeks later.

Hidrocystomas

Apocrine Hidrocystoma Most often arising about the eyes as a solitary clear to bluish nodule, an apocrine hidrocystoma may clinically resemble a blue nevus. Less frequent sites of occurrence include other areas of the face, ears, scalp, chest, and shoulders. This form of hidrocystoma is symptomless and grows slowly to less than 1.0 cm in diameter.

Management Apocrine hidrocystomas are best treated at an early stage because they most commonly arise about the cosmetically significant periorbital region. Simple excision with complete dissection of the cyst and primary closure may produce a good cosmetic result.

Eccrine Hidrocystoma These 0.1- to 0.3-cm cystic lesions are primarily localized to the cheeks and periorbital regions. Occasionally multiple, these yellow to blue cysts are generally singular and thus mimic apocrine hidrocystomas. Eccrine hidrocystoma can enlarge and increase in number with exposure to heat. Hence, these lesions tend to wax and wane during summer and winter months, respectively.

Management

1. Excision as described in the treatment section for apocrine hidrocystoma may be done.
2. Electrosurgical ablation of lesions can produce satisfactory cosmetic results with little chance of recurrence. Low-current electrodesiccation may be repeated as necessary.

Milium

Milia appear as white or yellow globoid papules that measure 0.1 to 0.2 cm. Multiple spontaneous milia may arise about the face, particularly on the cheeks and eyelids. Spontaneous or primary milia are thought to arise from the infundibulum of vellus hairs. Traumatic or secondary milia arise in association with blistering disorders, dermabrasion, and radiotherapy and within wounds that heal by secondary intention. The latter form may be more random in distribution about the affected areas compared with a spontaneous milium.

Management

1. A milium can be nicked with a No. 11 blade or a small-gauge needle. It can then be easily removed with the needle tip or expressed with a comedo extractor. Recurrence is uncommon, and the cosmetic results are generally excellent.
2. Light electrodesiccation can also be used, as can application of a keratolytic to peel the epidermis covering the cyst.

Steatocystoma Multiplex

These multiple, rounded cystic flesh-colored to yellowish lesions measuring 0.2 to 3.0 cm are located over the upper anterior chest and the proximal arms and legs. Autosomal dominant and spontaneous forms generally manifest in adolescence and progress with age. The cysts are filled with a clear yellow liquid or a cheesy white substance.

Management Management of steatocystoma multiplex lesions involves several considerations. The multitude of lesions precludes removal of all cysts. As this entity tends to progress with age, new lesions are destined to arise and the patient's overall well-being is not compromised by this benign condition.

If the patient wants a cosmetically significant lesion to be removed, the methods described in the management section for the epidermoid cyst may be employed.

Trichilemmal Cyst

Also known as *pilar* cysts, these lesions primarily arise on the scalp and are clinically indistinguishable from epidermoid cysts. Sometimes called *wens,* these round, smooth, firm nodules can be several centimeters in size, lobulated, and multiple.

Proliferating pilar cysts may mimic squamous cell carcinoma both clinically and histologically. Regional lymph node metastases have been known to occur.[10]

Management The methods described in the management section for the epidermoid cyst are generally applied, with the following considerations.

1. Piezosurgery and the punch biopsy method as described above should not be considered because the thicker although less adherent walls of trichilemmal cysts resist extraction through such a small incision.[11]
2. Proliferating cysts require a margin of excision since they tend to recur if tissue is left behind.

DERMATOFIBROMAS

These firm, smooth, freely movable nodules are common and benign. They can occur in any location; however, the extremities, particularly the lower extremities of women, are the most frequent site. Most measure a few millimeters, but some may reach several centimeters in size. The color varies from red to purple to dark brown. A diagnostic feature is central dimpling with the application of lateral pressure. The course of dermatofibroma is static, although spontaneous regression has been reported.[12]

Management

1. After adequate local anesthesia, excision to the superficial fat is the treatment of choice. Because the majority of lesions occur on the lower extremities of women, the resulting surgical scars may be out of proportion to the original lesions.
2. Excellent cosmetic responses can be obtained with cryotherapy. A cryoprobe one-half to two-thirds the diameter of the lesion is applied, and the tissue is frozen with a 1- to 2-mm rim. Repeat treatment may be necessary in 6 to 8 weeks. A different spray technique can be employed for large lesions. After the center of the lesion is punctured by a key punch, liquid nitrogen is sprayed into this site. The spray should be continued until a 1- to 2-mm rim of freeze is obtained.[13,14]

KERATOACANTHOMAS

Clinically, keratoacanthomas are sharply demarcated firm, smooth, dome-shaped nodules which possess a keratin-filled central crater. They are one of the most controversial tumors of the skin. Whether they are benign, malignant, or pseudomalignant is still under discussion. Characteristically, these flesh-colored to erythematous lesions evolve over a 6-week period, reaching a diameter of 1.0 to 2.5 cm or more. Most tumors involute in the following 2 to 6 months. Some lesions may persist longer than a year. Ulceration occurs infrequently, generally after infection or trauma, and can contribute to the depressed scarring associated with a spontaneously healing keratoacanthoma.

Because malignant transformation to squamous cell carcinoma has been reported,[15,16] these lesions require at least biopsy and, when appropriate, removal. Whether the original lesion is misdiagnosed as keratoacanthoma or whether true malignant degeneration occurs are beyond the scope of this chapter. Recurrent lesions, particularly those located on the lip, must be scrutinized for squamous cell carcinoma and possible metastasis.[17]

Management

Although spontaneous regression is apt to occur, treatment is advocated for several reasons. Clinical misdiagnosis would be disastrous, the resultant scar from spontaneous regression is often unacceptable, and the appearance of the lesion will undoubtedly make the patient anxious.

1. If the lesion is to be biopsied prior to complete removal, the surgeon must be aware that shave, punch, and pie-shaped wedge biopsies are often inadequate. A spindle-shaped incision through the center of the lesion, including normal tissue from both sides and subcutaneous fat from beneath the lesion, should be done.[18]
2. An elliptical excision with primary closure is frequently recommended. Curettage generally allows good healing, but some histopathologists object to basing a diagnosis on bits and pieces of the specimen.
3. Mohs micrographic surgery is excellent for recurrent keratoacanthoma, keratoacanthoma that arises on the lips and other mucosal surfaces, and giant keratoacanthoma.
4. Other treatment modalities include the following.

a. Intralesional 5-fluorouracil (5-FU) 50 mg/cm^2. 5-FU injections are repeated weekly until 70 to 80 percent involution occurs. Goette and Odom[19] reported that 40 of 41 lesions cleared in an average of 3 to 4 weeks.
b. Blunt dissection of the lesion can be accomplished with scissors and a blunt dissector. Monsel's solution is then used as a styptic.[20]
c. Radiotherapy may provide an alternative to radical surgery in multiple, giant, or progressive keratoacanthoma. A total dose of 4,500 to 5,000 rad divided into 15 to 20 doses can provide excellent results.[21]
d. Conservative therapy is advocated by some authors.[22,23] The diagnosis must be certain and the patient must be highly motivated, since close follow-up is required.

LENTIGENES

There are two benign forms of lentigenes: *simplex* and *solar* (senile).

Lentigo Simplex

These evenly pigmented brown-black macules measure 0.1 to 0.2 cm. The lesions arise in childhood and may increase in number with age. Lentigo simplex may arise on any mucocutaneous surface, remain static, become confluent, or regress.

Several syndromes have lentigo simplex as a characteristic feature, including Peutz-Jeghers syndrome, LEOPARD syndrome, and LAMB syndrome, as well as centrofacial lentiginosis.

Lentigo Solar

This form of lentigo arises as a consequence of exposure to ultraviolet irradiation. Thus the face, arms, and hands are common sites of predilection. Generally multiple, these tan to brown macules are irregular in shape and usually measure less than 0.5 cm; however, they may reach several centimeters in diameter. Lesions rarely arise before the fourth or fifth decade and are most commonly found on the dorsum of the hands.[24]

Management

1. Liquid nitrogen. Alternating cotton tip application, spray, or cryoprobe may be used. The freeze should extend just beyond the pigmented border. Thaw time should be about 20 to 30 s.
2. Trichloroacetic acid (TCA) in a concentration of 10 to 50% is applied until the lentigo achieves an "acid frost." Scarring is almost never seen.
3. CO_2 laser therapy has been used. A defocused mode at an energy level that will attain a slight opalescence of the pigmented lesion may produce an acceptable cosmetic result without scarring.

LIPOMAS

Lipomas are common, benign tumors composed primarily of adipose tissue. Most lipomas are localized to the subcutis; however, they may infiltrate the deeper soft tissues. Although lipomas may arise in any location, the trunk, nape of the neck, and arms are the most common sites. These subcutaneous nodules may occur as single or multiple tumors. Lipomas may be barely perceptible (less than 1.0 cm) or large enough to be quite evident (greater than 5.0 cm). Tangential lighting may aid in the localization of lipomas because they rarely alter the overlying integument. Palpation reveals a soft round to ovoid mass that may be lobulated and generally freely movable.

Angiolipomas are frequently multiple, slightly more firm than common lipomas, and occasionally painful. Histologically, mature adipose tissue is interspersed with varying degrees of vascularity.[25]

Management Incision and enucleation are the treatment of choice. If the fat encountered is atypical, a biopsy rather than complete removal should be performed.

1. The lesion is palpated, and its margins are outlined. Local anesthesia is infiltrated over the center of the lipoma, and a 2- to 3-mm incision is made over the lesion. A 2-mm cutting curette is then used to free and deliver the lipoma through the small incision. Sutures are not required with this method but are useful. Usually 2×2 squares under a pressure dressing are utilized.[26]
2. Larger lipomas may be approached in a similar manner, with the following additions. A small ellipse about 2 cm can accept small curved iris scissors and a small toothed hemostat. The fibrofatty mass is held and maneuvered with the hemostat while being freed with the scissors.

Some adhesions may be disrupted by rotation of the lipoma with the pickups; care should be taken to avoid twisting the instrument and disrupting the mass. Once it is free, the lipoma is delivered whole. A large dead space may be partially closed with buried absorbable suture, though this is rarely necessary. Closure of the ellipse removes some of the integumental slack produced by the mass effect of the lipoma. Pressure dressings help prevent hematoma formation. If hematoma does arise, evacuation, resuturing, and placement of a drain should be considered.

3. Lipomas arising in areas of aesthetic consequence may be approached by "excision from a distance." The length of the incision should approximate its distance from the lipoma. Preferred sites for these aesthetically acceptable incisions include the scalp, eyelids, preauricular region, nasolabial folds, oral mucosa, and inframammary folds. Tunneling requires assistance and good lighting. Hemostasis during this procedure is a must.[27] Other techniques described under item 2 should be followed.
4. Liposuction removal of lipoma may be considered (see Chap. 30).

Angiolipomas, being more vascular, may bleed slightly more than do common lipomas. This rarely complicates the procedures described above; however, it does alert the surgeon to the importance of hemostasis in surgical management of these lesions.

MELANOCYTIC NEVI

These benign lesions are composed of nevus cells. Dopa-positive staining is characteristic of nevus cells, just as with melanocytes. Nevus cells differ from melanocytes in their tendency to be arranged in clusters or "nests." Nevocytic nevi may appear flat, slightly elevated, papillomatous, dome-shaped, or pedunculated. The first three clinical forms are always pigmented, and the latter two may or may not appear pigmented. All forms of melanocytic nevi can be found on any cutaneous surface.

A prediction of histologic appearance can occasionally be made by clinical appearance, but exceptions are frequent. Junctional nevi have a proliferation of nevus cells at the dermal-epidermal (D-E) junction. Clinically, junctional nevi are flat, smooth, and pigmented. Compound nevi consist of nevus cells intradermally and at the D-E junction. Clinically, they appear slightly elevated to dome-shaped and may or may not appear pigmented. Intradermal nevi are composed solely of dermal nevus cells. Generally this form appears flesh-colored and dome-shaped.[28]

Management Nevi are usually brought to the dermatologist's attention by patients for one of four reasons. When there is irregular growth, change in color, ulceration, and/or bleeding, removal is suggested. Incisional biopsy through the thickest portion in large lesions and lesions located on cosmetically significant surfaces is an alternative.

Cosmetic and impaired function are other common presenting complaints. There are two surgical approaches to this problem.

1. Simple excision can achieve complete removal. Margins beyond the clinical lesion do not have to be included since melanocytic nevi tend to be anatomically confined to the clinical presentation. Depending on the location, excision may not be acceptable; in this case the approach described below may be followed.
2. Shave excision can produce excellent cosmetic results. The shave should be flush with the skin surface. Refer to the description of shave excision in the treatment section for angiofibroma for the technique. Since the entire lesion may not be removed by this method, the following complications should be explained to the patient.
   a. Irregular repigmentation and elevation may occur; excision is then curative.
   b. Scarring can alter future biopsy, confusing this benign entity with melanoma.

NEVUS SEBACEOUS OF JADASSOHN

Nevus sebaceous presents at birth or shortly thereafter as a well-circumscribed, smooth, waxy plaque that has an orange-yellow to chamois color. Most lesions occur on the hair-bearing scalp and in decreasing frequency on the face, arm, chest, and back.

Although composed of benign components, nevus sebaceous also possesses pluripotential cells which at puberty may evolve into syringocystadenoma papilliferum. Basal cell epithelioma can also occur within the lesion. These changes, although infrequent, occur most commonly at puberty. Other postpubertal changes include linear formation instead of round or irregular plaques, deepening of color, and the development of velvety, verrucous, or even nodular lesions.[29]

Because of the potential for malignant degeneration, nevus sebaceous is best removed before or shortly after puberty to eliminate the lesion prior to the development of secondary and possibly malignant changes.

Management Assessment of scalp laxity should be done prior to excision to assure that primary closure is feasible. Complete excision to the depth of the hair follicles (deep subcutaneous fat) is the treatment of choice. All margins of the lesion must be histologically evaluated to ensure complete removal.[30]

SEBACEOUS HYPERPLASIA

Lesions of sebaceous hyperplasia usually arise in individuals past middle age. Located primarily on the forehead and cheeks, they most commonly appear as small, grouped yellowish papules. Close examination invariably reveals a central follicular punctum. Telangiectatic vessels often accompany sebaceous hyperplasia, and so confusion with basal cell carcinoma may occur; however, clinical scrutiny allows differentiation. Biopsy of any suspicious lesions is recommended.

Management If the clinical impression is certain, treatment is purely cosmetic. The objective of electrosurgery or CO_2 laser surgery is to plane or flatten the lesions. These methods of removal should not be so aggressive as to leave a depressed scar. Repeat treatment may be required.

The treatment approach is based on the number of lesions.

1. A small number of lesions can be managed by simple excision or punch.
2. Light electrodessication followed by curettage provides good results.
3. A point cryoprobe placed in the central punctum with a 5- to 10-s freeze or a 1-mm rim is sufficient for most lesions. This approach can be effective in treating multiple lesions. A few test lesions should be evaluated first.[31]
4. Multiple sebaceous hyperplasia can be treated with dermabrasion.
5. CO_2 laser: For parameters, refer to CO_2 treatment in the section for treatment of angiofibroma.
6. Trichloroacetic acid (TCA) 10 to 20% can be used to peel down the lesion.

SEBORRHEIC KERATOSIS

Seborrheic keratosis occur primarily on the face and trunk. These sharply demarcated, brown to black, elevated lesions generally arise in middle to later life. Appearing "stuck on," most seborrheic keratoses measure 1.0 cm or less but may reach several centimeters in diameter. These lesions become increasingly apparent with advancing age, although they may have a congenital etiology, being dominantly inherited.

A soft fibroma may be confused with the pedunculated form of a seborrheic keratosis. This variant is frequently encountered about the neck and upper chest.

Dermatosis papulosa nigra is a condition arising in blacks consisting of multiple, 0.1- to 0.5-cm brown to black papules that are histologically identical to seborrheic keratoses. They are found about the face, neck, and upper trunk. Management methods 1 through 4 listed below provide the best cosmetic results.

Management

1. Curettage can be the simplest and most complete method of removal. The curettement should be done with a quick, firm rotational flick of the wrist followed by the application of a styptic. A local anesthetic may not be required in a stoic patient (Fig. 3). Pretreatment with liquid nitrogen can render larger soft lesions firm, allowing easier removal while providing anesthesia.
2. Pedunculated seborrheic keratoses can be removed by simple scissor excision.
3. Shave excision provides complete removal; however, local anesthesia is necessary.
4. Electrodessication can be used alone or in combination with curettage. Again, local anesthesia is advised.

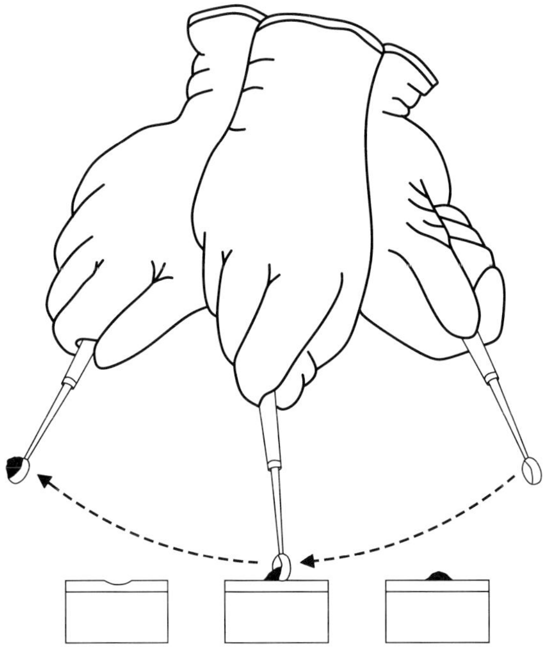

FIGURE 3

5. Although cryotherapy alone can provide excellent cosmetic results, incomplete removal is the rule, and curettage should follow freezing.
6. A keratolytic can be applied for several weeks. Salicylic acid (Keralyt) or a similar wart treatment chemical compound (Occlusal) can be used.

SYRINGOMAS

These yellow to flesh-colored papules arise most commonly in women at or shortly after puberty. Although singular lesions may occur, multiple, firm 0.1- to 0.3-cm papules usually arise about the lower eyelids in a bilaterally symmetrical pattern. Other areas of predeliction include the cheeks, neck, axillae, chest, umbilicus, and pubic region.

An eruptive form (eruptive hidradenoma of Darier and Jaquet) may arise in successive crops over the chest and abdomen. These syringomas can remain static or spontaneously resolve.[32] Therefore, observation rather than treatment is warranted initially in eruptive hidradenoma.

Management See the management section for angiofibroma.

TRICHOEPITHELIOMAS

Spontaneous singular and multiple autosomal dominant forms exist. Both types arise primarily on the face and neck, with multiple trichoepitheliomas commonly appearing symmetrically about the eyelids, cheeks, and nasolabial folds. Multiple types range from 0.2 to 0.8 cm in diameter, while the singular type may reach 2.0 cm.[33] Both types appear as firm elevated papules and nodules that are yellow to pink to flesh-colored. Telangiectatic vessels may be associated with these lesions, mimicking basal cell epithelioma.

A variant known as desmoplastic trichoepithelioma occurs most commonly in women. A single indurated plaque with a depressed center and a raised rolled border may be clinically confused with basal cell epithelioma or granuloma annulare.[34]

Management

1. A shave excision as described in the treatment section for angiofibroma can provide a good cosmetic result.
2. CO_2 laser and electrocautery may be used to plane these lesions. Refer to the treatment section for angiofibroma for the technique and parameters.
3. Simple excision of individual lesions may be adequate.

VERRUCAE

Warts represent clinical infection with one of the members of the human papillomavirus group. Each subtype, of which over 50 are known, has a distinct DNA genome that can be identified by radiolabeling and molecular hybridization.[35]

Verruca Plana

Flat warts occur most commonly on the face and the dorsum of the hands. They arise as multiple flat, slightly elevated flesh-colored to tan papules 0.1 to 0.3 cm in diameter. Shaving the infected beard area can lead to extensive autoinoculation and so represents a real problem.

An aggressive initial approach is not warranted with flat warts on the face.

Management

1. Topical tretinoin (retinoic acid, Retin-A) cream 0.025% is a nonaggressive means of treating facial flat warts. Daily application can achieve a variable response.
2. Application of 10 to 35% TCA in the office is effective. The process can be repeated every 1 or 2 weeks. Hypopigmentation is an occasional side effect of this technique as well as of the treatments described below, but scarring is unknown.
3. "Painting" the flat wart surface white with a Hyfercator tip can eradicate these lesions. The instrument should be turned to the "just on" position; a pointed tip works best. Lesions fall off in a few days.
4. Liquid nitrogen can be applied with alternating cotton-tipped applicators to maintain a 1- to 2-mm rim of "freeze" for 5 to 10 s.
5. Painting the lesions with a keratolytic or a wart compound can be efficacous after 4 to 8 weeks. Scarring is unknown.

Verruca Vulgaris

Common warts may arise at any site and at any age. Children under 12 are the most commonly infected, and the dorsum of the hand is the most frequent site. Periungal verrucae may be tender and difficult to treat. Other sites of infection are generally asymptomatic.

Clinically, these 0.1- to 2.0-cm firm, hyperkeratotic papular lesions are well circumscribed and can appear filamentous.

Management

1. Liquid nitrogen applied with alternating cotton-tipped applicators to produce a 1- to 2-mm ring of freeze is effective. Freeze times vary from 3 to 30 s, depending on the size of the lesions. Although the wart generally is shed with the blister roof (blisters arise in 12 to 24 h), new or recalcitrant lesions may occur, and retreatment may be necessary.
2. Multiple topical agents are available. Salicylic acid–impregnated films (40% salicylic acid plaster, Mediplast) are easier to confine to the lesion and are of greater concentration than are liquid preparations. The plaster is trimmed to the shape of the wart and covers it. Waterproof tape may then be used to keep the film in place. Every 2 to 5 days the plaster is removed. The wart is soaked in water, and the loose whitish tissue is gently rubbed away. A fresh tape is trimmed and reapplied.
3. Electrodessication and curettage are an excellent treatment modality for verrucae; local anesthesia is necessary. Smaller periungal extensions may be removed with a small curette while the nail is left intact.[36]
4. For recalcitrant periungal verrucae, a local anesthetic is followed by nail plate avulsion and wart electrodessication. A small cutting curette is used to remove the white puffy mass.
5. CO_2 laser, 5 to 10 W, in the continuous wave and defocused mode is effective. After multiple passes, the char is removed with peroxide.
6. Bleomycin in the sulfated salt form is available as a 15-unit vial with a potency of 1.2 to 1.7 U/mg. Reconstituted with saline, it is stable for 4 weeks if refrigerated. Verrucae are first cleansed with isopropyl alcohol. At each treatment session the total volume injected is limited to 2 ml of bleomycin reconstituted with saline. The amount injected in each lesion is determined by size. Warts smaller than 5 mm are treated with 0.2 ml, warts 5 to 10 mm are treated with 0.2 to 0.5 ml, and larger lesions are treated with the single largest dose per lesion of 1.0 ml. We suggest the use of a Luer-lock syringe with a 30-gauge needle. Follow-up in 2 weeks will determine whether a second and final treatment is necessary.[37]

XANTHELASMAS

These lesions appear as smooth, soft yellow papules and plaques about the medial canthi and eyelids. Approximately two-thirds of all persons with xanthelasma palpebarum have normal serum lipid levels. Several inherited lipid disorders, hepatobiliary disease, and prolonged cholestasis-related hypercholesterolemia can also manifest as xanthelasma.

Treatment

1. Simple excision with primary closure may provide an excellent cosmetic result.
2. Office application of 10 to 35% TCA may be effective. The process is repeated every 1 or 2

weeks. An occasional side effect is hypopigmentation. Recurrent and large xanthalasmas may resolve with office application of 50 to 100% TCA.[38]

3. Laser: CO_2 laser with continuous wave at 5 W and a 1- to 2-mm spot size has achieved a good response.

REFERENCES

1. Nickel WR, Reed WB. Tuberous sclerosis. Arch Dermatol. 1962;85:209–226.
2. Kopf AW, Popkin GL. Shave biopsies for cutaneous lesions (letter). Arch Dermatol. 1974;110:637.
3. Shelley WB. The razor blade in dermatologic practice. Cutis 1975;16:843–845.
4. Roenigk HH Jr. Dermabrasion: State of the art. J Dermatol Surg Oncol. 1985;11:306–314.
5. Epstein E, Epstein E Jr. Techniques in Skin Surgery. Philadelphia: Lea & Febiger, 1979:171–176.
6. Coleman WP, Andreassi L. Cysts, in Rook AJ, Parish LC, Beare JM (eds) Practical Management of the Dermatologic Patient, Philadelphia, Lippincott, 1986:40–43.
7. Strauss JS. Sebaceous glands, in Fitzpatrick TB, Eisen AZ, Wolff K, et al. (eds) Dermatology in General Medicine, 2d ed. New York: McGraw-Hill, 1979:437–458.
8. Shelley ED, Shelley WB. Piezo surgery: A conservative approach to encapsulated skin lesions. Cutis. 1986;38:123–126.
9. Witkowski JA, Parish LC. Taping of a cyst: A method to facilitate removal of a scalp cyst. Int J Dermatol, 1974; 13:226.
10. Holmes EJ. Tumors of the lower hair sheath: The common histogenesis of certain so-called "sebaceous cysts," adenomas, and "sebaceous carcinomas." Cancer. 1968;21: 234–248.
11. Bennett RG. Fundamentals of Cutaneous Surgery. St. Louis: CV Mosby, 1988:749.
12. Niemi KM. The benign fibrohistiocytic tumours of the skin (review). Acta Derm Venereol (Stockh). 1970:50(suppl 63):1–66.
13. Torre D, Lubritz R, Kuflik E. Practical Cutaneous Cryosurgery. Norwalk: Appleton & Lange, 1988:73–36.
14. Lubritz RR. Cryosurgery. Clin Dermatol 1987; 5:120–127.
15. Rook A, Whimster I. Keratoacanthoma: A thirty year retrospective. Br J Dermatol. 1979;100:41–46.
16. Poleksi S, Yeung KK. Rapid development of keratoacanthoma and accelerated transformation into squamous cell carcinoma of the skin. Cancer. 1978;41:12–16.
17. Schnur PL, Bozzo P. Metastasizing keratoacanthomas? The difficulties in differentiating keratoacanthomas from squamous cell carcinomas. Plast Reconstr Surg. 1978;62: 258–262.
18. Popkin GL, Brodie SJ, Hyman AB, et al. A technique of biopsy recommended for keratoacanthoma. Arch Dermatol. 1966;94:191–193.
19. Goette DK, Odom RB. Successful treatment of keratoacanthoma with intralesional fluorouracil. J Am Acad Dermatol. 1980;2:212–216.
20. Habif TP. Extirpation of keratoacanthoma by blunt dissection. J Dermatol Surg Oncol. 1980;6:652–654.
21. Farina AT, Leider M, Newall J, et al. Radiotherapy for aggressive and destructive keratoacanthoma. J Dermatol Surg Oncol. 1977;3:177–180.
22. Strane MF, Robertson GA. Conservative treatment of keratoacanthoma. Ann Plast Surg. 1979;2:525–530.
23. Wolinsky S, Silvers DN, Kohn SR, et al. Spontaneous regression of keratoacanthoma: Photographic documentation and histopathologic correlation. J Dermatol Surg Oncol. 1981;7: 897–901.
24. Hodgson C. Lentigo senilis. Arch Dermatol. 1963;87:197–207.
25. Howard WR, Helwig EB. Angiolipoma. Arch Dermatol. 1960;82:924–930.
26. Hardin FF. Surgical gem: A simple technique for removal of lipomas. J Dermatol Surg Oncol. 1982;8:316–317.
27. Peinert RA, Courtiss EH. Excision from a distance: Removal of benign subcutaneous lesions. Plast Reconstr Surg. 1983;72:94–96.
28. Beare JM, Koblenzer PJ. Nevi, melanocytic, in Rook AJ, Parish LC, Beare JM (eds) Practical Management of the Dermatologic Patient. 1986. Philadelphia: JB Lippincott, 1986; 138–142.
29. Mehregan AH, Pinkus H. Life history of organoid nevi. Arch Dermatol. 1965;91:574–598.
30. Schultz BC, McKinney P. Office Practice of Surgery. Philadelphia: WB Saunders, 1985:118–119.
31. Zacarian SA. Cryosurgery. St. Louis: CV Mosby, 1985:51–52.
32. Hashimoto K, Dibella RJ, Borsuk GM, et al. Eruptive hidradenoma and synringoma. Arch Dermatol. 1967; 96: 500–519.
33. Lever WF, Schaumburg-Lever G. Histopathology of skin, 7th ed. Philadelphia: JB Lippincott, 1990:582–586.
34. Brownstein MH, Shapiro L. Desmoplastic trichoepithelioma. Cancer. 1977;40:2979–2986.
35. Jablonska S, Orth G. Warts/human papillomaviruses. Clin Dermatol 1985;3:1–220.
36. Krull EA. Surgical gems: The "little" curet. J Dermatol Surg Oncol. 1978;4:656–657.
37. Shumer SM, O'Keefe EJ. Bleomycin in the treatment of recalcitrant warts. J Am Acad Dermatol. 1983;9:91–96.
38. Stegman SJ, Tromovitch TA. Cosmetic Dermatologic Surgery. Chicago: Year Book, 1984:20–21.

CHAPTER

7

Hemangiomas and Other Vascular Malformations

EDWARD GLASSBERG
GARY P. LASK
LAURENCE M. DAVID

HEMANGIOMAS

Hemangiomas are benign blood vessel tumors consisting of endothelial lined spaces. They are common developmental vascular abnormalities occurring in the skin, mucous membranes, or other soft tissues. They may present as nodules or tumors, or macular lesions consisting of dilated, ectatic blood vessels. Most tend to occur at birth or shortly thereafter,[1,2] commonly on the head or neck, although any portion of the body may be involved.

Capillary (Strawberry or Hypertrophic) Hemangioma

Capillary hemangioma, the most common of hemangiomas in young children, is often absent at birth and develops within days to months thereafter. A localized area of pallor may precede the development of a red to deep purple tumor with a smooth or nodular surface. Hemangiomas appear commonly on the skin of the head, although other locations, including mucous membranes or any part of the body, are affected. The hemangioma can continue to grow until the child is about 6 to 18 months of age, after which time gradual spontaneous involution (in 70 to 76 percent of cases) usually takes place with completion by 5 to 15 years of age.[3] There may be minimal residual skin changes or variable degrees of atrophy, wrinkling, fibrosis, or telangiectasias.[4]

Some authorities distinguish a more cellular variant (cellular hemangioma) composed of immature endothelial cells that are locally aggressive, have less tendency to involute, and present as soft smooth tumors in the dermis or subcutis shortly after birth.[5] Another variant is the mixed hemangioma, which is composed of both immature capillary elements and cavernous sinuses and behaves much like the typical strawberry hemangioma.[5]

TABLE 1
LASER TREATMENT OF CAPILLARY HEMANGIOMAS

Laser	Power (Watts)	Spot Size (mm)	F/D*	Pulse Duration (s)
Argon	1.0–2.0	1.0–5.0	(F)	0.2–Continuous wave
CO_2	5.0–15.0	0.2–1.0	(F/D)	Continuous wave
Nd:YAG	20.0–30.0	2.0–3.0	(D)	0.5–0.7

* F = focused, D = defocused

Cavernous Hemangiomas

Also known as angioma cavernosum, the cavernous hemanigioma is composed of mature dilated blood vessels or sinusoidal spaces. It usually occurs during childhood, with indolent but persistent growth, and little tendency toward spontaneous involution.[5] Clinically, it appears as a soft globular or multilobular tumor and ranges in color from blue to purple. Multiple cavernous hemangiomas occur in the "blue rubber bleb nevus syndrome"[6] and in Maffucci's syndrome.[7]

Management

A generally conservative approach to treatment is usually recommended for these hemangiomas; however, significant cosmetic and functional impairment (e.g., visual obstruction) may warrant early treatment.[8]

Laser Ablation Several lasers (Table 1) have been used, with varying success, on these hemangiomas.

All treatment modalities can be complicated by either flat or hypertrophic scarring. The argon laser is primarily used for capillary hemangiomas. This laser is more specific for oxyhemoglobin, and the minimal power necessary to blanch the lesion can be employed[9]; carbon dioxide (CO_2) and Nd:YAG lasers are relatively nonspecifically absorbed, requiring somewhat higher total energies overall. The CO_2 laser can be useful in excising either cavernous or capillary hemangiomas (focused mode) and for hemostasis by cautery (defocused mode).[10] The Nd:YAG sapphire tip contact probe is also effective for excisions.

When using the Nd:YAG laser (defocused) for ablation of thick (especially cavernous) hemangiomas, it is very helpful to compress the lesion with a glass slide and lase through it to allow an adequate depth of laser penetration[11] (Fig. 1). Some crusting and oozing usually occurs (with most laser modalities) and re-epithelialization is complete by about 2 to 4 weeks. Wound care in general consists of daily cleansing with hydrogen peroxide, topical antibiotic ointments, and optional dressings.

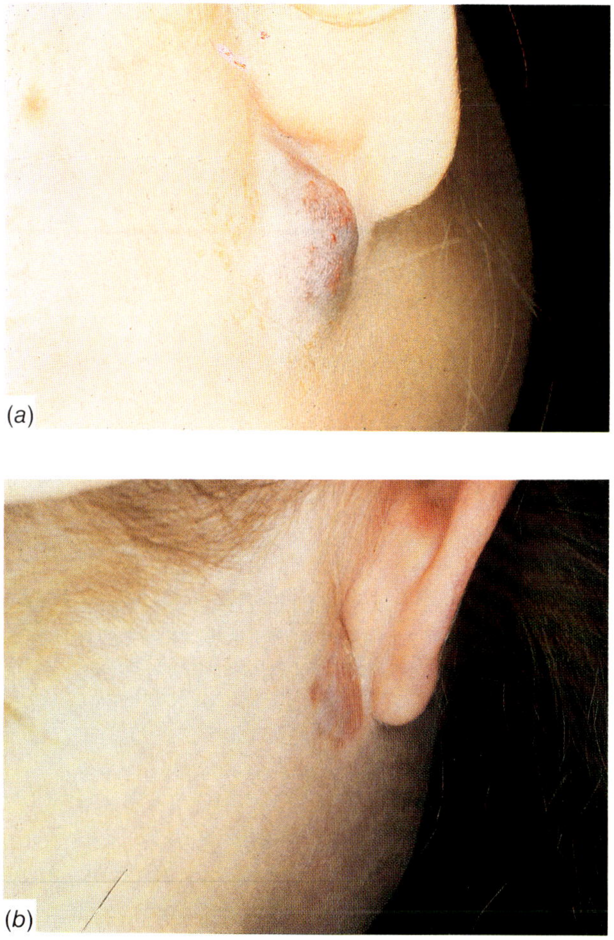

(a) (b)

FIGURE 1
Young child with a cavernous hemangioma in the inferior post-auricular region (A). Same patient several weeks after ablation with the Nd:YAG laser (B).

The 577nm/585nm pulsed dye laser may prove useful in aborting very early, developing hemangiomas that are still relatively flat. Studies defining the energy density parameters have yet to be undertaken. The argon laser has shown some success in treating very early capillary hemangiomas.[12,13]

Systemic Corticosteroids

Doses of 2.5 to 3.0 mg/kg of prednisone are recommended (or 5 mg/kg alternate day therapy) for 1 to 4 weeks, until growth is arrested and involution begins.[5,14] Gradual tapering over 4 to 8 weeks is then recommended.

Intralesional Corticosteroids

If risks are too high, or complications are encountered with systemic steroids, some studies have shown a very effective response from intralesional corticosteroids in periorbital lesions.[15,16] In one study, an injection of 40 mg triamcinolone acetate (Kenalog) (in 1.0 cc) and 6 mg of a 50/50 solution of betamethasone sodium phosphate and betamethasone acetate (Celestone Soluspan) (in 1.0 cc) was injected directly into the tumor in several separate sticks under brief, light general anesthesia.[15] Twice this amount can be used for very large tumors, and a repeat dose can be given if resolution is not complete by 6 to 8 weeks.

Surgery

Limited surgical excision may be helpful in treating small lesions, or lesions reduced by previous laser surgery. Complications have included scarring (as with any approach), infection, hemorrhage, and anesthesia-related risks.[17]

Cryosurgery

Much work has been done in the cryosurgical treatment of vascular lesions. Capillary hemangiomas and some (superficial) cavernous hemangiomas are very amenable to such therapy.[18] Using a prechilled, flat or round-tipped cryoprobe of the approximate diameter of the lesion, firm pressure is applied to the center of the lesion to freeze and compress blood out of the tissue. Decreased blood content allows a faster freeze and slower thaw. The probe is held in place until a halo of ice 1.0 to 1.5 mm beyond the visible tumor margin is seen (regardless of the time it takes).[19] When the probe is withdrawn, the lesion is flattened and about one-third to one-fourth its original size. Larger lesions (>3–4 cm) can be treated in sections.

The lesion will become edematous and larger in size, sometimes with hemorrhagic bullae, an oozing serous exudate, and development of a purplish to black color.[19] This will begin to subside after 3 or 4 days and complete healing takes 3 to 6 weeks. Wound care consists of soap and water, saline, or hydrogen peroxide washes followed by antibiotic ointment.

VASCULAR ECTASIAS

Salmon Patches

Also known as nevus flammeus nuchae, this congenital vascular malformation is seen in up to one-half of newborns[20,21] and presents as a pink to light red or violaceous patch on the nape of the neck, glabella, or upper eyelids. Many of these lesions fade with time, but those on the neck may persist to adulthood. Vascular lesions can be treated with argon or pulsed dye laser (Table 2).

Nevus Flammeus

Commonly known as a portwine stain (PWS) or hemangioma, this vascular malformation consists of ectatic capillaries and venules primarily in the superficial vascular plexus.[22] This lesion presents at birth as a pink, red, or red-purple macular area often unilaterally on the face (or any other area) and persists into adulthood with darkening, thick-

TABLE 2
LASER TREATMENT FOR PERSISTENT VASCULAR ECTASIAS

Laser	Power/Energy	Spot Size (mm)	Pulse Duration	Clinical Endpoint
Argon	0.5–1.5 W	1.0–5.0	0.2 CW	Skin blanch
577/585 nm pulsed dye	5.5–7.5 J/cm^2	3.0–5.0	450 μ sec	Gray-blue purpura

TABLE 3
LASER TREATMENT OF NEVUS FLAMMEUS

Laser	Power/Energy	Spot Size (nm)	(F/D)*	Pulse Duration
577/585 nm pulsed dye	5.5–8.0 J/cm^2	3.0–5.0	(F)	450 μ sec
Argon	0.6–1.0 W	0.2–2.0	(F)	0.2 sec to CW
Argon-pumped CW tunable dye	0.1–0.5 W	0.1	(F)	CW
CO_2	5.0–10 W	0.2–1.0	(D)	CW
Nd:YAG	20–30 W	~1.5–3.0 (2.0–3.0 cm from skin)	(D)	0.2–0.5 sec

* F = focused, D = defocused

ening, and/or development of papular and nodular areas. It can occur alone, or in conjunction with mental retardation and other congenital anomalies, as in the Sturge-Weber syndrome.[23] Nevus flammeus of an extremity can result in hypertrophy of the involved limb or area. Lesions of the face can cause facial asymmetry. Incidence is reported to be 0.3 to 1.0%[21,24] of the population.

Laser Treatment of Nevus Flammeus

Multiple laser modalities are currently in use for portwine stain treatment. With the proven efficacy of the 577 (or 585) nm pulsed dye laser, treatment of early, macular lesions in infants or children is possible with minimal risks. This, of course, would obviate the psychological trauma and social stigma associated with an obvious facial anomaly or asymmetry. The roles of argon, tunable dye, Nd:YAG, and CO_2 lasers in PWS treatment are discussed below (Table 3).

Pulsed Dye Laser Excellent results have been reported with the 577 or 585 nm pulsed dye laser,[17,25,26] with very minimal incidence of scarring (Figs. 2 and 3). This modality appears to work equally effectively in children and adults. The parameters noted in Table 3 are used, usually with a 5.0 mm spot size. Lower energy densities, 5.5 to 6.5 J/cm^2, are recommended for children. The le-

FIGURE 2
Portwine stain of posterior thigh of an adult female patient (A). Same patient after treatments with the 577 nm pulsed dye laser (B).

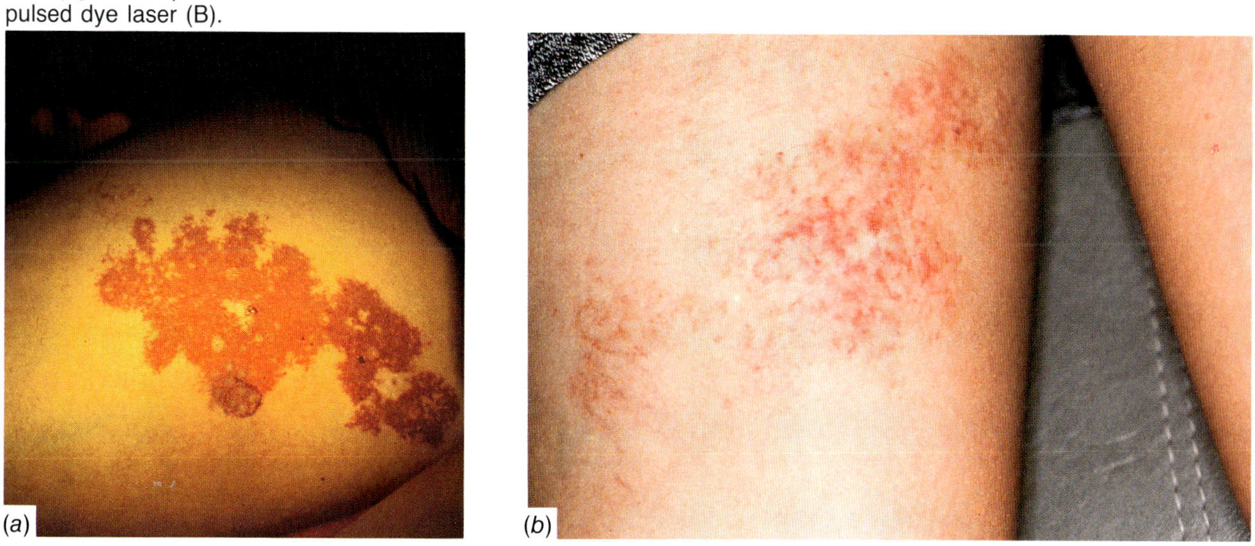
(a) (b)

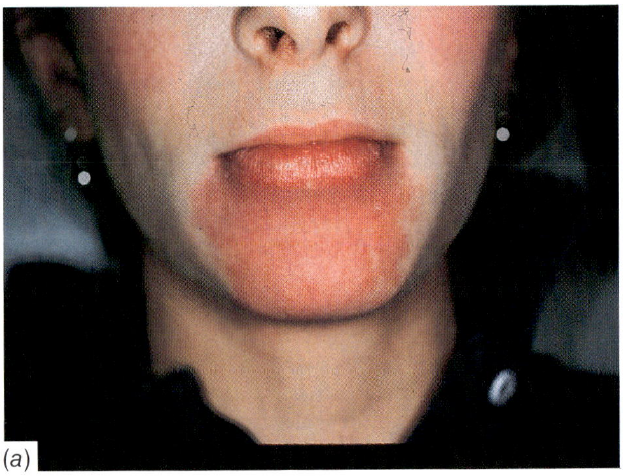

FIGURE 3
Adult female patient with portwine stain of chin area (*a*). Same patient about two months after treatment with the 577 nm pulsed dye laser (*b*).

sion is "dotted" with single pulses tangentially placed, with minimal overlap. Each pulse will be followed by a bluish-gray purpura either immediately or within minutes. After 6 to 8 weeks the reticulated "bridging" between initial treatment areas can be gone over with the laser to get even fading or clearing. A given area can be retreated several times if needed to obtain maximal fading. Postoperative care involves use of antibiotic ointment and optional telfa dressing. Occasional crusting occurs in the treated areas. The purpura may darken somewhat before they fade in 5 to 14 days. Maximal fading of the lesion occurs usually between 2 and 3 months after treatment, although some continued fading may occur beyond this time.

Argon Laser The argon laser, pulsed or continuous, also shows generally good results, particularly in adults, but scarring can occur. The best results with this laser are seen in patients in their mid-thirties or older, with violaceous, boggy lesions of the head and neck area (Fig. 4). The lesion is "painted" with consecutive, adjacent passes of the laser, using the minimal energy needed to induce visible blanching.[10] Meticulous wound care is recommended, as crusting and oozing may be prominent.

Tunable Dye Laser An argon-pumped continuous wave tunable dye laser tuned to 577 nm may also be used on macular portwine stains. A very small

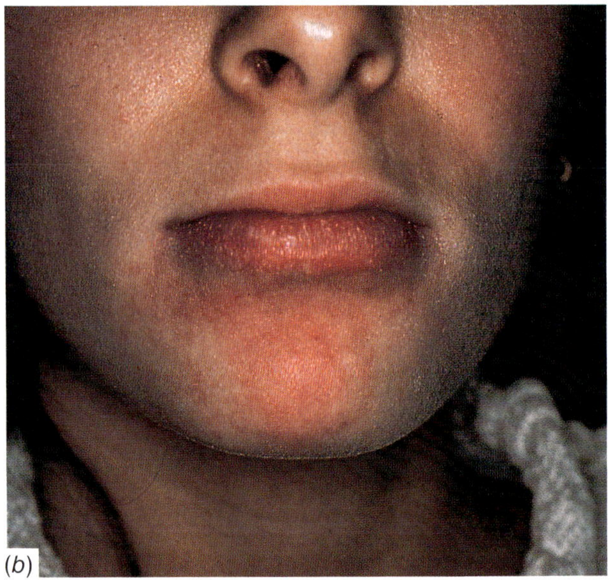

FIGURE 4
Adult male patient with a mature portwine stain of the malar area (*a*). Same patient several months after argon laser therapy (*b*).

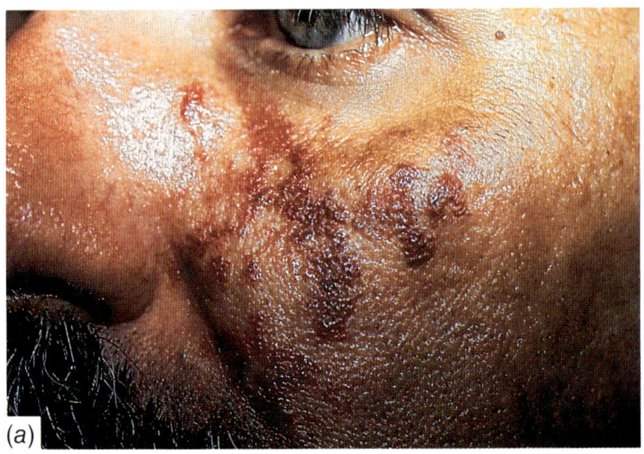

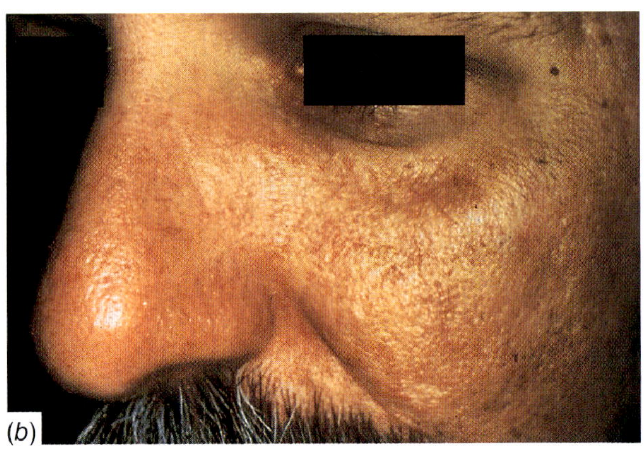

TABLE 4
LASER TREATMENT OF VENOUS LAKE

Laser	Power/Energy	Spot Size (mm)	(F/D)*	Pulse Duration
577/585 nm pulsed dye	7.0–8.0 J/cm^2	3.0–5.0	(F)	450 μ sec
Argon	0.6–1.0 W	1.0–2.0	(F)	0.2 sec–CW
CO_2	5.0–10.0 W	0.2–1.0	(D)	CW

* F = focused, D = defocused

spot (0.1 mm) size is employed in the focused mode and is used to "trace" individual vessels within the lesion, causing their ablation. A section about one square centimeter in diameter is treated and then one moves on to another area of the lesion, because surrounding erythema may impair distinction of surrounding vessels. Excellent results can be obtained, but the work can be time consuming and tedious, and results depend on the skills and experience of the operator.

CO_2 and Nd:YAG Lasers Carbon dioxide and Nd:YAG lasers can be useful in hypertrophic, mature lesions with prominent nodules or blebs, although the risk of hypertrophic scarring may be increased.[10,11,27] Blebs may be excised with the CO_2 laser (as described earlier) or ablated using the Nd:YAG laser in combination with glass slide compression[11] for thicker areas. These modalities may be combined with argon or dye lasers, which are used to treat more macular parts of the PWS lesion.

Venous Lake

Sometimes called venous varix or senile ectasia, the venous lake is a small (1- to 5-mm) dark blue, soft, compressible nodule that occurs most commonly in older people on the lips, face, ears and neck.[5] It is composed of dilated venules in the upper dermis and usually blanches with pressure.

Laser Therapy

Results with the argon and CO_2 lasers are more consistently favorable, whereas the pulsed dye laser is rather variable, although complications are minimal with this modality (Table 4).

Electrodessication These lesions may also be lightly electrodessicated under local anesthesia using a Bircher Hyfrecator. Results are generally very good with this method of treatment.

PYOGENIC GRANULOMA

This common, acquired vascular (granulation tissue) proliferation (also known as septic granuloma or pregnancy tumor) can occur at any age on mucous membranes or skin,[28] commonly on the fingers, face, and gingiva (especially in early pregnancy). It usually presents as a solitary red to red-brown pedunculated lesion (~1/2 to 2 cm) that is soft, friable, and bleeds easily after trauma, though usually is not painful. A collarete of epithelium is commonly seen at the constricted base. The lesion may undergo rapid growth or spontaneous necrosis and shrinkage.[29]

Curettage and Electrodessication

After appropriate local anesthesia with lidocaine 1% the lesion is shaved flush with the skin surface using a scalpel and then curetted, or directly curretted if feasible. Cautery of the base is used to achieve hemostasis. Care must be taken to avoid overly aggressive cauterization, especially in cosmetically sensitive areas on the face, as unsightly scars may occur.

Surgical Excision

The base is infiltrated with lidocaine 1% with or without epinephrine 1:100,000 (as appropriate). The entire lesion is excised with a full-thickness elliptical incision using a scalpel with a No. 15 blade. The defect can usually be closed primarily with interrupted 5.0 or 6.0 nylon sutures after bleeding is controlled.

Laser Therapy Laser therapy is usually effective (Table 5).

TABLE 5
LASER THERAPY OF PYOGENIC GRANULOMA

Laser	Power (w)	Spot Size (mm)	(F/D)*	Pulse Duration
Argon	1.0–2.5	0.2–2.0	(F)	0.2s–CW
CO_2	5.0	1.0	(D)	CW

* F = focused, D – defocused

TABLE 6
LASER TREATMENT OF SENILE ANGIOMA

Laser	Power/Energy	Spot Size (mm)	(F/D)*	Pulse Duration	Clinical Endpoint
Argon	1.0 W	0.2–1.0	(F)	0.2–CW	Minimal Power needed to blanch
CO_2	5.0–10.0 W	~1.0	(D)	CW	Blanching
577/585 nm pulsed dye	6.0–7.5 J/cm^2	3.0–5.0	(F)	450 μ sec	Gray purpura

* F = focused, D = defocused

Cryosurgery

If biopsy confirmation is needed, local anesthesia is given, then the lesion is shaved flush with a scalpel. A flat cryoprobe the same diameter as the base of the lesion is used to induce freezing with a 1- to 2-mm halo of ice around the probe.[19] Very good results can be achieved with this method.

SENILE ANGIOMA

Commonly referred to as a cherry angioma or capillary angioma, this superficial proliferation of dilated capillaries appears as a deep-red papular or nodular lesion usually a few millimeters in diameter.[30] They occur primarily on the trunk and arms during middle age (but can occur earlier) and are usually multiple. They may be secondary to weakening of the connective tissue surrounding and supporting the capillary walls.[31]

Laser Treatment

Senile angioma can be treated with the argon, CO_2, or 577 nm pulsed dye laser (Table 6).

Electrodessication

Infiltrate the lesion with lidocaine 1%. Lightly electrodessicate with a Bircher Hyfrecator until blanching of the lesion occurs.

CONCLUSION

Hemangiomas and other vascular malformations can usually be treated with various lasers. Electrodessication, surgery, and cryosurgery can also be used in some cases with good results, but the laser offers the greatest hope for the best treatment for the majority of these kinds of lesions.[32]

REFERENCES

1. Carsteno PJB. The Weibel-Palade in the diagnosis of endothelial tumors. Ultrastruct Pathol. 1981; 2:315–325.
2. Ladapo AA. Hemangioma of the cheek. Oral Surg. 1981; 39:778–779.
3. Bowers RE, Graham EA, Tomlinson K. The natural history of the strawberry neavus. Arch Dermatol. 1960; 82: 667–680.
4. Simpson JR. Natural history of cavernous hemangiomata. Lancet. 1959; 2:1057–1059.
5. Pasyk KA. Classification and clinical histopathological fea-

tures of hemangiomas and other vascular malformations, in Ryan TJ, Cherry GW, (eds) Vascular Birthmarks. Oxford: Oxford Medical, 1987:1–54.
6. Fretzin DF, Potter B. Blue rubber bleb nevus. Arch Intern Med. 1965; 116:924–929.
7. Andersen IF. Mafucci's syndrome: Report of a case with review of the literature. S Afr Med J. 1965; 39:1066–1070.
8. Thernson G, Ward CM, Crawford JS, et al. Hemangiomas of the eyelid: Visual complications and prophylactic concepts. Plast Reconstr Surg., 1979; 63:641–647.
9. Apfelberg DB, McBurney E. Use of the argon laser in dermatologic surgery, in Ratz JL. Lasers in Cutaneous Medicine and Surgery. Chicago: Year Book, 1986:31–71.
10. Apfelberg DB, Maser MR, Lash H, et al. Past, present, and future usage of lasers in plastic surgery, dermatology and podiatry, in Apfelberg DB, (ed) Evaluation and Installation of Surgical Laser Systems. New York: Springer-Verlag, 1987:210–228.
11. Shapshay SM, David LM, Zeitels S. Neodymium-YAG laser photocoagulation of hemangiomas of the head and neck. Laryngoscope. 1987; 97:323–330.
12. Hobby LW. Further evaluation of the potential of the argon laser in the treatment of strawberry hemangiomas. Plast Reconstr Surg. 1983; 71:481–485.
13. Apfelberg DB, Greene RA, Maser MR, et al. Results of argon laser exposure of capillary hemangiomas of infancy—Preliminary Report. Plast Reconstr Surg. 1981; 67:188–193.
14. Bartoshesky LE, Bull M, Feingold M. Corticosteroid treatment of cutaneous hemangiomas: How effective? Clin Pediatr. 1978; 17:625–638.
15. Kushner BJ. The treatment of periorbital infantile hemangioma with intralesional corticosteroid. Plast Reconstr Surg. 1985; 76:517–524.
16. Nelson LB, Melick JE, Harley RD. Intralesional corticosteroid injections for infantile hemangiomas of the eyelid. Pediatrics. 1984; 74:241–245.
17. Tan OT, Gilchrest BA. Laser therapy for selected cutaneous vascular lesions in the pediatric population; A review. Pediatrics. 1988; 82:652–662.
18. Torre D, Lubritz R, Kuflik E. Practical Cutaneous Cryosurgery. Norwalk: Appleton and Lange, 1988:61–86.
19. Castro-Ron G. Cryosurgery of angiomas and birth defects, in Zacarian SA (ed) Cryosurgery for Skin and Cutaneous Disorders. St. Louis: CV Mosby, 1985:77–90.
20. Alper JC, Holmes LB. The incidence and significance of birthmarks in a cohort of 4,641 newborns. Pediatr Dermatol. 1983; 1:58–68.
21. Jacobs AJ. Walton RG. The incidence of birthmarks in the neonate. Pediatrics. 1976; 58:218–222.
22. Noe JM, Barsky SJ, Geer DE, et al. Port wine stains and the response to argon laser therapy: Successful treatment and the prospective role of color, age and biopsy. Plast Reconstr Surg. 1980; 65:130–136.
23. Butterworth T, Strean LP. Clinical Genodermatology. Baltimore: Williams and Wilkins, 1962.
24. Pratt AG. Birthmarks in infants. Arch Derm Syph. 1953; 67:302–305.
25. Glassberg E, Lask GP, Tan EML, et al. The flashlamp-pumped 577nm pulsed tunable dye laser: Clinical efficacy and in vitro studies. J Dermatol Surg Oncol. 1988; 1200–1208.
26. Tan OT, Sherwood K, Gilchrest BA. Treatment of children with portwine stains using a flash lamp pulsed tunable dye laser. N Engl J Med. 1989; 320:416–421.
27. Landthaler M, Diether H, Reinhold B, et al. Neodymium-YAG laser therapy for vascular lesions. J Am Acad Dermatol. 1986; 14:107–177.
28. Cooper PH, Helwig EG. Intradermal and subcutaneous pyogenic granuloma: Study of 40 cases (abstract). Lab Invest. 1979; 40:249.
29. From L, Assaad D. Vascular neoplasms, pseudoneoplasms, and hyperplasias, in Fitzpatrick TB, Eisen AZ, Wolff K, et al. (eds) Dermatology in General Medicine, 3d ed. New York: McGraw-Hill, 1987:1059–1077.
30. Lever FL, Schaumburg-Lever G. Tumors of vascular tissue, in Histopathology of the Skin. London: JB Lippencott, 1983:623–651.
31. Shah KC, Shah AC, Shah PC. Campbell de Morgan spots in diabetes mellitus. Br J Dermatol. 1966; 78:493–495.
32. Dover JS, Arndt KA, Geronemus RG, et al. Illustrated Cutaneous Laser Surgery. East Norwalk, CT: Appleton & Lange, 1990:1–142.

CHAPTER 8

Keloids and Hypertrophic Scars

A. PAUL KELLY

Surgical intervention for aesthetic improvement may result in the development of hypertrophic scars, keloids, or both, although most of these unwanted lesions are secondary to unplanned cutaneous trauma and noncosmetic surgical procedures. Some people develop spontaneous keloids, i.e., those which arise without any apparent precipitating trauma. Regardless of origin, hypertrophic scars and keloids are considered unattractive and unwanted by most patients, with the exception of some tribes in Africa, where raised scars are induced for cosmetic enhancement.

DEFINITION

Keloids are benign proliferative lesions of dermal connective tissue that usually result from an excessive tissue response to cutaneous trauma in predisposed individuals. Keloids expand beyond the boundaries of the original wounds, develop for many months to years, and persist for years or even for life. *Hypertrophic scars,* on the other hand, remain within the boundaries of the precipitating wound, progress for a few months, and usually regress in a few years.

Histologically, keloids are characterized by thick glassy collagen bundles, an abundance of mucinous ground substance, minimal to no foreign body reaction, and a few fibroblasts.[1] Hypertrophic scars have frequent foreign body reactions and numerous fibroblasts but few glassy collagen bundles and scanty mucinous ground substance. In normal scars and hypertrophic scars, collagen fibers are oriented parallel to the long axis of the scar, whereas in keloids, collagen is arranged in a haphazard pattern.[2] Humans are the only animals that form keloids, although lesions similar to keloids and hypertrophic scars have been seen in horses, cattle, and dogs and on the feet of vultures and eagles.[3] These lesions in animals differ from those in humans in that the growth clears when the tissue insult ceases.[4]

Jean Louis Alibert (1768–1837) introduced into

the French dermatologic literature the word *cheloide* (derived from the Greek *chele,* meaning "crab's claw," and *-oid,* meaning "like"), a term that was later changed to *keloid.* The first description of keloidlike scars, however, can be found in the Smith papyrus. The Yorubas also recorded their awareness of keloids 10 centuries before Alibert.[5] In 1854, Thomas Addison (1793–1860) introduced the term *true keloid* (arising spontaneously) and labeled Alibert's lesions *false keloids* (arising at sites of trauma). Because the lesions Addison described were probably morphea or scleroderma, his nomenclature should be discarded.

Blacks have an incidence of keloids 2 to 20 times greater than that of whites; however, once keloids develop, the recurrence rate is the same in all races. Hypertrophic scars occur with approximately the same incidence in all races. The male/female ratio has been found to be equal by some investigators, whereas others have reported a higher incidence in women. This difference may reflect the more frequent use of aesthetic procedures (ear piercing) in women.

Keloids and hypertrophic scars may be found anywhere on the body (Figs. 1 through 3) but occur most often on the chest, upper part of the back, and shoulders, which are areas of increased skin tension. Keloids are also very common on the earlobes (Fig. 4), and hypertrophic scars are more likely to develop in scars that cross joint spaces or are perpendicular to skin creases. Keloids may develop rarely on the scalp, eyelids, genitalia, palms, soles,

FIGURE 1
A large keloid of the left flank.

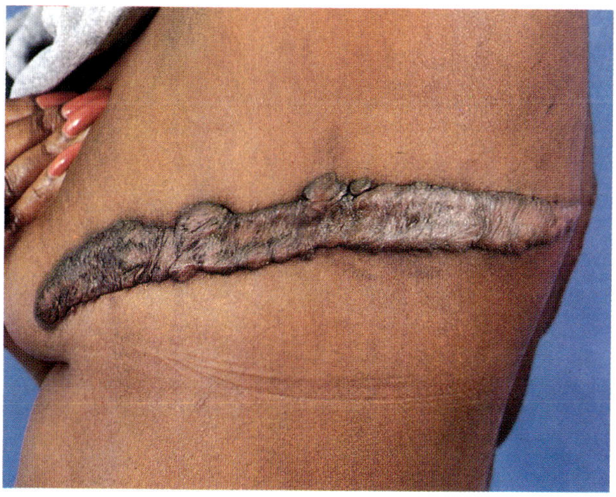

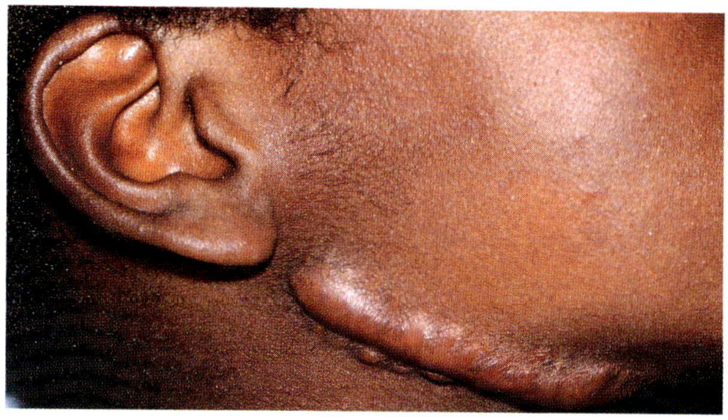

FIGURE 2
A keloid of the right submandibular area.

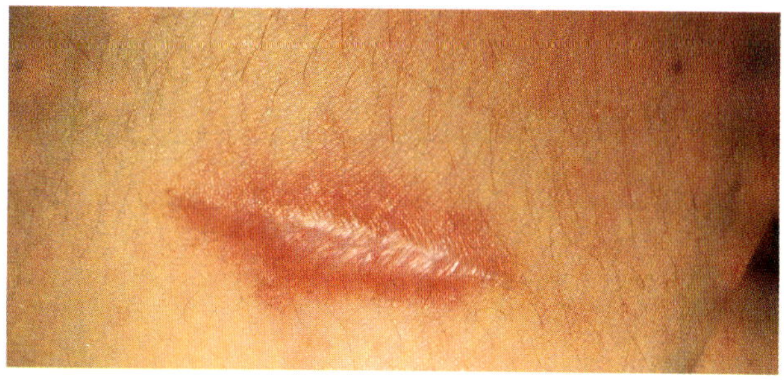

FIGURE 3
A hypertrophic scar of the left forearm.

FIGURE 4
A keloid on the upper border of the helix of the right ear.

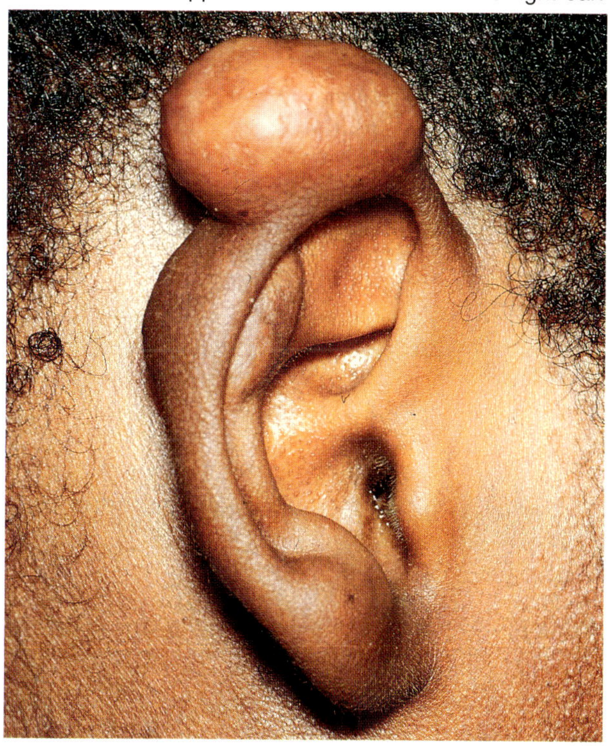

and mucous membranes. The relative absence of keloids and hypertrophic scars on the penis, even when circumcision is delayed until puberty, is puzzling considering the number of times the procedure is performed. Pregnancy seems to cause some keloids to enlarge and may have a similar effect on hypertrophic scars; however, the perineum never develops keloids, even after repeated episiotomies. Keloids rarely develop during infancy and early childhood or later years, whereas hypertrophic scars may arise at any age, although they are less common in older patients.

ETIOLOGY

The etiology of keloids and hypertrophic scars is not known, although trauma is the provoking factor in most patients. Many different kinds of injury, such as ear piercing, surgical wounds, burns, vaccinations, chronic deep cutaneous inflammation, tattoos, severe acne vulgaris, and chickenpox, have been implicated. Increased tension of surgical wounds, intradermal sebum secretion, foreign body reactions, endocrinologic factors (thymus, parathyroid, ovary, thyroid, and pituitary alone or in combination), sex hormones, decreased vasculature, decreased collagen degredation, and increased activity of melanocyte-stimulating hormone (MSH) have all been incriminated in the pathogenes of keloid formation. There is a definite familial predisposition to keloids, especially in persons with multiple lesions. The incidence of HLA-B14 and HLA-BW16 in white patients with keloids has been found to be significantly greater than it is in those without keloids.[6] In a study of HLA typing and keloids in Nigeria, HLA-BW35 and HLA-BW21 were statistically higher in keloid patients than in controls, whereas HLA-A28 and HLA-BW5 were significantly lower in keloid patients.[7]

Most keloids occur within a year of the precipitation trauma, although some take 20 or more years to develop. The incubation period is usually much shorter in keloids that occur after excision. Initially keloids are usually erythematous and become brownish red before turning pale or hyperpigmented as they mature. Hair follicles and other functioning adnexal glands are usually absent. Once keloids are present, the clinical course varies. Most continue to grow for weeks to months and sometimes for years. Growth is usually slow and steady but sometimes proceeds rapidly. Once keloids stop growing, they remain stable or involute slightly. They rarely regress spontaneously. They are smooth and vary in consistency from doughy to rubbery hard. Keloids on the ears, neck, lower part of the abdomen, and pubic area tend to be pedunculated, while those on the chest and extremities are usually raised with a flat surface. Most keloids are round, oval, or oblong with regular margins; however, some have a clawlike configuration (Fig. 5) with irregular borders. Hypertrophic scars are usually smooth erythematous nodules confined to the area of cutaneous trauma, although in British nomenclature, the term *hypertrophic* refers to a widespread depressed scar.[8] Both keloids and hypertrophic scars may be tender, painful, and/or pruritic, but most patients seek medical or surgical intervention for cosmetic relief.

FIGURE 5
A midchest keloid with pseudopod-like extensions.

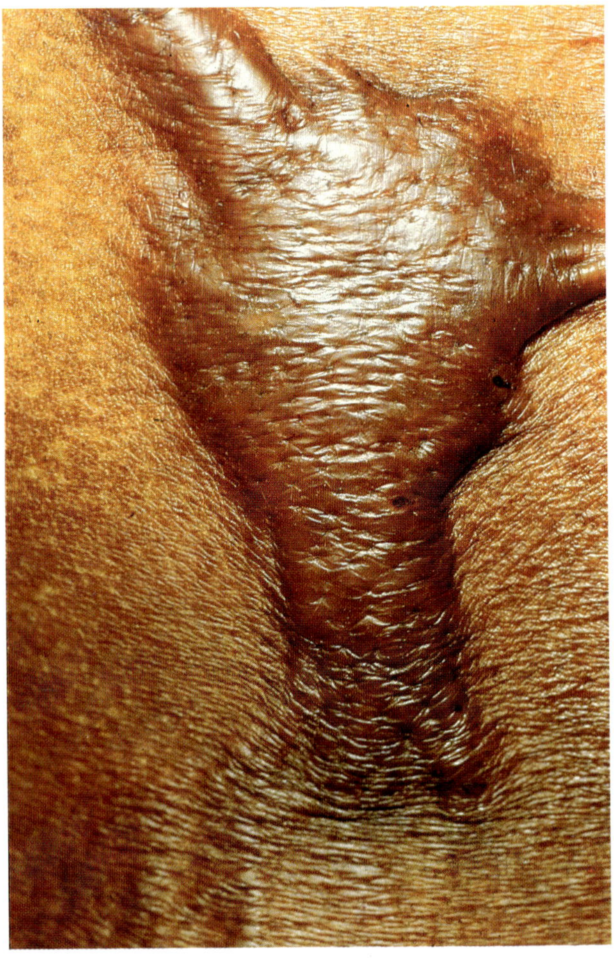

MANAGEMENT

The first rule of therapy for hypertrophic scars and keloids is prevention. Nonessential cosmetic surgery should be withheld from known keloid formers (persons with only earlobe keloids who do not have a family history of keloids are not considered keloid formers). All surgical wounds should be closed with minimal tension. If possible, incisions should not cross joint spaces and should follow skin creases, and midchest incisions should be avoided. A pressure gradient elastic garment or apparatus for applying pressure should be worn or used for 4 to 6 months after burns, surgical procedures, or major skin trauma by known hypertrophic scar or keloid formers.

Therapeutic alternatives for hypertrophic scars are as follows.

1. Patience and reassurance that the scars will eventually flatten. The lighter one's skin, the more erythematous the scars will appear.
2. Application of a class I or II topical steroid (Temovate, Diprolene, Topicort) twice a day.
   - **a.** Faster results may be achieved with steroids under occlusion (especially with Actiderm).
   - **b.** Persons with fair skin will have more residual erythema after long-term topical steroid therapy with occlusion.
3. Application of a mixture of topical tretinoin (retinoic acid; Retin-A), available in liquid, gel, or cream, and a class I or II steroid twice a day until it resolves or becomes asymptomatic.
4. Injection of glucorticoids [especially triamcinolone acetonide (Kenalog), 10 mg/cc] every 2 or 3 weeks until flattening. Three or four injections may be sufficient but not always.
   - **a.** An insulin syringe or a 27-gauge needle on a Luer-lock syringe makes injecting easier.
   - **b.** Triamcinolone acetonide (40 mg/cc) often "puddles" in the injection site, producing yellowish cutaneous deposits which may have to be incised and/or curetted for optimum cosmetic results.
   - **c.** Patients with fair skin often have residual erythema and telangiectasia in the injected sites.
5. Surgical removal with adequate undermining to prevent tension on the postoperative site. The cosmetic appearance of the scar may be enhanced by changing the direction of the scar with a Z-plasty or W-plasty procedure.
6. An Ace bandage, a Jobst pressure gradient garment, or another method of sustained pressure usually causes the lesions to regress much faster. For best results, pressure should be applied 16 to 20 h a day.
7. When hypertrophic scars resolve with or without therapy, there may be residual erythema, telangiectasia, hyperpigmentation, hypopigmentation, or any combination of these conditions. Many of these cutaneous blemishes clear with time, but this may take months to years. Dermablend is an excellent cutaneous cover for masking the residual sequelae of hypertrophic scars.

No single therapeutic modality is best for all keloids. The location, size, and depth of the lesion; the age of the patient; and the patient's past response to treatment determine the type of therapy to be used. Types of therapy are outlined below.

1. The treatment of choice for most earlobe keloids as well as those in locations other than the midchest is the combined liquid nitrogen, intralesional steroid, and surgical approach.
   - **a.** To decrease the discomfort and increase the ease of injecting steroids, a 10- to 15-s freeze of the lesion with liquid nitrogen is recommended. Liquid nitrogen causes tissue edema and may provide some local anesthesia.
     - **(1)** Freezing longer than 25 s in patients with dark skin may result in hypopigmentation which usually lasts 6 to 18 months.
     - **(2)** Shorter freezing, especially in patients with brown or black skin, may cause postinflammatory hyperpigmentation lasting 6 to 12 months.
   - **b.** Corticosteroids are injected into the keloid every 2 to 3 weeks at least four times before surgery. (If the lesion is too large to be reduced with intralesional steroids or the injections are unduly painful, preoperative injections are waived.) Triamicinolone acetonide (Kenalog; 10 mg/cc) is preferred. Early keloids respond better to corticosteroid injections than do older ones.
     - **(1)** If the keloid is large enough to require multiple injections, 10 mg/ml triamcinolone acetonide is diluted with equal parts of 2% lidocaine. The lidocaine does not relieve the initial pain of injection but usually allows one to perform multiple injections with minimal discomfort and

prevents most postinjection pain.

(2) Because triamcinolone acetonide in strengths of 3 mg/ml or stronger may cause hypopigmentation of injected sites, all patients receiving steroid injections should be informed of this sequela and told that the hypopigmentation may remain for 6 to 12 months (Fig. 1).

(3) For large lesions, mechanical injectors (Derma-Jet, Mada-Jet) are easier to use and often are less painful. Injection of keloids is enhanced if at the time of purchase the manufacturer is asked to set the tension higher for keloid injection.

c. If the response to 10 mg/ml of triamcinolone acetonide is minimal to absent after two or three injections or if the keloids have been injected previously with no decrease in hardness or size, triamcinolone diacetate (Aristocort, 25 mg/ml) or triamcinolone acetonide (Kenalog-40; 40 mg/ml) is recommended.

(1) A Luer-lock or fixed-needle syringe is necessary to prevent separation of the needle from the syringe during injection.

(2) To prevent clogging of the injection needle with the triamcinolone acetonide suspension, nothing smaller than a 27-gauge needle should be used.

d. Sometimes the base of the keloid is so fibrotic that it is almost impossible to inject. In these cases, where a needle and syringe are preferred to a pressure injection apparatus, the needle is inserted into the keloid and the steroid is injected into the needle tract as the needle is slowly withdrawn.

(1) To prevent steroid leakage at the insertion site, the area is painted with tincture of benzoin and covered with a piece of waterproof tape.

(2) The steroid should be injected only into the keloid, because injecting into the surrounding area may cause atrophy of normal tissue and cause the keloid to sink down to skin level but not flatten or become softer.

e. The highest potency topical steroids (clobetasol proprionate; Temovate) can reduce keloids and hypertrophic scars, probably because of the side effect of atrophy.

2. If there is no significant response after several injections, the keloid is too large to inject, the keloid no longer responds to injections, or the pain of injection cannot be tolerated, surgical removal is recommended. The surgical method varies according to the size and location of the lesion.

a. For keloids with narrow bases and those amenable to primary closure without excess wound tension or distortion of the anatomic site, a simple excision followed by undermining the base and closing with interrupted sutures will suffice. Before closing, the base of the wound is injected with triamcinolone acetonide or triamcinolone diacetate.

b. For posterior pedunculate earlobe keloids where cosmetic appearance is not important, shaving the lesions at the base followed by pressure hemostasis is a simple and efficient method. The spring-type clothes pin is an ideal apparatus for providing hemostasis.

c. For pedunculated keloids with a wide base or large nonpedunculated earlobe keloids and for wide-base keloids on other anatomic areas, removal is more complex.

(1) First, a half-moon-type incision approximately one-fourth to one-fifth the size of the lesion is made from one border into the part of the keloid with the smoothest and flattest-looking skin surface. The remaining part of the keloid is then excised, and the keloid tissue is dissected from the lip of skin created with the half-moon incision. The wound edges are undermined, and the lip of skin is approximated to the undermined borders with 6.0 nylon interrupted sutures. Sometimes 6.0 nylon sutures are used to tack down the overlying skin because owing to its thinness, it is essentially a split-thickness graft (Figs. 6 and 7).

(2) The sutures are left in for 10 to 14 days because earlier removal may cause wound dehiscence. This slow healing may be caused by the injection of triamcinolone acetonide into the base of the postoperative site.

(3) One week after suture removal, the postoperative site is injected with triamcinolone acetonide for the first time. Injections are repeated every 2 or 3 weeks. A total of four postoperative injections is usually sufficient to prevent recurrence.

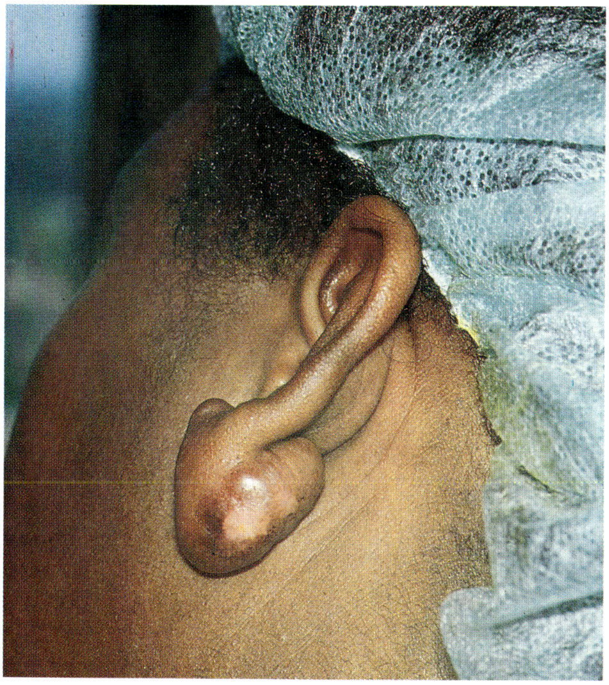

FIGURE 6
Preoperative view of a keloid on the right earlobe.

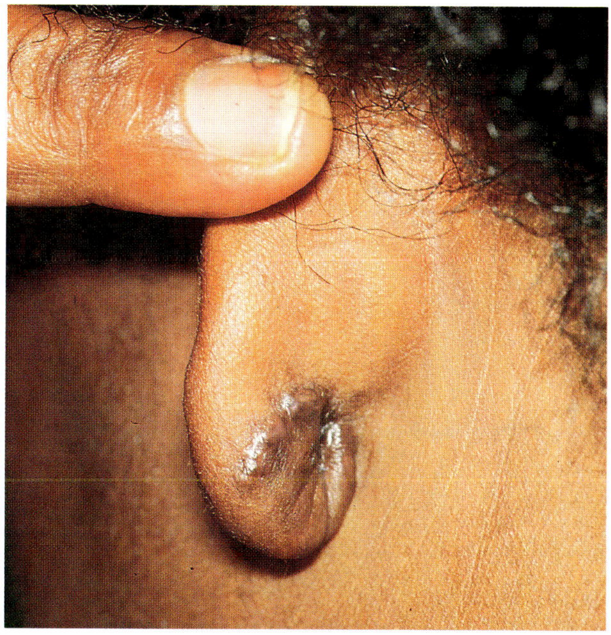

FIGURE 7
Postoperative view of a keloid on the right earlobe after saving the overlying tissue to close the excision site. The natural contour of the ear was preserved.

(4) Another adjunct for preventing recurrence is a pressure gradient garment on the postoperative site for at least 8 h but preferably for 16 to 20 h a day for 4 to 6 months.

(5) Wearing pressure earrings helps prevent the recurrence of earlobe keloids. The earrings should be worn continuously for 4 to 6 months.*

d. Another adjunct for preventing recurrence after surgery is postoperative x-ray therapy. Although many regimens have been proposed, we prefer 300 to 400 rad given within the first week after surgery and every 2 to 3 days thereafter for a total of 1200 rad.[9]

3. Ligatures may be used for pedunculated keloids when surgery is either contraindicated or refused by the patient. A 4.0 nonabsorbable suture is tightly tied around the base of the lesion, and a new suture is applied every 2 or 3 weeks.

a. The sutures gradually cut into the base of the keloid and strangulate it, causing autoamputation.

b. Some patients find the tight sutures too painful and uncomfortable to tolerate.

4. Topical tretinoin (retinoic acid) in a gel, cream, or liquid applied twice a day sometimes alleviates pruritus and other keloid symptoms and may cause various degrees of keloid regression.[10] Topical tretinoin is often more successful if combined with equal parts of a class I or class II topical steroid.

5. Colchicine, one tablet 3 times a day for 3 to 4 months after surgical removal of keloids, may prevent recurrence.[11] Colchicine is thought to increase collagenase production and inhibit the release of histamines from mast cells.

a. The colchicine should be initiated at the time of suture removal, because starting it earlier may retard wound healing.

b. Colchicine does not soften or flatten keloids that are already present.

6. Laser therapy has had mixed reviews in the treatment of keloids. Kantor et al.[12] claimed success with carbon dioxide laser excision. The author has found that carbon dioxide (Neodymium:Yitrium Aluminum Garnet, Nd: YAG) laser therapy is a quick way of removing keloids but does not prevent recurrence unless

* Pressure earrings can be purchased from H & A Enterprises, Inc., Whitestone, New York, or Pagent Instrument Co., Kansas City, Missouri.

the base of the keloid is injected with 40 mg/ml triamcinolone acetonide immediately after surgery.[12] Once the postoperative site heals, 4 to 6 months of pressure therapy and/or 2 to 3 weeks of injections with 10 mg/ml triamcinolone acetonide four times daily usually prevents recurrence.

7. If triamcinolone injections and/or pressure is used postoperatively, the keloids reccur rapidly. Onwukewe[13] reported success with surgical excision combined with methotrexate. The methotrexate is given orally or parentally, starting 1 week before surgical excision and continuing for 3 to 4 months. Fifteen to twenty milligrams of methotrexate is given in a single dose every 4 days. (This is not currently FDA approved.)[13]
8. Intralesional interferon may be successful against keloids: in a recent study,[14] intralesional injections of interferon alpha-2b into a progressively enlarging keloid resulted in a 41 percent reduction of its area. Also, keloid fibroblast persistently produced normal or subnormal amounts of collagen and normal levels of collagenase after interferon alpha-2b injections.
9. Other medications and therapeutic approaches such as asiaticoside (asiatic acid), penicillamine. 3-aminopropionitrile, β-aminopropionitrile), ultrasound, and antihistamines have been advocated but have proved to be less effective than the previously mentioned modalities. Also, as with hypertrophic scars, Covermark or another product to camouflage skin blemishes is often an excellent adjunct to enhance the cosmetic appearance of keloids, sites of keloid resolution, and postoperative sites.

REFERENCES

1. Blackburn WR, Cosman B. Histological basis of keloid and hypertrophic scar differentiation. Arch Pathol Lab Med. 1966; 82:65–71.
2. Holmstrand K, Longacre JJ, de Stefano GA. The ultrastructure of collagen in skin, scars, and keloids. Plast Reconstr Surg. 1961; 27:597–607.
3. Cosman B, Crikelair GF, Ju MC, et al. The surgical treatment of keloids. Plast Reconstr Surg. 1961; 27:335–358.
4. Cohen IK, McCoy BJ. Keloid: Biology and treatment, in Dineen P, Hildick-Smith G (eds), Surgical Wound. Philadelphia: Lea & Febiger; 1981:123–131.
5. Kelly AP. Keloids, in McDonald CJ, Scott DA (eds) Dermatologic Clin (Dermatology in Black Patients). Philadelphia: WB Saunders, 1988; 6:413–424.
6. Laurentaci G, Diaguardi D. HLA antigens in keloids and hypertrophic scars. Arch Dermatol 1971; 113:1726.
7. Oluwasanmi JO, Nwabuebo IO, Otusanya MO. Human leucocyte antigens (HLA) and keloids. W Afr J Med. 1983; 2:127–130.
8. Crikelair GF, Ju DMC, Cosman B. Scars and keloids, in Converse JM (ed) Reconstructive Plastic Surgery, 2d ed, vol. 1. Philadelphia: WB Saunders, 1977:413–441.
9. Enhamre A, Hammar H. Treatment of keloids with excision and postoperative x-ray irradiation. Dermatologica. 1983; 167:90–93.
10. Janssen DeLimpens AMP. The local treatment of hypertropic scars and keloids with topical retinoic acid. Br J Dermatol. 1980; 103:319–323.
11. Peacock EE. Pharmacologic control of surface scarring in human beings. Am Surg. 1981; 193:592–597.
12. Kantor GR, Wheeland RG, Balin PL, et al. Treatment of earlobe keloids with carbon dioxide laser excision: A report of 16 cases. J Dermatol Surg Oncol. 1985; 11:1063–1067.
13. Onwukewe MF. Surgery and methotrexate for keloids. Schoch Lett. 1978; 24:4.
14. Berman B, Duncan MR. Short-term keloid treatment in vivo with human interferon alpha-2b results in selective and persistent normalization of keloid fibroblast collagen, glycosaminoglycan, and collagenase production in vitro. J Am Acad Dermatol. 1989; 21:694–701.

CHAPTER 9

Malignant Lesions

FREDERIC E. MOHS
STEPHEN N. SNOW

The inclusion of a chapter on malignant skin lesions may seem odd when the discussion is to be focused on aesthetic dermatology. Unlike the removal of benign tumors where the purpose is the relief of symptoms or the improvement of appearance, the management of skin cancer takes on a more serious focus. A basal cell cancer rarely kills a patient but it can leave a highly destructive path; hence, the rodent ulcer. A squamous cell cancer should not be considered a benign prickle cell epithelioma, for it can metastasize and cause the death of the patient. A malignant melanoma is so serious a tumor that little attention can be given to details other than saving the patient. Other malignancies, such as sarcomas or metastatic lesions, are beyond the scope of this text.

There are many conventional methods for ridding the skin of a malignancy. These range from curettage and electrodesiccation to laser therapy, and from cryosurgery to radiotherapy. Unfortunately, all of these modalities do not address the problem of unpredictable small-caliber outgrowths that occur as a result of the countless variations in structural or nutritional conditions in the tissues.[1]

Micrographic surgery was devised to provide a means for managing these silent outgrowths. With this method, cutaneous cancers can be excised under complete microscopic control.[2] The method is based upon the simple concept of excising the suspected tissues layer by layer and examining frozen sections of the entire undersurface of each layer in the microscope until a completely cancer-free level is reached. The technique ensures eradication of the grossly invisible malignant outgrowths, and it does this with minimal loss of normal tissue because the excisions are abruptly stopped in areas that are seen to be free of cancer.

The total microscopic control provided by micrographic surgery can be achieved by the fresh-tissue technique, in which the layers of tissue are excised and inspected in a fresh, unfixed state, and by the fixed-tissue technique, in which the tissues are subjected to chemical fixation *in situ* prior to excision of the successive layers.[3,4]

CONVENTIONAL TREATMENT OF SKIN CANCER

Basal Cell Carcinoma

Several different modalities are perfectly acceptable for the treatment of basal cell carcinomas and give good to excellent cosmetic results. No one procedure can be certified as the perfect procedure; location of the lesion and operator experience influence the choice.[5,6,7]

The most popular therapy is *curettage and electrodesiccation.* Under local anesthesia, the lesion is vigorously curetted until no friable material remains. The base and the adjoining tissue to several millimeters is electrodesiccated. Some dermatologists prefer to repeat the procedure to ensure elimination of the tumor.

Good cosmetic results can be anticipated for lesions less than 15 mm. A white atrophic scar forms in about two to three weeks. Unfortunately, removal of lesions on the trunk may lead to hypertrophic scars following surgery. Cure can be anticipated in over 90 percent of the lesions treated. When the lesions are larger than 15 mm or located in the paranasal area or periorbital region, micrographic surgery should be considered.

Scalpel and suture surgery has its proponents. The lesion can be excised with a no. 15 scalpel. The area may be closed with a 4.0 silk or nylon suture on the body, left in place for 7 to 10 days, or with 6.0 silk or nylon suture on the face, removed after 3 to 5 days. Again, cosmetic results can be excellent.

Excising a margin of up to 5 mm may be sufficient to ensure no recurrence. Generally, in lesions larger than 15 mm, the use of micrographic surgery will give the surgeon more confidence, before repairing the area with grafts and flaps.

A *carbon dioxide* (CO_2) *laser* can be used, once histologic confirmation has been obtained. Along with CO_2 treatment for noncontrolled distribution of this tumor, 5 to 10 watts on a continuous wave mode can also be employed.

Cryosurgery has its advocates. Appropriate probes with thermocouples must be used. Once over lightly with a swab or a spray of liquid nitrogen cannot be condoned. For basal cell carcinoma, a thermocouple temperature between −40°C and −50°C and a halo thaw time of 3 min or longer is recommended.

Radiotherapy, given with 50 to 150 kv units, can give excellent aesthetic results on the face. Treatment is given in divided doses, 4500 to 5500 rad over 12 sessions. The resulting scar can be almost invisible. However, in some cases, atrophy and telangiectasia can result over time.

The use of *topical 5-fluorouracil* still has some proponents. Although the resulting appearance can approach that of normal skin, there is the danger that the tumor has not been destroyed and that a rodent ulcer may become apparent in a short time.

Micrographic surgery will be discussed thoroughly later in the chapter.

Squamous Cell Cancer

Squamous cell cancer and its variants, Bowen's disease and squamous cell cancer *in situ,* can be treated in similar ways. Actinic keratoses of a more superficial nature are discussed in Chapter 6, and keratoacanthomas are covered in Chapter 5.

Curettage and electrodesiccation will give equally good results. Because of the possibility of metastases, vigorous currettage is needed. This procedure is particularly recommended for the so-called grade ½ squamous cell cancers, Bowen's disease and squamous cell cancer in situ.

Scalpel and suture surgery can be accomplished with good results, particularly in larger lesions. Unfortunately, the surrounding tissue may be quite fragile because of the sun damage that may have instigated the primary tumor in the first place.

The CO_2 laser can be used in the way it is used for the treatment of basal cell carcinoma. Appropriate cryosurgery can be used with very good results. Radiotherapy generally is not recommended for these tumors. Except in unusual circumstances, topical chemotherapy will not be helpful.

MICROGRAPHIC SURGERY OF SKIN CANCER

Fresh-Tissue Micrographic Surgery for Carcinomas

The fresh-tissue technique is used for more than 95 percent of cutaneous carcinomas. In preparation for excision with fresh-tissue micrographic surgery, local anesthesia is produced by injecting 1% lidocaine with epinephrine 1:100,000 around the small basal cell carcinoma (BCC) on the nasal ala (Fig. 1*a*). The main mass is excised with a scalpel, and if the pearly tissue is obviously BCC, as in the

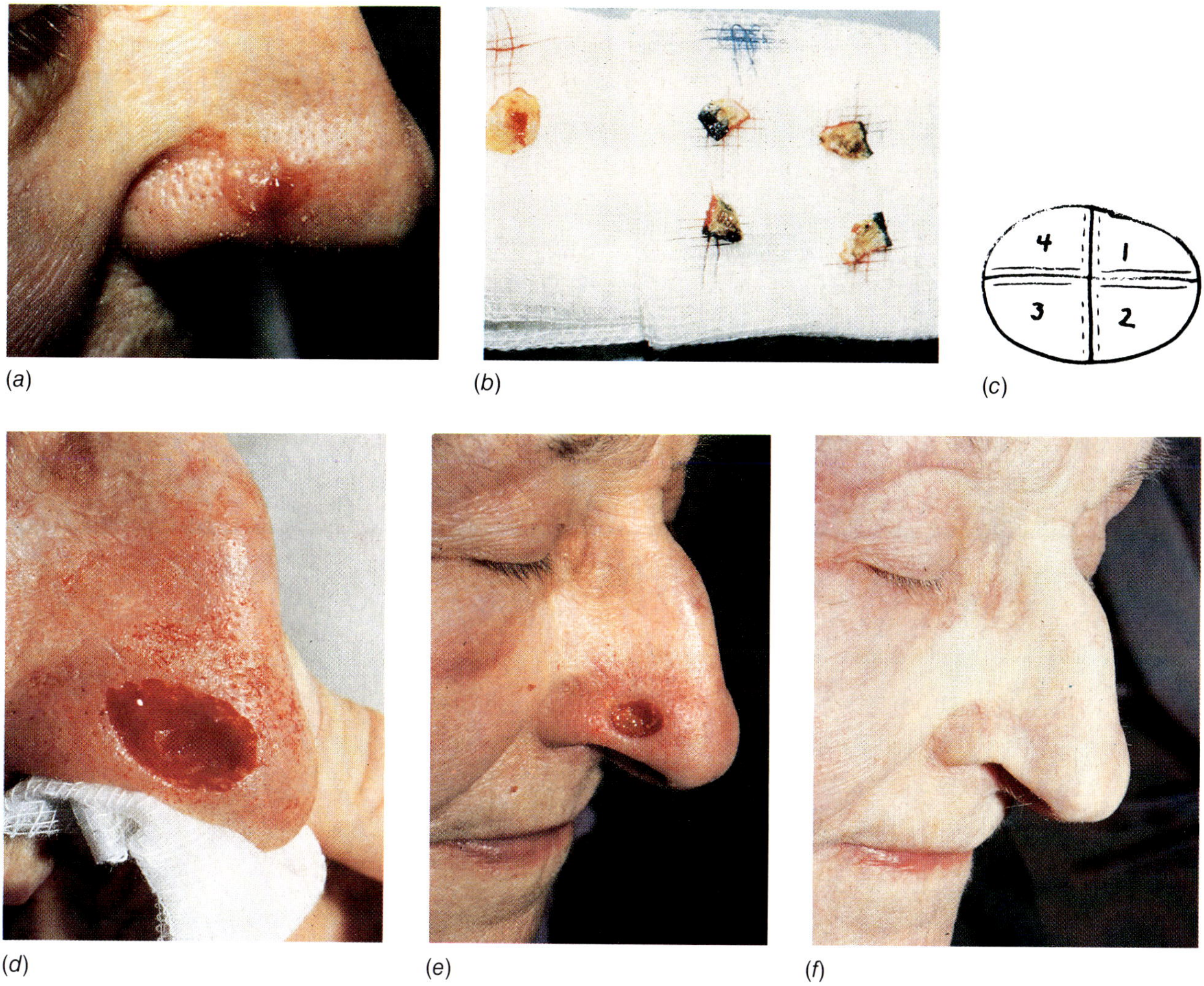

FIGURE 1
(*a*) Basal cell carcinoma limited to the nasal ala. (*b*) Specimen of first layer on left and the four specimens of the second layer with red and blue orientation markings on two edges. The skin is the marker for the third edge. (*c*) Map of the second layer. (*d*) Wound before the application of oxidized cellulose (Oxycel cotton) for hemostasis. (*e*) Healing wound after the removal of the Oxycel crust after 10 days. (*f*) Appearance after 2 years. No recurrence in 10 years. (*Reproduced with permission from FE Mohs.*[7])

figure, a second layer is excised immediately. The flat specimen is divided into four specimens and two edges of each specimen are color-coded with permanent red and blue dyes (Fig. 1*b*). A map is drawn to show the location of each of the four specimens (Fig. 1*c*). An hour later the frozen sections, which have been stained with hematoxylin and eosin, are ready for examination by the operator. The vertically cut section of the first layer shows BCC, but scanning the sections through the undersurface of the second layer reveals no cancer; this is indicated by a negative sign (Fig. 1*c*). If any cancer had been seen, its location would have been marked on the map in red pencil, and the next excision would have been limited to the areas of cancer. The process would be repeated until a cancer-free level was reached.

Oxidized cellulose (Oxycel cotton) is applied to the bleeding wound (Fig. 1*d*) to achieve hemostasis. When the crust is removed in 10 days, healing by granulation is under way (Fig. 1*e*). After 2 years, no notching of the rim is seen and the scar is barely visible (Fig. 1*f*).

In a given anatomic area the management of a

defect varies with its extensiveness. When cartilage is not involved, as in Fig. 1, healing by granulation gives a good result. If a deeper lesion requires the removal of some cartilage, a simple closure often can avoid a defect, but if there is a larger full-thickness defect, repair with a composite earlobe graft is preferable.[8]

A larger defect on the bridge and root of the nose with exposure of the septal cartilage and nasal bone and with incision through the mucosa on both sides of the septum requires prompt closure (Fig. 2*a*). Because of previous unsuccessful treatment of this patient with electrodesiccation, topical 5-fluorouracil, and plastic surgery, there was con-

FIGURE 2

(*a*) Defect following micrographic surgical excision of a basal cell carcinoma that recurred after electrosurgical excision, topical 5-fluorouracil treatments, and plastic surgery. (*b*) Partial closure brings the subcutaneous tissues over the exposed bone, cartilage, and mucosal defect. (*c*) Healed lesion after 6 months shows minimal scarring. (*d*) The profile is good. No recurrence in 5 years. (*Reproduced with permission from FE Mohs.*[7])

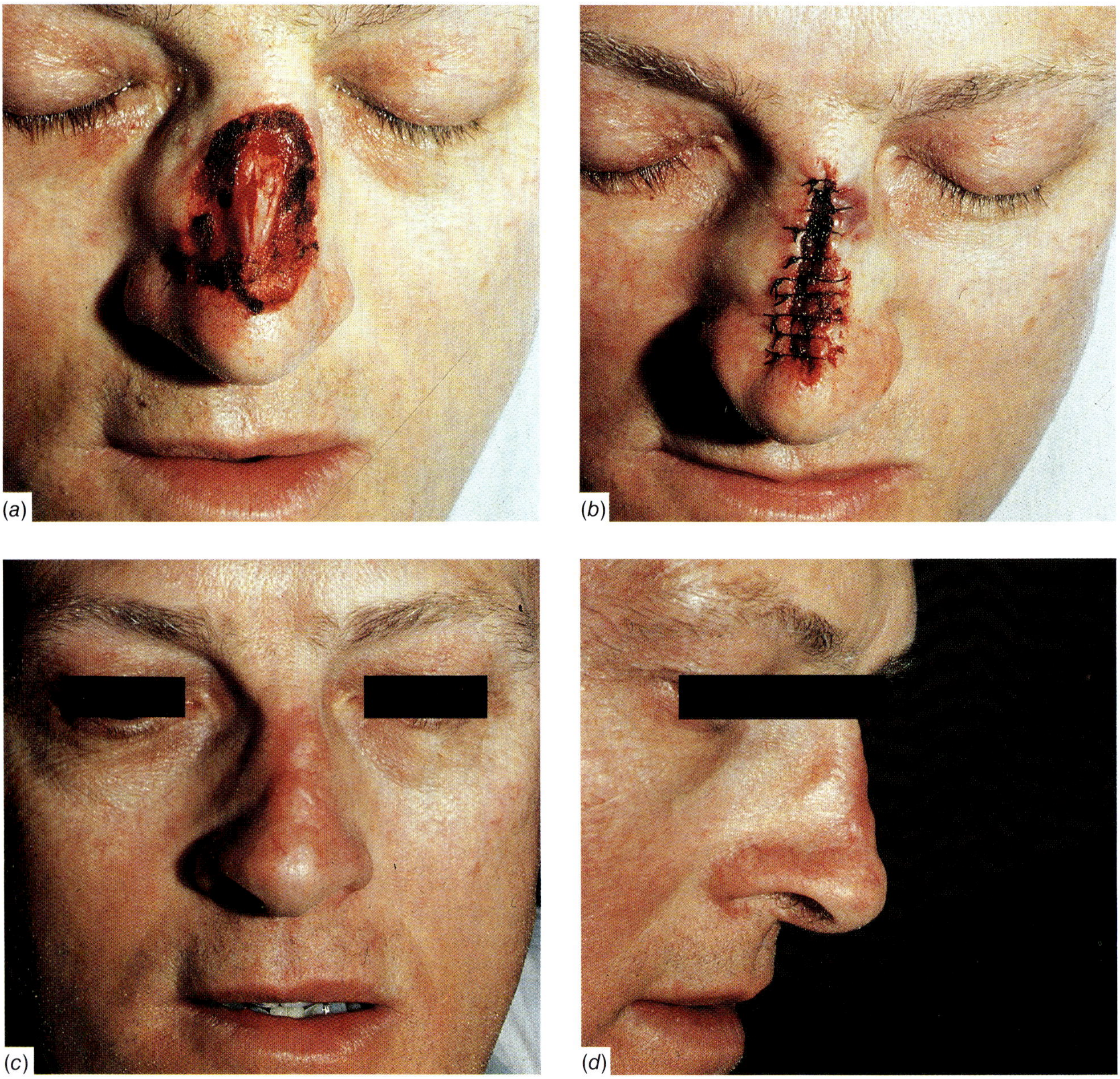

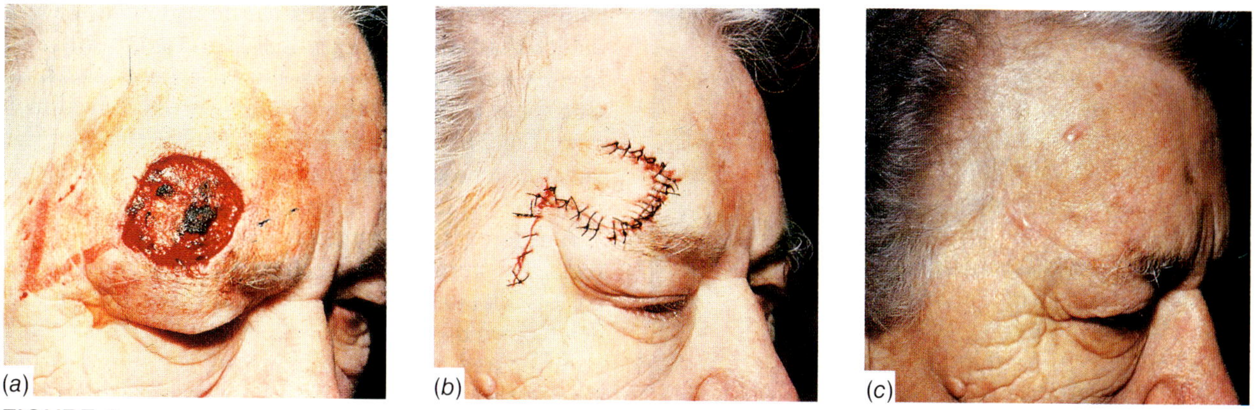

FIGURE 3
(*a*) Defect from removal of a basal cell carcinoma that involved part of the eyebrow. (*b*) Covering the defect with a rhomboid flap to avoid a scar that could pull up the lateral eyebrow. (*c*) Appearance after 5 months. No recurrence in 3 years.

cern that these treatments had resulted in outlying cancerous foci that were not contiguous with the main neoplastic mass. To avoid concealing these foci, a simple vertical partial closure was used rather than covering the defect with a flap (Fig. 2*b*). The skin grew across the small remaining defect in 10 days. There was no desiccation necrosis of the exposed cartilage or bone, and the mucosal defect closed spontaneously. The scar is now barely visible (Fig. 2*c*), and the profile is not impaired (Fig. 2*d*).

Although healing by granulation or by partial closure may be preferable in some cases, as in Fig. 1 and 2, the use of a flap or graft often is indicated because of the size or location of the defect. For example, if a defect above the lateral brow is left to heal by secondary intention, the resultant scar can be quite noticeable and the scar contraction can elevate the eyebrow (Fig. 3*a*). These complications can be avoided by using a rhomboid flap from the temple (Fig. 3*b*). The final result in this patient was satisfactory (Fig. 3*c*).

A large defect from the removal of a BCC on the cheek (Fig. 4*a*) can be covered satisfactorily by a bilobed flap (Fig. 4*b*). The scar, though long, is not noticeable (Fig. 4*c*).

Although skin grafts can be quite noticeable because of a poor match with facial skin, there are places where a full-thickness graft provides a good cosmetic result. For example, a BCC that extends

FIGURE 4
(*a*) Defect from the removal of a basal cell carcinoma. (*b*) Closure with a bilobed flap. (*c*) Appearance after 10 months. No recurrence in 4 years.

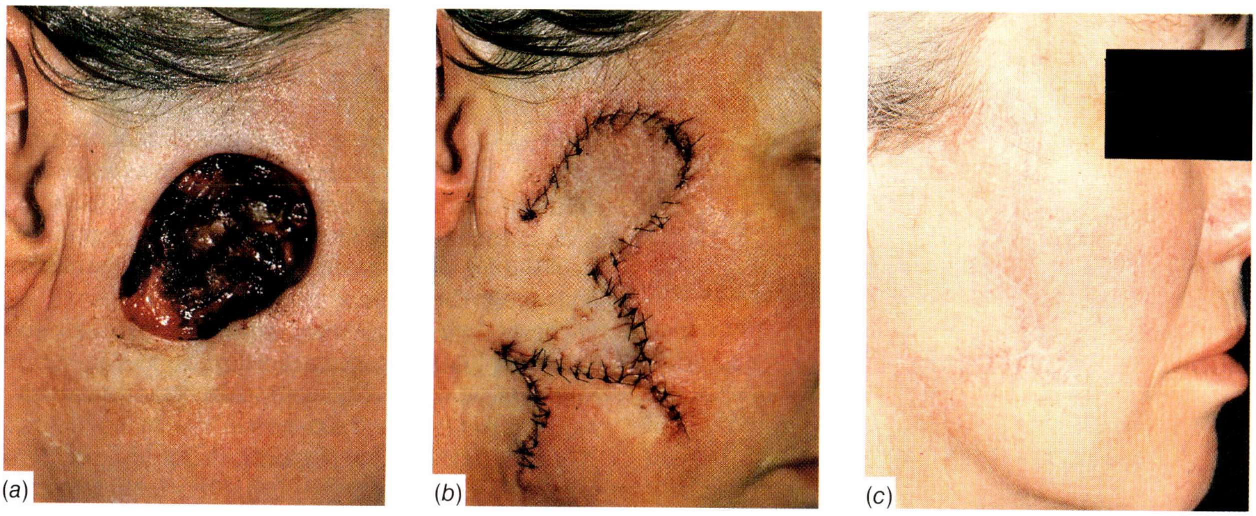

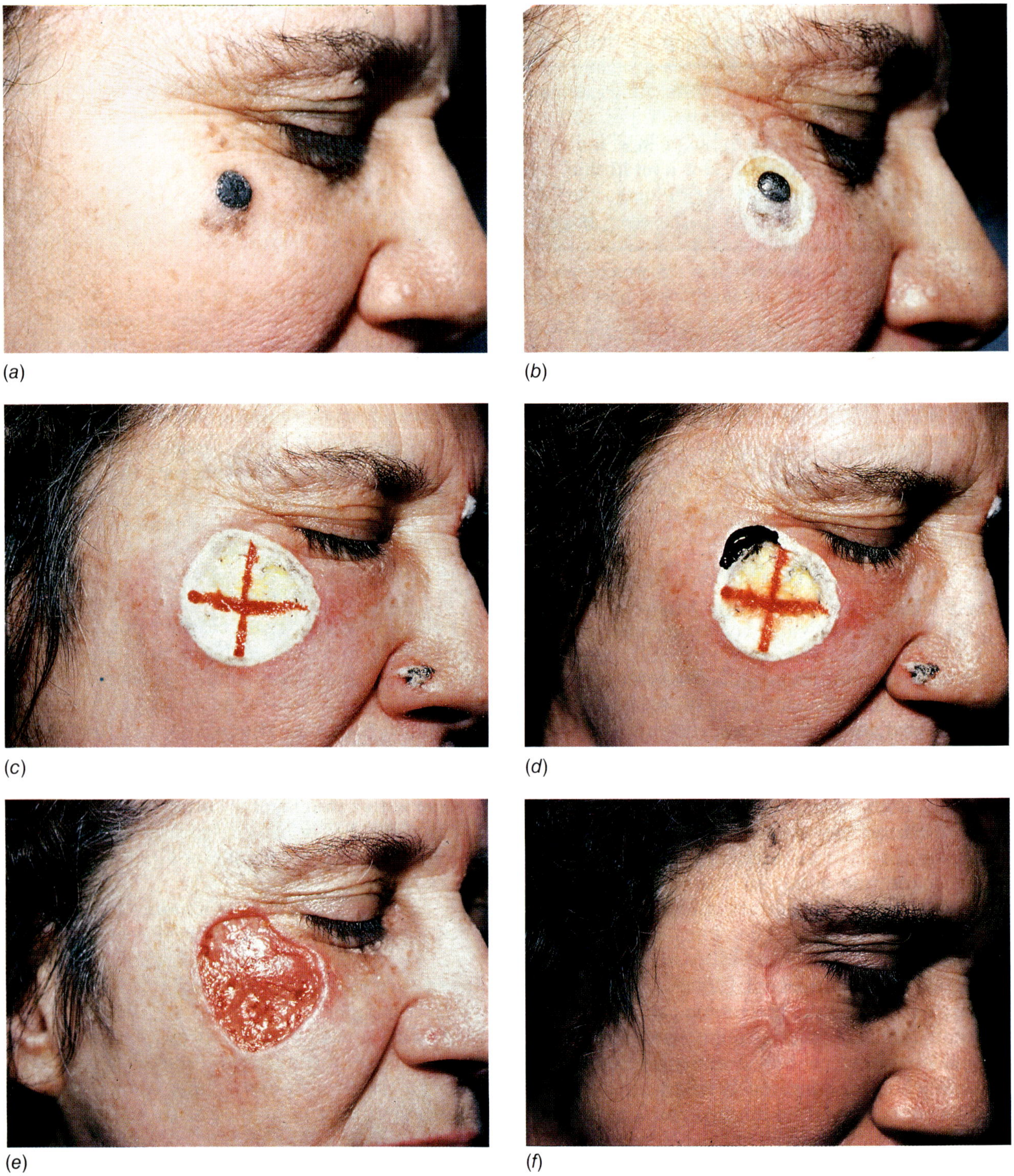

FIGURE 6
(*a*) Lentigo maligna melanoma arising in a patient with lentigo maligna. (*b*) Whitening produced by dichloroacetic acid except over the black melanoma. (*c*) White fixed tissue with red dye marks showing the source of each specimen. (*d*) Fixative is applied to the one remaining area of lentigo maligna at the upper edge. (*e*) Granulations after separation of the final layer of fixed tissue after 10 days. (*f*) Appearance 2 months later. No recurrence in 5 years.

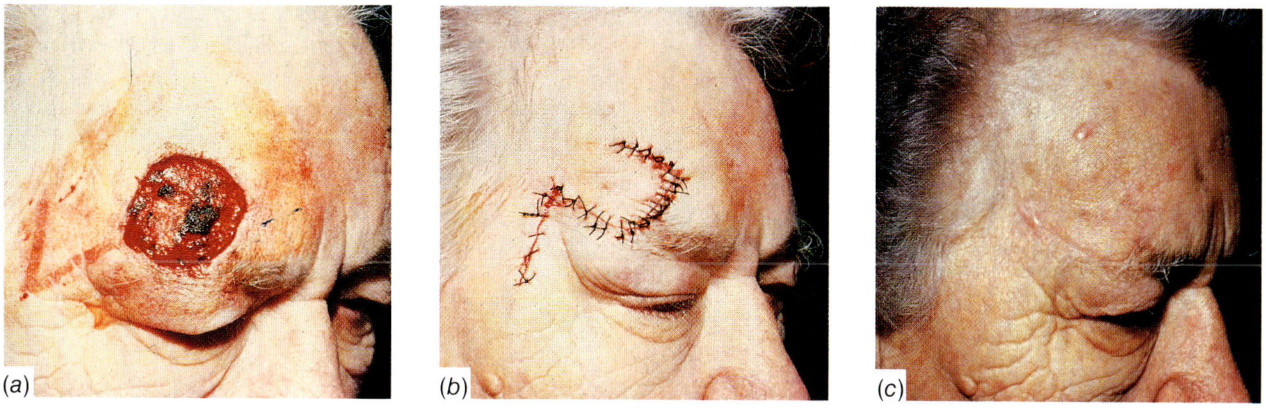

FIGURE 3
(*a*) Defect from removal of a basal cell carcinoma that involved part of the eyebrow. (*b*) Covering the defect with a rhomboid flap to avoid a scar that could pull up the lateral eyebrow. (*c*) Appearance after 5 months. No recurrence in 3 years.

cern that these treatments had resulted in outlying cancerous foci that were not contiguous with the main neoplastic mass. To avoid concealing these foci, a simple vertical partial closure was used rather than covering the defect with a flap (Fig. 2*b*). The skin grew across the small remaining defect in 10 days. There was no desiccation necrosis of the exposed cartilage or bone, and the mucosal defect closed spontaneously. The scar is now barely visible (Fig. 2*c*), and the profile is not impaired (Fig. 2*d*).

Although healing by granulation or by partial closure may be preferable in some cases, as in Fig. 1 and 2, the use of a flap or graft often is indicated because of the size or location of the defect. For example, if a defect above the lateral brow is left to heal by secondary intention, the resultant scar can be quite noticeable and the scar contraction can elevate the eyebrow (Fig. 3*a*). These complications can be avoided by using a rhomboid flap from the temple (Fig. 3*b*). The final result in this patient was satisfactory (Fig. 3*c*).

A large defect from the removal of a BCC on the cheek (Fig. 4*a*) can be covered satisfactorily by a bilobed flap (Fig. 4*b*). The scar, though long, is not noticeable (Fig. 4*c*).

Although skin grafts can be quite noticeable because of a poor match with facial skin, there are places where a full-thickness graft provides a good cosmetic result. For example, a BCC that extends

FIGURE 4
(*a*) Defect from the removal of a basal cell carcinoma. (*b*) Closure with a bilobed flap. (*c*) Appearance after 10 months. No recurrence in 4 years.

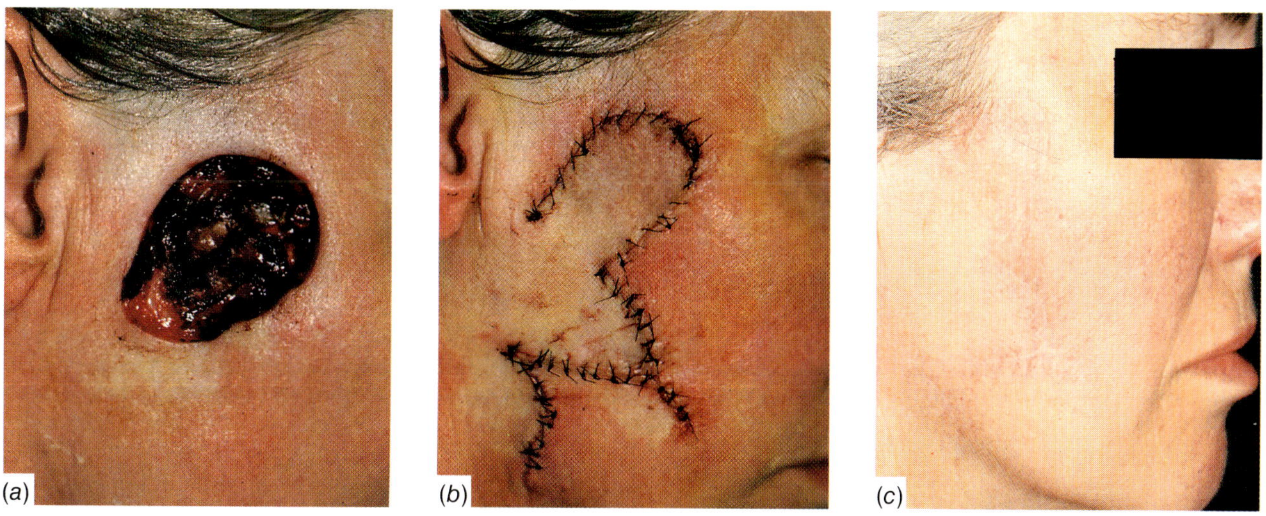

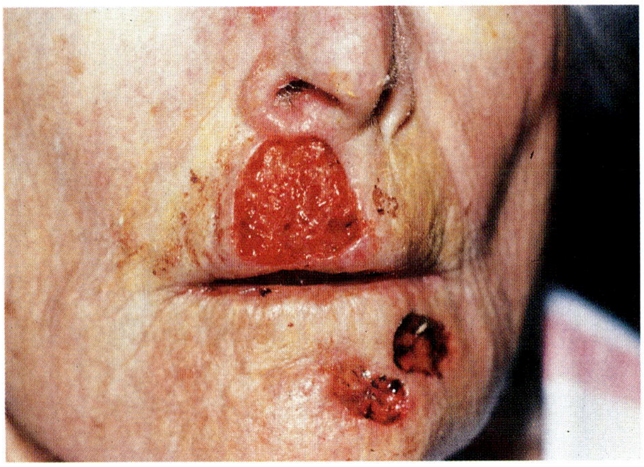
(a)

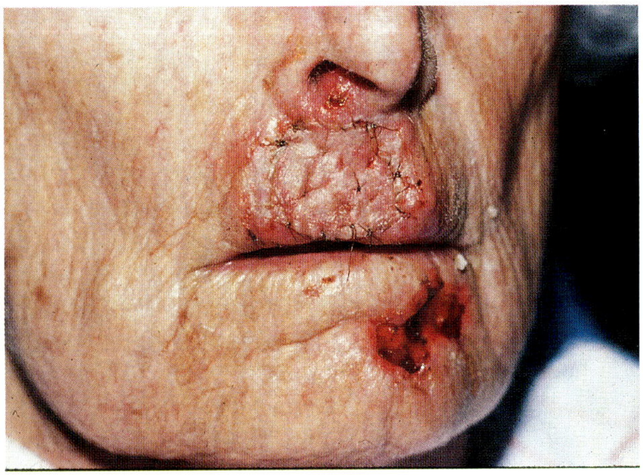
(b)

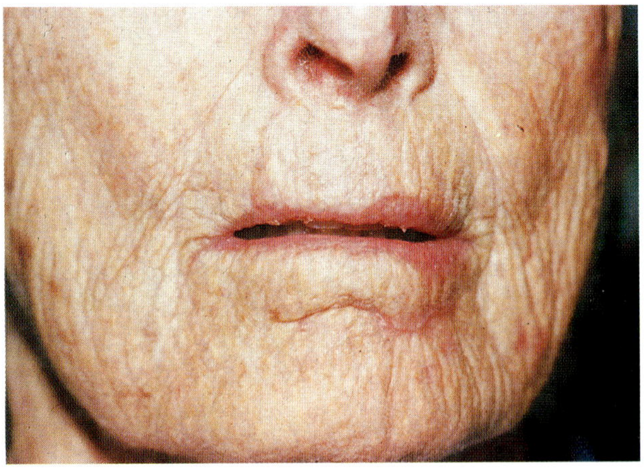
(c)

FIGURE 5
(a) A defect after the removal of a basal cell carcinoma. (b) A good take after the removal of sutures 5 days after the placement of a full-thickness graft from the neck. (c) Appearance after 4 months. No recurrence in 3 years.

from the vermilion border to the nose can leave a defect that is a good candidate for a graft (Fig. 5*a*). In this patient there was a total take of the full-thickness graft, and the sutures were removed in 5 days (Fig. 5*b*). There was no upward traction on the vermilion border, and there was a good color match (Fig. 5*c*).

A micrographic surgeon can manage many defects by permitting healing by granulation, by partial closures with guiding sutures to prevent defects, and by simple flaps and grafts. More complicated procedures requiring general anesthesia are the province of plastic surgeons, microsurgeons, oculoplastic surgeons, otolaryngologists, head and neck surgeons, and other specialists, depending on the nature and location of the defect.

In general, the simplest possible repair is best, especially if there has been previous unsuccessful treatment that might have resulted in outlying noncontiguous deposits of malignant cells that can be disseminated if transected. When it is realized how well a small defect on a lid margin can correct itself by the hammocklike contraction of the scar and how well canthal lesions can heal by granulation,[9,10] one is motivated to avoid overly complicated surgical repairs. With defects on the lower lip after removal of a squamous cell carcinoma, a simple anteroposterior closure often yields excellent cosmetic and functional results; if the defect is too deep for this procedure, the lesion can be converted to a simple V-closure.[11] Such uncomplicated repairs are often feasible because of the sparing of normal tissue that is possible when removal of the cancer is done under complete microscopic control.

CONVENTIONAL TREATMENT OF MALIGNANT MELANOMA

Malignant melanoma is so dangerous that elimination of the tumor overshadows concern for aesthetic results. This does not mean that mutilation is recommended for a superficial melanoma, but it does indicate that great concern must be given for destroying the tumor.

The malignant melanoma must be graded clinically and histologically according to various criteria. Table 1 gives the composite grading recommended by Zina and Sanderson.[12]

In low risk lesions, the tumor should be excised with a 10 mm margin of normal tissue. In interme-

TABLE 1
MALIGNANT MELANOMA GRADING

Low risk:	Tumor thickness <0.76 mm Clark's level I or level II thin
Intermediate risk:	Tumor thickness 0.76–1.5 mm Clark's level II thick or level III thin
High risk:	Tumor thickness >1.5 mm Clark's level III thick or level IV to V thin

Source: G. Zina and K.V. Sanderson,[12] p. 125, with permission.

diate risk lesions, a 3 to 5 cm margin of normal tissue should be included. In high risk lesions, a 5 cm margin of normal tissue should be taken into account. The defect would then require skin grafting.

A variety of chemotherapeutic agents can be employed. These include such drugs as DTIC (dacarbazine), vincristine, thiotepa, melphalan, and bleomycin, singularly or in combination. More details are to be found in the melanoma literature.[13]

Fixed-Tissue Micrographic Surgery for Melanoma

Melanomas, in common with carcinomas of the skin, often spread contiguously as silent outgrowths that may extend well beyond the clinically visible and palable borders.[14] In contrast with carcinomas, melanomas can also spread noncontiguously as emboli that lodge in the lymphatics to form satellites less than 5 cm from the primary tumor) or in-transit metastases (5 cm or more from the primary tumor but in the same lymphatic drainage pattern). In addition, melanoma cells are highly transplantable. Therefore, with conventional surgery there is a possibility that if either the contiguous or the noncontiguous melanomatous foci are transected, the melanoma cells can be disseminated during undermining to permit primary closure or can be concealed under a graft or flap until they become dangerously enlarged. Of course, this danger is recognized by surgeons who excise a wide margin of apparently normal tissue to reduce the likelihood of transecting any melanomatous foci. This procedure is quite successful in areas where a wide surgical margin poses no problem, but in areas such as the face, where there is strong motivation to spare tissue around an eye, ear, or nose, the danger of cutting into live melanoma tissue increases.

The rationale of fixed-tissue micrographic surgery is that the silent outgrowths from the main melanomas can be accurately located and selectively followed to their terminations by incisions through fixed (killed) tissue. Furthermore, outlying microsatellites that are not visible to the naked eye are not disturbed or disseminated and can be safely removed with the fixed-tissue technique when they become clinically visible.

Another safety feature of fixed-tissue micrographic surgery is that after the melanoma has been removed, the wound is permitted to heal by granulation. This avoids dissemination from melanomatous foci that might have resulted from a previous excisional biopsy or from clinically invisible satellites or in-transit metastases. When a residual melanoma becomes grossly visible, it can be removed with the fixed-tissue technique. With conventional surgery, by contrast, the wound is usually closed or is covered with a graft or flap; during this period any melanomatous foci can be transected, disseminated, and hidden from view for some time.

The fixed-tissue technique can be illustrated by a case of lentigo maligna melanoma (LMM) that arose in a patient with lentigo maligna (LM) (Fig. 6*a*). Dichloroacetic acid is applied until the skin turns white, indicating penetration through the keratin layer that otherwise would form a barrier to the zinc chloride fixative (Fig. 6*b*). The fixative paste[3] is applied in a thickness of 3 mm and is covered with a thin layer of cotton to hold the fixative in place. For occlusion, an overlapping petrolatum-spread cotton layer is taped in place. A suitable analgesic is prescribed.

Four hours later a layer including most of the LMM is excised. Frozen sections cut perpendicular to the surface show LMM, Clark's level III, in the center, surrounded by LM. (See Table 2.) The fixative is reapplied.

The next morning a layer is excised, using care not to incise the underlying unfixed tissue. The layer is divided into four specimens, and the source of each specimen is marked with merbromin on the white fixed tissue (Fig. 6*c*). Two edges of the specimens are colored with red and blue permanent dyes for purposes of orientation as the sections are systematically scanned in the microscope. In this patient no LMM is observed, but the LM extends farther than the grossly visible pigmentation at the upper edge. The fixative is applied to that area (Fig. 6*d*), and sections taken the next

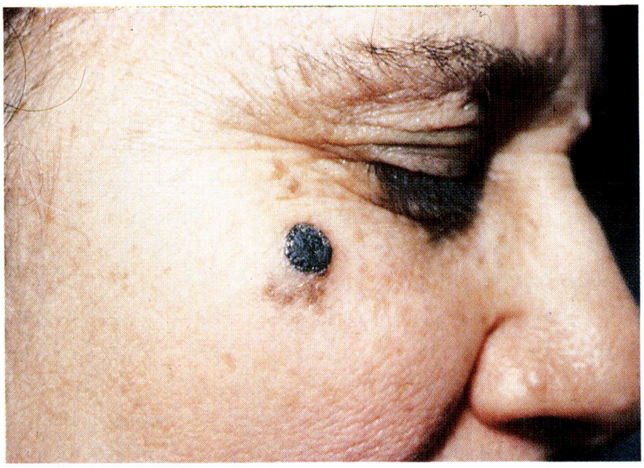

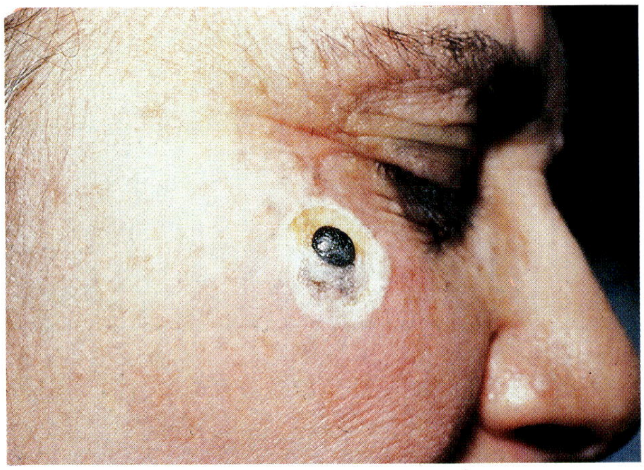

(*a*) (*b*)

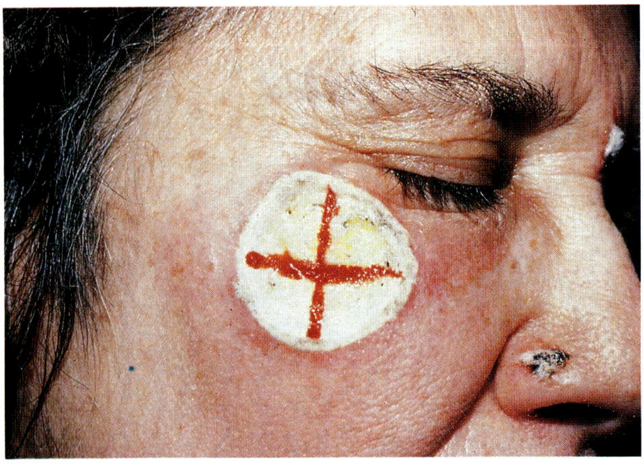

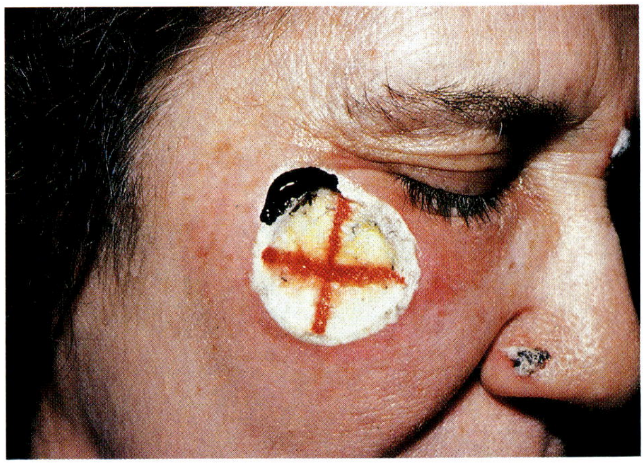

(*c*) (*d*)

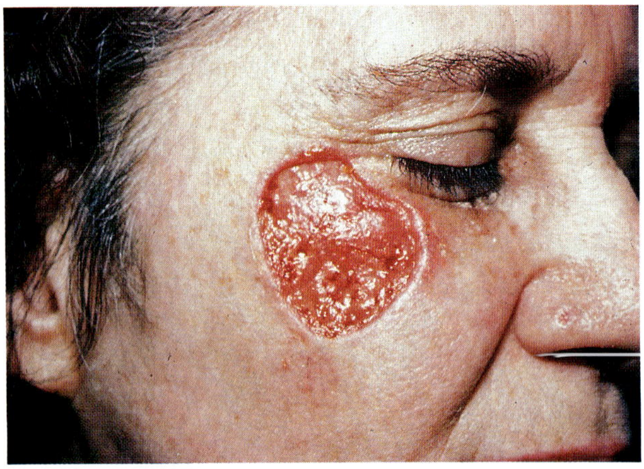

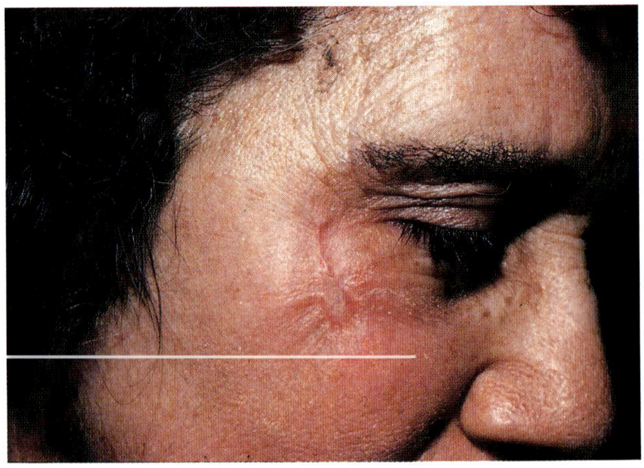

(*e*) (*f*)

FIGURE 6
(*a*) Lentigo maligna melanoma arising in a patient with lentigo maligna. (*b*) Whitening produced by dichloroacetic acid except over the black melanoma. (*c*) White fixed tissue with red dye marks showing the source of each specimen. (*d*) Fixative is applied to the one remaining area of lentigo maligna at the upper edge. (*e*) Granulations after separation of the final layer of fixed tissue after 10 days. (*f*) Appearance 2 months later. No recurrence in 5 years.

TABLE 2
CLARK'S GRADING OF MELANOMAS

Level I:	intraepidermal confinement
Level II:	papillary invasion
Level III:	superficial vascular plexus involvement
Level IV:	reticular dermis invasion
Level V:	subcutaneous tissue involvement

day are negative. Ten days later the final layer of fixed tissue separates and is removed by snipping a few strands, revealing a well-vascularized granulating base (Fig. 6*e*). The lesion is left to heal by granulation, and after 2 months the scar is satisfactory (Fig. 6*f*).

In cases of melanoma in the periorbital area, the advantage of a tissue-sparing technique is obvious.[15] A complicated structure such as the ear is much easier to repair if a generous amount of normal tissue can be spared.[16] The same holds true for melanoma in the nasal area[3,20] and, to a lesser degree, for melanoma in other facial areas.[17,18]

There is controversy about whether to do a prophylactic dissection of the regional nodes or to carefully follow the patient so that the nodes can be removed before they are 1 cm in diameter. We usually prefer the latter course because in some cases the positive nodes appear in the backwaters of the lymphatic drainage system and can be missed by the usual node dissection.[3]

Satellites and in-transit metastases are adverse occurrences but should not necessarily cause one to give up; in some cases a cure can be achieved by removing the lesions with the fixed-tissue technique.[19]

CONCLUSIONS

The first thought in cancer surgery is the elimination of the tumor. Surgical intervention does not always have to be mutilating, particularly if the physician takes into account the clinical morphology, the histologic picture, and the natural history of the disease. A superficial basal cell cancer does not require devastating surgery, nor does a large malignant melanoma permit quick freezing.

REFERENCES

1. Mohs FE, Lathrop TG. Modes of spread of cancer of skin. Arch Dermatol. 1952; 66:427–439.
2. Mohs FE. Chemosurgery: A microscopically controlled method of cancer excision. Arch Surg. 1941; 42:279–295.
3. Mohs FE. Chemosurgery: Microscopically controlled surgery for skin cancer. Springfield, IL: Charles C Thomas, 1978; 5:225–248.
4. Mohs FE. Chemosurgery for skin cancer: Fixed tissue and fresh tissue techniques. Arch Dermatol. 1977; 112: 211–215.
5. Gross PR, Kerdel-Vegas F. Tumors, malignant: Basal cell cancer and squamous cell cancer, in Rook A, Parish LC, Beare JM, Practical Management of the Dermatologic Patient. Philadelphia: JB Lippincott, 1986:205–208.
6. Ketcham AS, Moffat FL. Cancer of the skin and the surgical oncologist, in Epstein E, Epstein E, Jr: Skin Surgery. Philadelphia: WB Saunders, 1987:140–152.
7. Mohs FE. Chemosurgery. Clin Plast Surg. 1980; 7:349–360.
8. Davenport G, Bernard FG. Improving the take of composite grafts. Plast Reconstr Surg. 1959; 24:175–182.
9. Mohs FE. Micrographic surgery for the microscopically controlled excision of eyelid cancers. Arch Ophthalmol. 1986; 901–909.
10. Mohs FE. Micrographic surgery for the microscopically controlled excision of eyelid cancer: History and development. Adv Ophthalmol Plast Reconstruct Surg. 1986; 5:381–408.
11. Mohs FE, Snow SN. Microscopically controlled surgical treatment for squamous cell carcinoma of the lower lip. Surg Gynec Obstet 1985; 160:37–41.
12. Zina G, Sanderson KV. Melanoma, in Rook A, Parish LC, Beare JM: Practical Management of the Dermatologic Patient. Philadelphia: JB Lippincott, 1986:124–127.
13. Balch CM, Milton GW. Cutaneous Melanoma. Philadelphia: JB Lippincott, 1985:1–538.
14. Mohs FE. The width and depth of the spread of malignant melanoma as observed by a chemosurgeon. Am J Dermatopathol 1984; 6 (suppl l):123–126.
15. Mohs FE. Microscopically controlled surgery for periorbital melanoma: Fixed-tissue and fresh-tissue techniques. J Dermatol Surg Oncol. 1985; 11:284–291.
16. Mohs FE. Fixed-tissue micrographic surgery for melanoma of the ear. Arch Otolaryngol Head Neck Surg. 1988; 114:625–631.
17. Mohs FE. Chemosurgical treatment of melanoma: A microscopically controlled method of excision. Arch Dermatol Syphilol. 1950; 62:269–279.
18. Mohs FE. Chemosurgery for melanoma. Arch Dermatol. 1977; 113:285–291.
19. Mohs FE. Micrographic surgery for satellites and in-transit metastases of malignant melanoma. J Dermatol Surg Oncol. 1986; 12:471–476.
20. Mohs FE, Snow SN, Larson PO. Mohs micrographic surgery fixed-tissue technique for melanoma of the nose. J Dermatol Surg Oncol (in press).

CHAPTER

10

Pigmentary Changes

JEAN-PAUL ORTONNE

Normal skin color results from a mixture of several colored pigments, including oxygenated and reduced hemoglobin, carotenoids, and melanins; however, the melanins are most responsible for skin color.[1] Melanins are regarded as a fairly heterogeneous group of pigments including eumelanins (brown-black), pheomelanins (yellow-red), and mixed-type melanins. These pigments vary in their chemical and physical properties. They are produced by highly specialized dendritic cells—the *melanocytes*—which are found in the basal layer of the epidermis. Melanins are synthesized and packaged in specialized organelles called *melanosomes.* These granules are transferred to epidermal and follicular *keratinocytes* and transported to the skin surface. Normal skin color is a function of the number, size, and distribution of the melanosomes.[1]

Melanin pigmentation is a complex multistep process involving active cooperation between melanocytes and keratinocytes. This functional unit has been termed the *epidermal melanin unit.* Its activity is under genetic control but is also modulated by environmental (light) and internal (hormones) factors.[1] Many processes can disturb the function of the epidermal melanin unit, leading to pigmentary abnormalities.

CLASSIFICATION OF MELANIN PIGMENTARY DISTURBANCES

There are three categories of pigmentary disturbances: *leukodermas* (mild to marked decrease in normal skin color), *melanodermas* (mild to marked brown darkening), and *cerulodermas* (mild to marked gray, slate, or blue discoloration). In some instances these abnormalities may be unrelated or only partly related to the melanin pigmentary system[2] (Figs. 1 and 2).

Most leukodermas are due to hypomelanosis, which may be subdivided into hypomelanosis with a reduction or absence of melanocytes (*melanocytopenic hypomelanosis*) and hypomelanosis

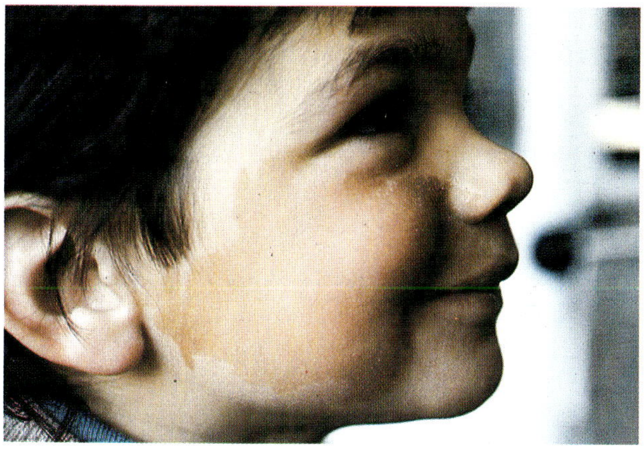

FIGURE 1
Extensive café au lait spot on the face.

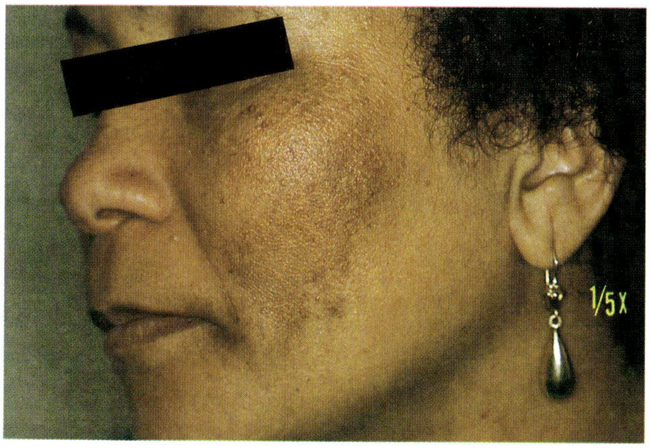

FIGURE 2
Typical melasma.

with a normal number of melanocytes but an absence of or reduction in melanins (*melanopenic hypomelanosis*). The subdivision of melanotic disease (normal number of melanocytes but increased melanin pigment) and melanocytic disease (increased number of melanocytes) applies to melanoderma and ceruloderma.[2]

Some of these disorders are very common and represent everyday practical problems for most dermatologists. Although these dermatoses do not limit physical activities or pose a threat to the life of the individual, some of them may have an important effect on personality, in some cases constituting a psychosocial disaster because of alteration of appearance.[3] Thus, physicians need to be especially alert to the psychological effects of pigmentary disorders and should not underestimate the consequences of cosmetic disfigurement.

Apart from the patient history and a careful examination of the individual, examination under a Wood's light is of prime importance in classifying melanin pigmentary disorders, both hypomelanoses and hypermelanoses, and should be part of the evaluation in all these patients. Examination can help distinguish epidermal from dermal hypermelanoses. Epidermal or brown hypermelanosis is accentuated, and dermal melanosis may disappear or at least become less obvious. For hypomelanoses, the greater the loss of epidermal pigmentation in comparison to normal skin, the more marked the contrast on Wood's light examination. Wood's light examination is most helpful in fair-skinned individuals to identify the presence and location of hypomelanotic macules.

Skin biopsy is exceptionally useful in the diagnosis of most common pigmentary disorders. In the classification of melanin pigmentary disorders, there are two main theoretical situations by which the therapist is confronted.

1. There is too much melanin or too many melanocytes in the skin. The aim of treatment is to destroy or discolor the melanins or to reduce the number of melanocytes, mostly by means of destruction. Bleaching and depigmenting agents are used hopefully to achieve these goals.
2. There is not enough melanin or melanocytes in the epidermis and/or hair follicles. The aim of treatment is to stimulate the appearance of melanins and/or melanocytes in the hypomelanotic areas or to use covering agents or dyes to reduce the contrast between involved and uninvolved skin. At present, only photochemotherapy with photoactive drugs allows one to repigment melanocytopenic macules to any extent.

Among the hypomelanoses, the most common disorders for which patients seek treatment are vitiligo, idiopathic guttate hypomelanosis (Fig. 3),

FIGURE 3
Idiopathic guttate hypomelanosis, close-up view.

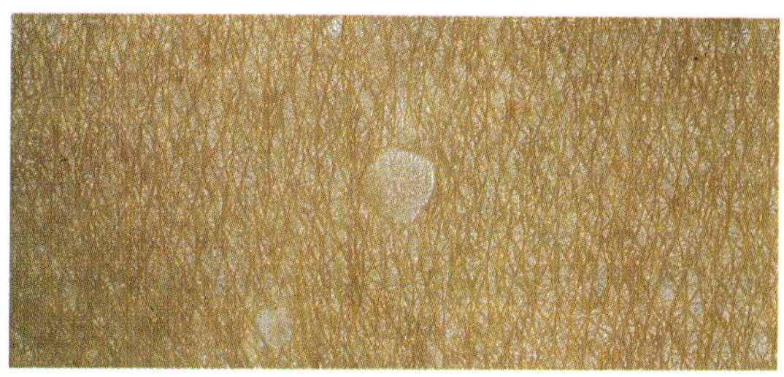

postinflammatory hypomelanosis or pityriasis alba, and hypomelanotic tinea versicolor.

Among the hypermelanoses, the most common disorders include ephelides, melasma, actinic and senile lentigines, café au lait spots, postinflammatory hypermelanosis, and Becker's nevus.

Facial melanosis in women is a common dermatological problem in Japan. Cosmetics have been considered causal agent, and the name *pigmented cosmetic dermatitis* has been proposed for these facial pigment disorders.[4] However, the causative role has not been firmly established.

MANAGEMENT OF HYPERMELANOSES

Depigmenting Agents

A large number of chemical compounds induce depigmentation of the skin in humans.[2,5,6] Only a small number, including hydroquinone and its derivatives, have been employed in the treatment of various pigmentary disorders.

Hydroquinone For nearly 20 years hydroquinone has been used in patients with hypermelanoses.[7] It is probably the most widely used depigmenting agent. Hydroquinone is used at a 2 to 5% concentration. It is a useful treatment for patients with melasma, hypermelanosis of cosmetic origin, ephelides, and postinflammatory hypermelanoses; however, it is more effective for hypermelanoses of epidermal origin. Several months of treatment are required to obtain a cosmetically acceptable result in 70 to 90 percent of patients. The preparation should be used twice daily or only once daily if burning sensations occur. Concomitant use of sunscreen with a high sun protection factor (SPF) is recommended. It is unusual to be able to induce a complete disappearance of hypermelanosis; depigmentation must be considered temporary and reversible. There is no difference in reactivity between blacks and whites. Increasing the concentration of hydroquinone increases the effectiveness of the drug but also increases its irritancy. Indeed, hydroquinone is a mild primary irritant and may provoke sensitivity and contact dermatitis. Thus, it is unwise to use hydroquinone at concentrations higher than 5%.[8] There is almost no adverse reactivity to 2% hydroquinone, 30 percent reactivity to 5% hydroquinone, and constant irritancy to 10% hydroquinone. The most frequently observed side effects are irritancy, sensitization, postinflammatory hyperpigmentation which gradually fades, hydroquinone-induced ochronosis, occasionally brown discoloration of the fingernails, and confetti-like depigmentation in a few cases.[2,7,9]

Several attempts have been made to increase the potency of hydroquinone and to reduce its side effects. The following formula was proposed by Kligman and Willis[10]:

Hydroquinone	5.00%
Tretinoin (retinoic acid)	0.10%
Dexamethasone 21-acetate	0.10%
Ethanol, 95%	47.40%
Propylene glycol	47.40%

The vehicle may also be a hydrophilic ointment and another steroid may be used in place of dexamethasone. The guidelines for the use of this depigmenting solution or cream are as follows[11]:

The preparation should be applied twice daily every day for several months.
The preparation should not be more than 30 days old because it may deteriorate.
No other treatment should be used concomitantly on the treated site except a protective agent before exposure to the sun.
The preparation should be kept out of sunlight in a cool, fresh site.
Alteration in the color of the cream or solution results from chemical alteration and is thus associated with decreased depigmenting activity.

Complete depigmentation of normal skin in adult black men has been produced by the daily application of hydroquinone for 5 to 7 weeks. During the first weeks of treatment, erythema and desquamation usually precede depigmentation. In clinical use, 60 to 90 percent of patients with melasma, ephelides, and postinflammatory hyperpigmentation achieved a satisfactory response. Yet senile lentigines were resistant to this therapy. Depigmentation was less satisfactory in fair-skinned individuals than in blacks.

Either alone or included in Kligman's formula, hydroquinone is the only relatively safe and effective treatment for lightening human skin.[10]

Hydroquinone Derivatives Monobenzyl ether of hydroquinone (monobenzone, or MBEH) has also been employed in treating human beings. This agent is known to produce excessive depigmentation at sites distant from its application. Furthermore, in some patients the leukoderma continues to progress for several months after application.[12] For these reasons, MBEH should not be used to treat hypermelanotic disorders such as melasma, ephelides, and postinflammatory hypermelanosis. MBEH also should be prohibited for use in cosmetic preparations. The endpoint of MBEH-induced hypopigmentation cannot be reliably predicted or controlled, and a vitiligo-like depigmentation may occur. The only clinical use of MBEH is for vitiligo patients who wish above all to be one color and who can accept the emotional and physical limitations of being totally amelanotic[12,13] (Fig. 4).

Permanent chemical depigmentation of uninvolved skin in patients with vitiligo may be achieved with twice-daily applications of 20% MBEH in an ointment base. The depigmentation usually takes several months to appear and a year to complete and is effective in almost every patient. The incidence of side effects, including a burning sensation and itching, erythematous eruption, dryness, contact dermatitis, and edema, is high.

Although occasional macules of repigmentation may occur, the patient must be made to understand that the depigmentation is usually irreversible. Thus, the following guidelines have been proposed for this treatment[13]:

- Desire for permanent depigmentation in a patient with vitiligo
- Age over 40
- More than 50 percent of the skin depigmented
- Willingness to accept the fact that repigmentation will no longer be possible

This treatment can be used only in a very limited number of carefully selected patients. Appropriate use generally gives fair results, and most patients are pleased with the results.

Monomethyl ether of hydroquinone (MMEH) is used in Europe and Africa because it is more effective and less irritating than hydroquinone.[14] This compound may be used in a 10% concentration. MMEH is capable of producing confetti-like hypopigmentation indistinguishable from that of MBEH. Thus, the same restrictions should be applied to the use of MBEH. This agent should not be used to treat hypermelanosis in human beings.

In summary, hydroquinone is the only agent available for clinical use. At present, it represents the least disappointing treatment for hypermelanotic disorders.

The mechanisms by which hydroquinone and its derivatives produce their effects are not known with certainty. The following mechanisms have been proposed: selective destruction of melano-

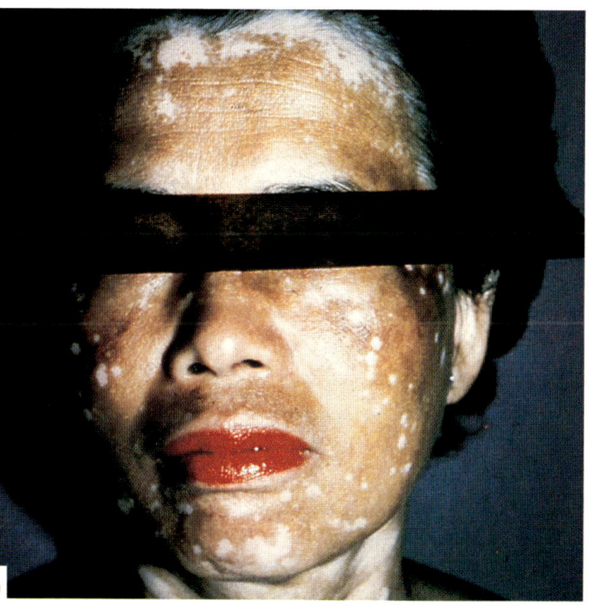
(a)

FIGURE 4
(*a*) Vitiligo-like hypomelanosis of the face in a patient using monobenzone to treat melasma. (*Courtesy J. Thivolet, M.D., Lyon, France; with permission.*) (*b*) Vitiligo-like hypomelanosis in the same patient, remote from the sites of direct application.

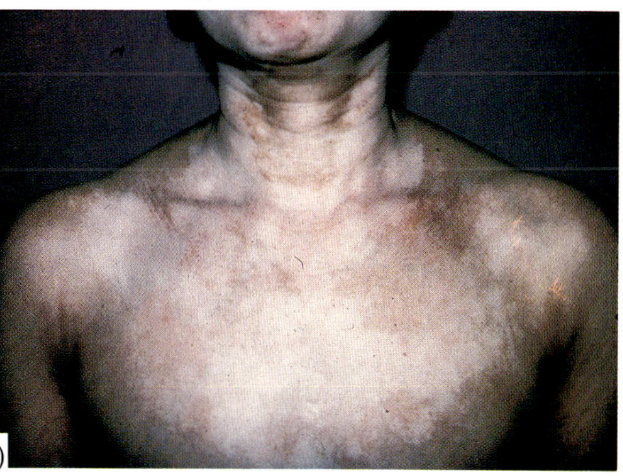
(b)

cytes, inhibition of melanosome function and alteration of melanosome structure, inhibition of tyrosinase biosynthesis, inhibition of melanin formation, interference with the transfer of melanosomes to keratinocytes, chemical effect on melanin or enhancement of melanin degradation, and conversion of hydroquinone and its derivatives to highly toxic free radicals that cause melanocyte death.

Azelaic Acid Azelaic acid (AA)[15] is a naturally occurring C_9 dicarboxylic acid. Because of its inhibitory effect on tyrosinase, the key enzyme in melanogenesis, it has been suggested that azelaic acid could be involved in the hypochromia of pityriasis versicolor (the fungus *Pityrosporum*, the etiological agent of the disease, is capable in culture of oxidizing oleic acid to AA) and could act as a depigmenting agent.

Creams with 10% or 20% AA have been prepared, but very little is known about the formula. This cream has no effect on normal skin. Applied twice daily for several months, it was shown to have a beneficial effect in the treatment of melasma, postinflammatory hypermelanoses, and hypermelanoses caused by physical or photochemical agents. Controlled clinical trials on the effect of AA are in progress, and further data are needed to confirm the initial findings. Several investigators have reported a beneficial effect of AA in the treatment of lentigo maligna melanoma.

There is, however, still some controversy about the activity of AA in hypermelanotic disorders. It is known that the type of formulation significantly affects the penetration of AA into the skin and thus affects the activity of the cream. This may explain the discrepancies in the therapeutic results obtained in different centers. Thus standardized formulations and regimen of application are needed for a precise evaluation of this drug.

The mechanism of action is unknown. AA does not have a selective effect on melanocytes. It may operate by reversibly inhibiting essential oxidoreductive enzymes. Additional data are required before it can be concluded that AA is useful in the treatment of hypermelanoses.

Other Drugs Many other drugs have been employed to lighten the skin. Mercurials have been widely used. Because cutaneous absorption of mercury may cause nephrotoxicity, their use should be banned.[12] The same conclusion should apply to topical corticosteroids. Indeed, their depigmenting properties are very mild. The well-known side effects associated with the long-term use of these compounds have limited their prescription as depigmenting agents. Furthermore, depigmentation is never total and always regresses after the discontinuation of therapy.

Bleaching Agents Bleaching agents[15] are used for hair lightening; they do this by oxidizing melanin pigments. If carried to extremes, this can lead to total solubilization and elimination. A variety of bleaching products are available. They contain hydrogen peroxide alone, with ammonia, or mixed with oxidizing products such as peroxy salts or peroxides. They are available in solutions, emulsions, creams, shampoos, powders, pastes, and oils.[16]

Physical and Chemical Treatments

These methods are used only for treating localized pigmented spots. Melanocytes are particularly susceptible to destruction by freezing. This treatment should never be used in dark-skinned people because of the risk of permanent depigmentation. The freezing agent must be applied gently to avoid blistering and skin necrosis.

Chemabrasion using trichloroacetic acid (TCA) is another therapeutic modality for removing freckles, solar lentigines, and other localized patches of pigmentation. The following procedure has been proposed[17]:

A single application of a 25% solution of TCA on a test site. In case of burning sensation, the area is washed with soap and water and rubbed with a soap-impregnated cloth.

If a 25% solution produces inadequate effects or results, 50% and even 75% solutions are tested on subsequent areas.

The concentration that produces desquamation and loss of the lesion without excessive injury is used as the treatment of choice. The solution is applied rapidly on the lesion by the physician, using a cotton-tipped swab, and washed off if a burning sensation occurs.

This procedure usually is effective in removing spotty hyperpigmentation. However, it should be used with extreme caution because concentrated TCA may cause instantaneous necrosis of the epidermis, and postinflammatory hyperpigmentation frequently occurs in patients with skin types V and VI. See Chapter 5.

Grafting and Transplantation of Melanocytes

Several "surgical" procedures for treating depigmented skin of vitiligo have been reported to be effective. These include grafting of suction-blistered epidermis within the white macules, thin thiersch grafts, or minigrafts.[18] Transplantation of *in vitro* cultured epidermis bearing melanocytes has also been used successfully. Another possibility of future technology is the use of *in vitro* cultured melanocytes. These techniques may represent an alternative for treating localized vitiligo, particularly when medical treatment has failed.

MANAGEMENT OF HYPOMELANOSES

Psoralen Photochemotherapy

Psoralen photochemotherapy (PUVA) is the most successful (or least disappointing) mode of current therapy involving the use of psoralens and subsequent exposure to long-wave ultraviolet A irradiation. Although, numerous psoralens have been identified,[19] only a few, including methoxsalen (8-methoxypsoralen), 4,5′-8-trimethoxypsoralen, and more recently bergapten (5-methoxypsoralen), have been used, almost exclusively for the treatment of vitiligo[12,20–22] (Figs. 5 and 6).

Psoralens are given mostly by oral administration, but they may also be applied topically. The guidelines for oral psoralen photochemotherapy[12,21,23] are summarized in Tables 1 and 2.

Khellin Photochemotherapy

Khellin, a furochrome which used to be prescribed for the treatment of angina pectoris and which has some structural similarities with methoxsafen (8-MOP), has been used to treat vitiligo in combination with natural sunlight or artificial UVA.[24–26] In a double-blind clinical study, 5 and 7 of 30 patients

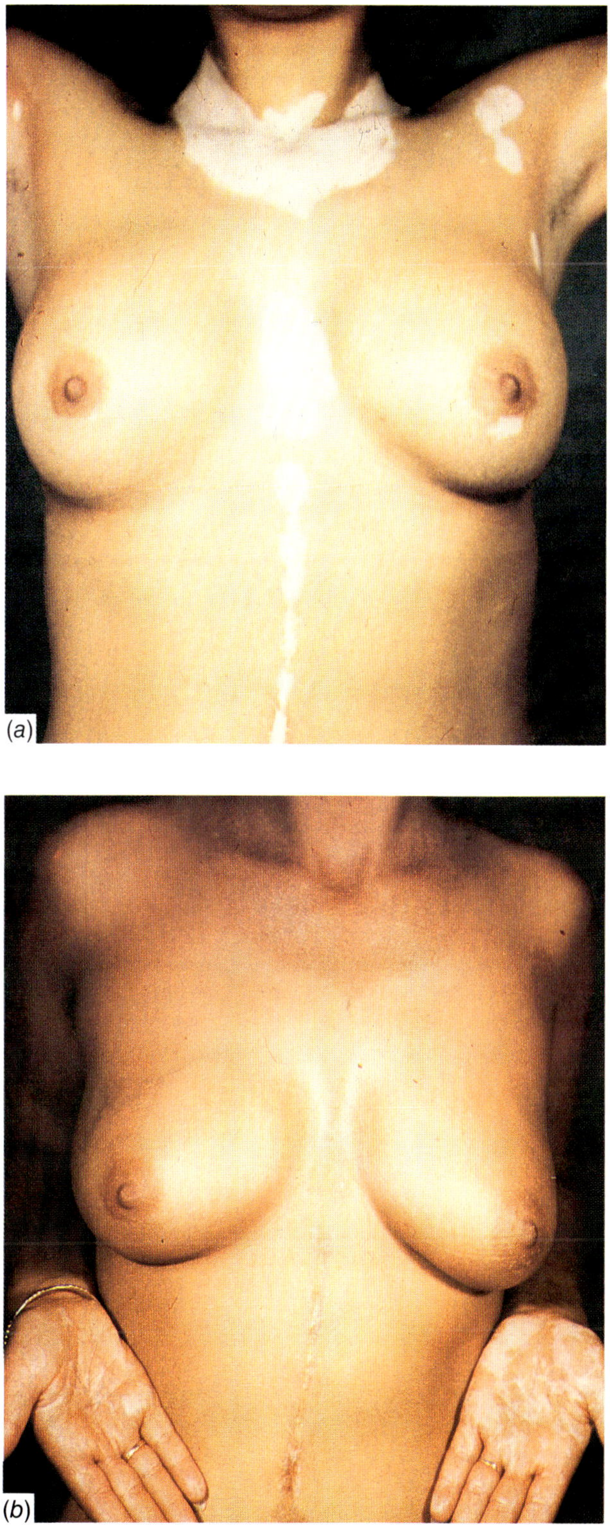

FIGURE 5
Psoralen photochemotherapy of vitiligo with an excellent result. (*a*) Before treatment; (*b*) after treatment.

TABLE 1
GUIDELINES FOR ORAL PUVA

Patient selection
- Only highly motivated patients
- Contraindications (absolute and relative)
  - History of cutaneous malignant tumors
  - History of exposure to carcinogenic agents (arsenic, Grenz-ray or x-ray therapy)
  - History of photosensitivity or photomediated disorders
  - Cataracts and aphakia
  - Severe cardiovascular, hepatic, or renal disease
  - Pregnancy, lactation
  - Age under 12
- Clinical parameters with prognostic significance for response to PUVA
  - Poor response
    - Segmental vitiligo with a dermatomal or zoosteriform distribution of macules
    - Acral and mucosal involvement
    - Presence of leukotrichia
  - Good response
    - Face, neck, trunk, proximal arms and legs
    - Presence of multiple perifollicular macules

Variables of treatment
- Drug
  - TMP less erythematogenic than 8-MOP (methoxsalen) for outdoor treatment and/or patients with skin types I through III
  - 8-MOP in a controlled therapeutic environment or in patients with skin types IV to VI
  - Relative responsiveness individually variable
- Dose
  - 8-MOP 0.3 to 0.6 mg/kg
  - TMP 0.6 to 1.2 mg/kg
  - Ingestion 2 h before anticipated exposure; avoid unnecessary exposure to sunlight throughout remainder of day and wear blocking sunglasses with an appropriate ultraviolet (UV) absorbing power
- UV radiation source
  - Sunlight preferably between 11:00 a.m. and 2:00 p.m. or high-intensity UVA sources
- Dosimetry of UV radiation
  - Sunlight: 5 to 10 min of summer sun with gradual increase until a maximum of 30 to 45 min is reached
  - Artificial UVA: 60 to 70 percent of the minimum phototoxic dose or starting dose in correlation with the skin phototype (type I: 0.5 J/cm^2; type II: 1 J/cm^2; type III: 1.5 J/cm^2; type IV: 2 J/cm^2; type V: 2.5 J/cm^2; type VI: 6 J/cm^2); maximum treatment exposure 8 to 12 J/cm^2 reached by successive increments of 0.5 to 1 J/cm^2
- Frequency of treatment
  - Daily treatment not necessary; two to three times a week; ideal frequency: one irradiation every third day; phototoxic reactions may cause more depigmentation (Koebner's phenomenon); persistent erythema not required for repigmentation
- Duration
  - Twelve months or more, as continuously as possible, for best results
- Permanence
  - Fully repigmented macules stay filled in; subtotal repigmentation may be reversed if treatments are discontinued

Source: Ortonne et al.[12]

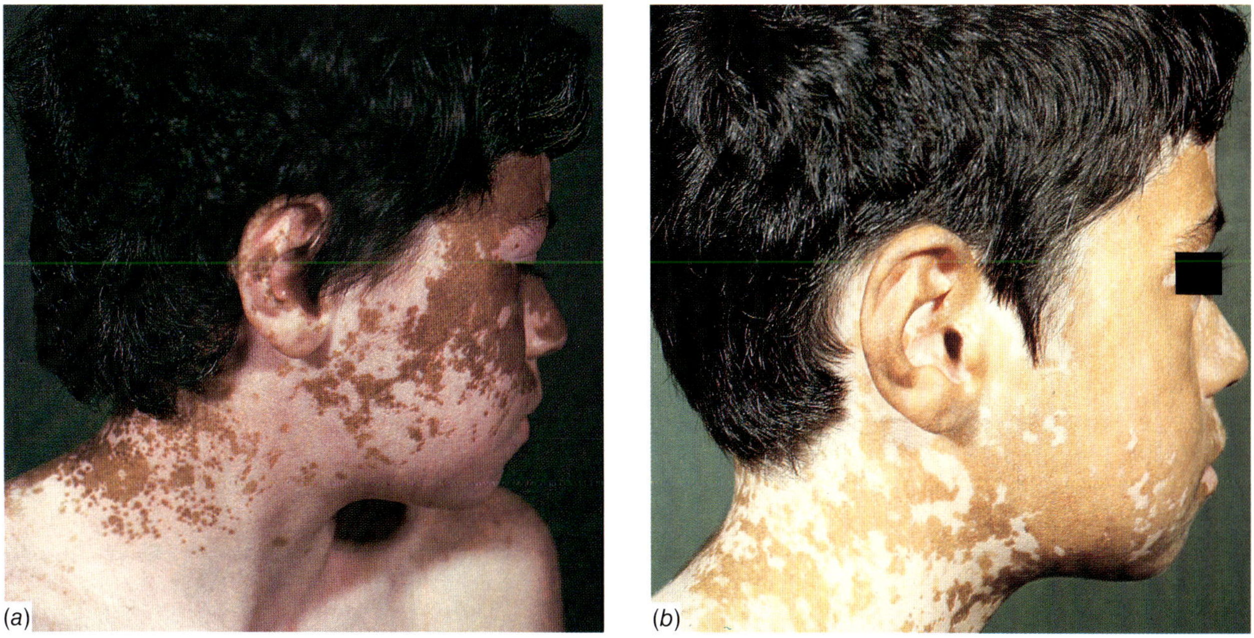

FIGURE 6
Psoralen photochemotherapy of vitiligo. Although this patient obtained good repigmentation, the result cannot be considered aesthetic. (*a*) Before treatment; (*b*) after treatment.

TABLE 2
GUIDELINES FOR TOPICAL PUVA

Patient selection
- Localized involvement
- Patients highly cooperative and compliant due to extreme photosensitivity of topical psoralens

Variables of treatment
- Drug
  - 8-MOP (methoxsalen) 0.1% dilution of commercially available lotion with a 1:1 mixture of ethanol and propylene glycol
- Dose
  - A careful application delivers about 0.25 ml to a macule of about 50 cm^2; casual application exposes patient to risk of phototoxic reactions and hypermelanosis; application should be restricted to lesional skin only 30 to 45 min prior to exposure; washing of treated areas with soap and water after exposure and application of a broad-spectrum sunscreen
- UV radiation source: artificial UVA or sunlight
- Dosimetry
  - Initial exposure minimal (0.25 J/cm^2 of UVA or 30 to 60 s of sunlight between 11:00 a.m. and 2:00 p.m.); increments of 0.25 J/cm^2 UVA or 30 s of sunlight with each exposure; maximum dose: 2 to 3 J/cm^2 UVA or 10 min sunlight
- Frequency of treatments
  - No more than every other day; ideal frequency: one irradiation every third day
  - High risk of severe phototoxic reaction
- Duration: repigmentation usually apparent after 10 to 20 treatments

Source: Mosher et al.[21] with permission.

showed 90 to 100 percent and 50 to 60 percent repigmentation, respectively, of the vitiliginous areas treated. This was achieved after a 4-month treatment period, with the patients receiving an oral daily dose of 100 mg of khellin in tablet form.[24] The repigmentation was stable for a period of 1 year after the discontinuation of treatment. Interestingly, no adverse side effects, including phototoxic erythema, were observed. Another study reported that khellin photochemotherapy is as effective as psoralen photochemotherapy.[26]

Short-term side effects include nausea, hypotension, and loss of appetite in about 30 percent of patients. The side effects usually do not lead to discontinuation of treatment. A more serious effect may be an asymptomatic elevation of transaminases, which appears in one-third of patients during the first 2 or 4 weeks of treatment. No long-term side effects have been observed after 1 or 2 years of therapy.

Further evaluation of khellin photochemotherapy in the treatment of vitiligo is required, but this treatment may represent a valuable alternative to the use of psoralens provided that the drug-induced hepatotoxicity is proved to be harmless.

Phenylalanine

Phenylalanine, orally administered (50 mg/kg body weight) in combination with UVA, has induced repigmentation in about one-fourth of vitiligo patients undergoing treatment.[27,28] Additional controlled trials are needed to confirm these findings. Interestingly, phenylalanine increases the phototolerance of vitiliginous skin and the tanning ability of uninvolved skin.

Hair Dyes

Colorants may be used for coloring diffuse gray hair or a white or gray lock. Because of the penetration of the dye into both gray and pigmented hair, making the pigmented hair darker, it is advisable to choose a shade that is somewhat lighter than the natural hair color.[29]

CAMOUFLAGING

Cosmetic products may also be used to camouflage cosmetic deficits due to hypermelanosis or hypomelanosis.[30] This may be helpful with lesions in exposed areas such as the face and the dorsal hands. Lotions containing dihydroxyacetone and certain aniline dyes (Vitadye, Dy-O-derm) produce good camouflage of hypomelanotic areas, but they gradually wash out and must be reapplied every few days.

Opaque cosmetics such as Dermablend, Covermark, and Continuous Coverage are available in various shades, allowing a perfect match to normal skin color in most patients. These agents combine a broad-spectrum sunscreen with a water-resistant opaque base. They are helpful in hyperpigmented disorders in which sunlight plays an aggravating and perpetuating role and in hypomelanoses. With practice, some patients can completely hide their vitiligo.

Oral β-carotene and canthaxanthin (Phenoro, β-carotene 10 mg and canthaxanthin 15 mg per capsule) have also been used to treat the cosmetic aspect of vitiligo. In one study,[31] 56 patients with vitiligo received an initial dose varying from 90 to 120 ml/day, according to body weight, over the course of 10 days. The maintenance dose was 30 to 60 ml/day for several weeks. Canthaxanthin was rated very satisfactory by 10 percent of the patients using it, satisfactory by 35 percent, and unsatisfactory by 54 percent. The treatment was more effective for light-skinned patients. By darkening vitiliginous skin, they decrease the contrast between involved and normally pigmented skin. Good cosmetic results are obtained mostly in vitiligo patients with skin types I and II. Unfortunately, xanthoderma is apparent on normally pigmented skin. An improved resistance to exposure to sunlight with canthaxanthin has also been reported in patients with vitiligo.[31] The eyes of patients taking canthaxanthin should be monitored regularly because retinopathy due to the drug has been reported.

REFERENCES

1. Quevedo WC Jr, Fitzpatrick TB, Szabo G, et al: Biology of the melanin pigmentary system, in *Dermatology in General Medicine,* 3d ed, Fitzpatrick TB, Eisen AZ, Wolff K, et al. (eds.) New York, McGraw-Hill, 1987:224–258.
2. Mosher DB, Fitzpatrick TB, Ortonne JP, et al. Disorders of melanocytes, in *Dermatology in General Medicine,* 3d ed, Fitzpatrick TB, Eisen AZ, Wolff K, et al. (eds.) New York, McGraw-Hill, 1987:818–821.

3. Porter J, Beuf AH, Nordlund JJ, et al. Psychological reaction to chronic skin disorders: A study of patients with vitiligo. *Gen Hosp Psychiatry,* 1979; 15:73–77.
4. Toda K, Ota M. Female facial melanosis, in *Biology and Diseases of Dermal Pigmentation,* Fitzpatrick TB, Kukita A, Morikawa F, et al. (eds.) Tokyo, University of Tokyo Press, 1981:225–229.
5. Gellin GA, Maibach HI: Chemically induced depigmentation, in *Models in Dermatology,* Maibach HI, Lowe N (eds.) Basel: Karger, 1985; 2:282–286.
6. Scarpa A, Guerci A: Depigmenting procedures and drugs employed by melanoderm populations. *J Ethnopharmacol,* 1987; 19:17–66.
7. Fitzpatrick TB, Arndt KA, El Mofty AM, et al: Hydroquinone and psoralens in the therapy of hypermelanosis and vitiligo. *Arch Dermatol,* 1966; 93:589–599.
8. Boyle J, Kennedy CT. Hydroquinone concentrations in skin lightening creams. *B J Dermatol,* 1986; 114:501–504.
9. Tidman MJ, Horton JJ, MacDonald DM: Hydroquinone-induced ochronosis—light and electron-microscopic features. *Clin Exp Dermatol,* 1986; 11:224–228.
10. Kligman AM, Willis I: A new formula for depigmenting human skin. *Arch Dermatol,* 1975; 111:40–48.
11. Rouault A, Thomas P: Les troubles de la pigmentation, in *Manuel Pratique de Médecine Esthétique*, Bartoletti CA, Legrand JJ (eds.) Paris, J. Med. Esthet. 1987, XIV:19–33.
12. Ortonne JP, Mosher DB, Fitzpatrick TB: *Vitiligo and Other Hypomelanosis of Hair and Skin.* Monograph in Topics in Dermatology. Parrish JA, Fitzpatrick TB (ser. eds.) New York, Plenum, 1983.
13. Mosher DB, Parrish JA, Fitzpatrick TB: Monobenzylether of hydroquinone: A retrospective study of treatment of 18 vitiligo patients and a review of the literature. *Br J Dermatol,* 1977; 97:669–679.
14. Boyle J, Kennedy CTC: Leucoderma induced by monomethyl ether of hydroquinone. *Clin Exp Dermatol,* 1985; 10:154–158.
15. Nazzaro-Porro M: Azelaic acid, in *Dermatology in Five Continents.* Proceedings of the XVII World Congress of Dermatology, Berlin, 1987:194–202.
16. Zviak C: Hair bleaching, in *The Science of Hair Care,* Zviak C. (ed.) New York, Marcel Dekker, 1986:213–233.
17. Nordlund JJ. Postinflammatory hyperpigmentation. *Dermatol Clin,* 1988; 6:185–192.
18. Falabella R: Grafting and transplantation of melanocytes for repigmenting vitiligo and other types of leukoderma. *Int J Dermatol,* 1989; 28:363–369.
19. Pathak MA, Kramer DM, Fitzpatrick TB: Photobiology and photochemistry of furocoumarins (Psoralens®) in *Sunlight and Man: Normal and Abnormal Photobiologic Responses.* Fitzpatrick TB, Pathak MA, Harber LC, et al. (eds.) Tokyo, University of Tokyo Press, 1974:335–368.
20. Fitzpatrick TB, Parrish JA, Pathak MA: Phototherapy of vitiligo (idiopathic leucoderma), in *Sunlight and Man: Normal and Abnormal Photobiologic Responses,* Fitzpatrick TB, Pathak MA, Harizer LC, et al. (eds.) Tokyo, University of Tokyo Press, 1974:783–791.
21. Mosher DB, Pathak MA, Fitzpatrick TB. Vitiligo: Etiology, pathogenesis, diagnosis and treatment, in *Update: Dermatology in General Medicine,* Fitzpatrick TB, Eisen AZ, Wolff K, et al. (eds.) New York, McGraw-Hill, 1983:205–225.
22. Pathak MA, Mosher D, Fitzpatrick TB: Safety and therapeutic effectiveness of 8-methoxypsoralen, 4,5′,8-trimethylpsoralen and psoralen in vitiligo. *Natl Cancer Inst Monogr,* 1984; 66:165–173.
23. Ortonne JP, Sannwald C, Thivolet J: La photochimiothérapie orale du vitiligo. *Ann Dermatol Venereol,* 1978; 105:617–624.
24. Abdel-Fattah A, Aboul-Enein MN, Wassel GM, et al: An approach to the treatment of vitiligo by Khellin. *Dermatologica,* 1982; 165:136–140.
25. Honigsmann H, Ortel B: Khellin photochemotherapy of vitiligo. *Photodermatol,* 1985; 2:193–194.
26. Ortel B, Tanew A, Honigsmann H: Treatment of vitiligo with Khellin and UVA. *J Am Acad Dermatol* 1988; 18:693–701.
27. Cormane RH, Siddiqui AH, Westerhof W, et al: Phenylalanine and U.V.A. light for the treatment of vitiligo. *Arch Dermatol Res* 1985; 277:126–130.
28. Cormane RH, Siddiqui AH. L-Phenylalanine and UVA/sunlight for vitiligo. *Arch Dermatol Res* 1985; 277:509.
29. Corbett JF: Hair coloring. *Clin Dermatol* 1988; 6(3):93–101.
30. Benmaman O, Sanchez JL. Treatment and camouflaging of pigmentary disorders. *Clin Dermatol* 1988; 6(3):50–61.
31. Gupta AK, Haberman JHF, Pawlowski D, et al: Canthaxanthin. *Int J Dermatol* 1985; 24:528–592.

CHAPTER

11

Scars: Traumatic and Factitial

GIOVANNI MICALI
UMBERTO M. REALI

The scar represents the final event in the biological phenomenon of *wound healing*. The aim of this process is the recovery of skin integrity; from this view point, it is a favorable event which leads to the healing of wounds of different natures, whether surgical or accidental. The scar may be either an aesthetic or a functional problem, depending on the site and seriousness of the trauma, the constitution of the patient, and the abnormal evolution of the tissue repair process.

DEFINITION OF THE PROBLEM

A complex homeostatic process leads to the healing of tissue wounds. It is characterized by the replacement of destroyed or lost tissue with new tissue through a series of cellular and tissue events involving the connective tissue, vessels, and epidermis. These events can be summarized in three fundamental phases.

Exudative or Inflammatory Phase

Inflammation represents the typical tissue reaction to any trauma; it develops within 24 h of the traumatic event.[1] In the area surrounding the wound, vasoconstriction of the terminal arteriola and an increase of vasopermeability and vasodilatation due to the release of chemical mediators sequentially occur. Exocytosis of neutrophils and then of lymphocytes and monocytes occurs. In normal conditions, a fibrin coagulum develops, forming a framework that wraps red blood cells, white blood cells, platelets, and plasma proteins, thus creating a mechanical basis for tissue repair.

In this process, which is fundamental in wound healing, a complex series of interdependent biochemical steps favors chemotaxis, cellular migration, phagocytosis, and reepithelialization.[2–7]

Proliferative Phase

Between 4 and 20 days after the trauma, keratinocytes and fibroblasts proliferate, with consequent collagen synthesis and neoangiogenesis. This phase is characterized by the formation of granulation tissue made of blood cells, fibroblasts, collagen, newly formed vessels, and ground substance. The neutrophils release hydrolytic enzymes; monocytes and macrophages release a factor (macrophage-derived fibroblast stimulating activator, or MFSA) that stimulates fibroblast proliferation and collagen is synthesized,[8,9] thus establishing a feedback mechanism which modulates wound healing.

Capillary vessels close to the wound area produce solid cords, penetrating the damaged area and forming highly anastomosed capillary lumina. Endothelial cell proliferation is active by day 2, while neoangiogenesis is completely evident at day 7.[3,10,11]

Fibroblasts differentiated from local precursors or from monocytes[8,9] are found in the heart of the lesion at day 4 or day 5. Macrophagic and lymphocytic factors as well as elevated PO_2 favor fibroblastic proliferation and collagen synthesis.

Collagen synthesis starts with the production of protocollagen; prolin hydroxylization and hydroxylysine glycosylation are fundamental stages in collagen synthesis. Protocollagen-derived microfibrils form immature collagen (type III); they are thin, are not oriented in bundles, have a gel-like consistency, have only a slight resistance to traction, and are acid-soluble.[5] Mature collagen (type I) has an improved resistance to traction as a result of inter- and intrafibrillar "cross links."

Remodeling Phase

During the synthesis and afterward, for a period of 2 to 12 months, the collagen is continuously modified in a remodeling process.

The contraction of the collagen bundles causes a volume reduction up to 80 percent of the initial volume. This process varies according to the type, shape, site, and dimension of the lesion; the process, which begins at day 5, goes on at a rate of 0.1 to 0.6 mm per day.[12] The cell population responsible for this process is assumed to be myofibroblasts, specifically differentiated fibroblasts with contractile microfilaments. These cells, which are numerous in the beginning of the contraction process, afterward diminish progressively.[13]

CLINICAL MANIFESTATIONS

The clinical features of scars depend on several factors, including age, sex, individual characteristics of the healing process, possible complications (hematomas, infection, necrosis), anatomic site and kind of trauma, and amount of tissue loss. A systematic description of the various clinical manifestations of scars is beyond the scope of this chapter. From a general point of view, either quantitative (number, width, thickness) or qualitative (color, shrinkage, distortion of neighboring tissues, trophism, and possible neoplastic transformation) parameters should be taken into consideration.

Scars following acne or viral infections such as varicella or herpes zoster are characteristically multiple, small, and depressed (Fig. 1), whereas

FIGURE 1
Acne scarring of the cheek.

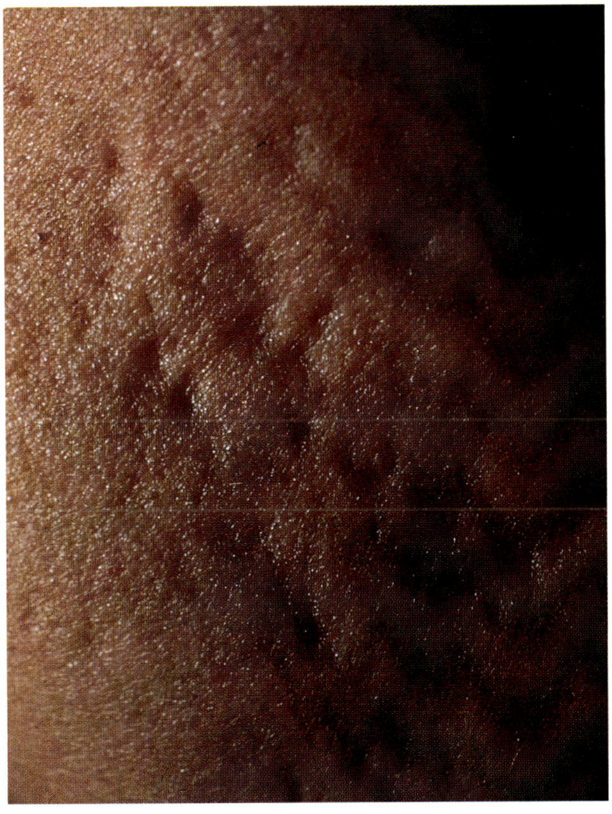

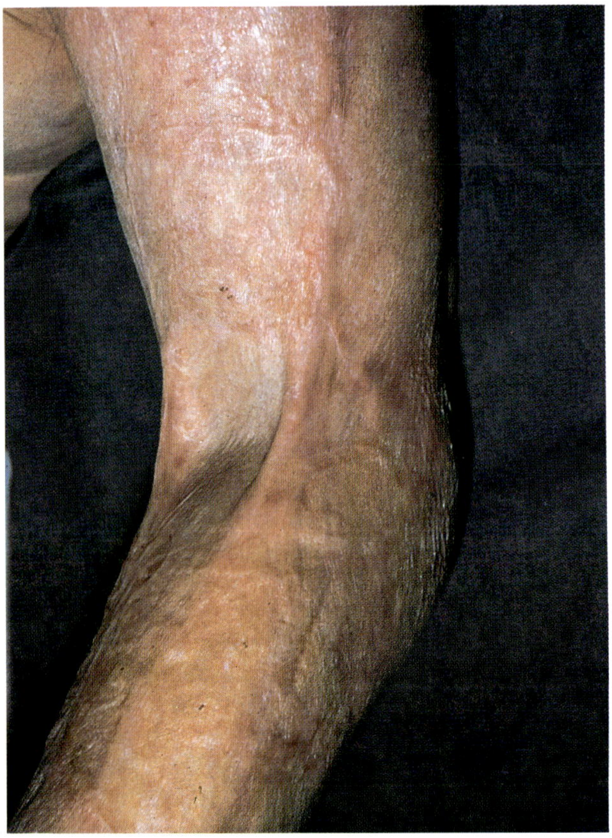

FIGURE 2
Burn scars and contracture of the elbow.

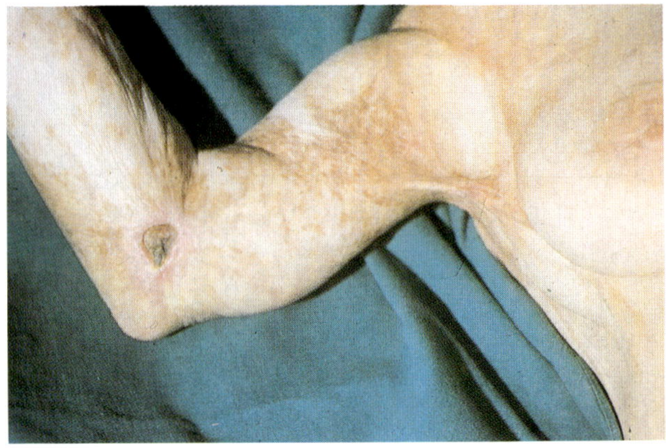

FIGURE 3
Chronic ulcer of the elbow and distortion of the breast with a broad burn scar.

FIGURE 4
Chronic ulcer due to mechanical (walking) tension.

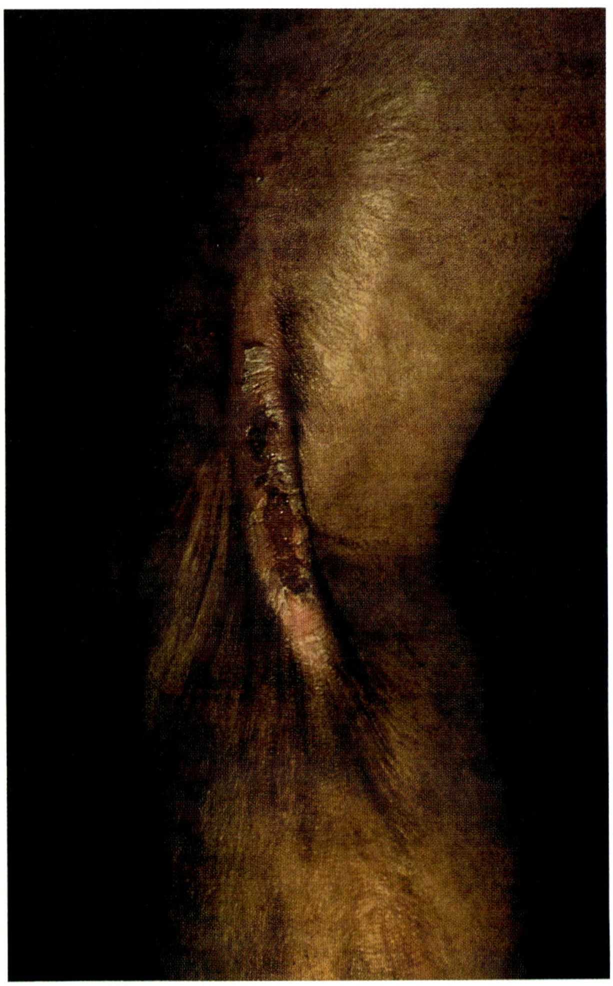

those due to deep burns (thermal, chemical, and electrical agents) appear as large plaques, are often hypertrophic or quite keloidlike, and usually are shrunken (Fig. 2). Multiple scars are observed frequently in self-inflicted lesions or following automobile injuries. When large tissue masses are lost, scars cause distortion of the surrounding areas (Fig. 3).

Although all the factors cited here may influence aesthetics and function, trophism is the most important factor in the evolution of scars. Wide and shrunken scars undergo mechanical tension that causes skin ulcerations followed by further cicatrization processes that may eventually result in a persistent ulcer (Fig. 4) over which a squamous cell carcinoma may arise. This is especially frequent with large scars caused by burns incurred during childhood (Fig. 5) or by osteomyelitis. For these reasons, such scars require surgical management.

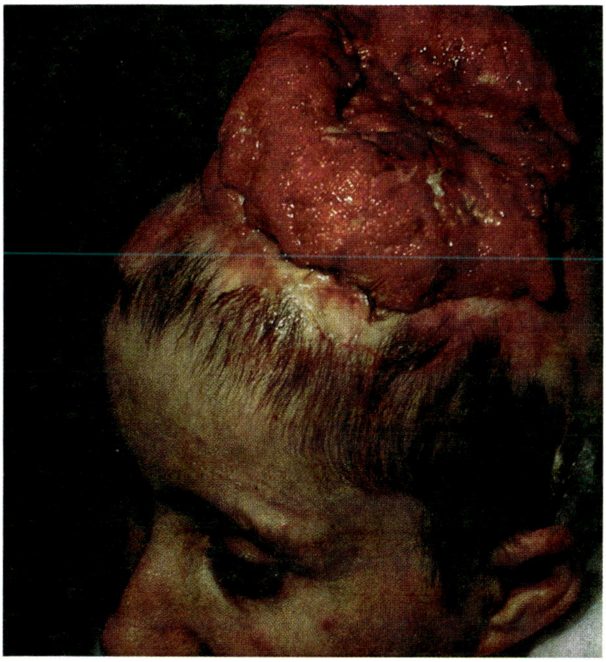

FIGURE 5
Squamous cell carcinoma in a burn scar. The 32-year-old patient suffered a scalp burn during childhood.

TECHNIQUES

From the viewpoint of functional and overall aesthetic recovery from damage consequent to a scar, one must consider whether the healing process is concluded. Indeed, during the healing process a spontaneous improvement of the scar usually occurs, in fact, while an early healed scar appears reddish and raised on the skin surface, after the remodeling process has been completed, it becomes pale and flat. Meanwhile, topical administration of moistening creams or triamcinolone can be useful. Surgical therapy is recommended when scars show certain negative characteristics.

Psychotherapy may help improve the patient's self-image; it is certainly helpful in removing the causes leading the patient to self-damage.[14]

The therapeutic approach to scars can be summarized as follows.

Medical Therapy

Medical therapy is advisable in the remodeling phase, especially for small scars. It is based on the topical application of drugs such as steroid-containing creams and the intralesional injection of enzymes (hyaluronidase) and corticosteroids (triamcinolone) to hinder the formation of excess collagen. Elastic pressure therapy is useful in preventing elevation and shrinkage of scars (Chap. 8).

Physiokinesiotherapy may be employed to reduce functional impairments due to old, wide scars. Intralesional injection of collagen or gelatin matrix implant is advisable in the treatment of small depressed scars (Chap. 26).

Surgical Therapy

Surgical therapy is generally performed once scars are fully mature. It may also be used in the early healing phases to prevent severe functional impairment which is thought to be likely. In these cases, repeated surgical interventions are usually needed.

A general rule in surgical therapy for scars suggests complete removal and careful reconstruction of all that was destroyed, with the transfer of adequate tissues. Several surgical techniques may be employed. They are described below in succession, from the easier to the more complex ones. The surgeon should perform the simplest technique that is capable of achieving the best results.

Dermabrasion Dermabrasion (Chap. 14) is advisable for reducing the evidence of scars, because it attenuates the differences between the scar and the surrounding normal skin.

Simple Excision Surgical excision is preferable in cases of moderately extended but not shrunken scars caused by rather small tissue loss, small depressed scars, tattooed scars (for instance, those due to asphalt tar particles in road accidents), and scars following improper suturing of wounds (suture marks, erroneous juxtaposition of margins). The cutting direction depends on the shape of the scar; when possible it should follow the relaxed skin tension lines (Fig. 6). After excision of all the scar tissue in both width and depth and hemostasis, the surgical wound, which should be as sharp as possible, is sutured. To obtain an accurate juxtaposition of the margins, subcutaneous tissues should be sutured separately with absorbable material, and the cutis with nonabsorbable material. Alternatively, one can join the lower portion of the dermis with interrupted catgut sutures and join the

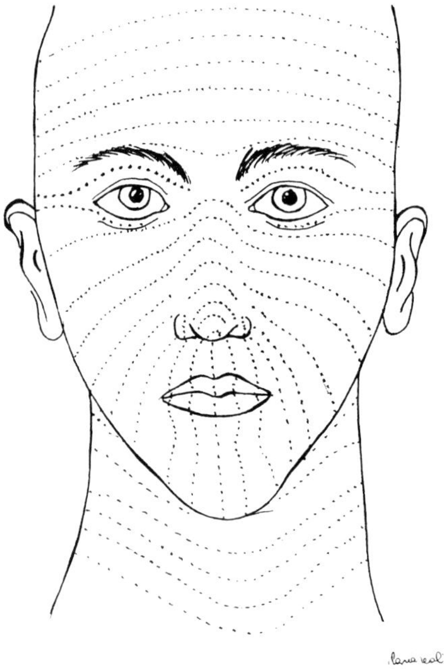

FIGURE 6
Relaxed skin tension lines.

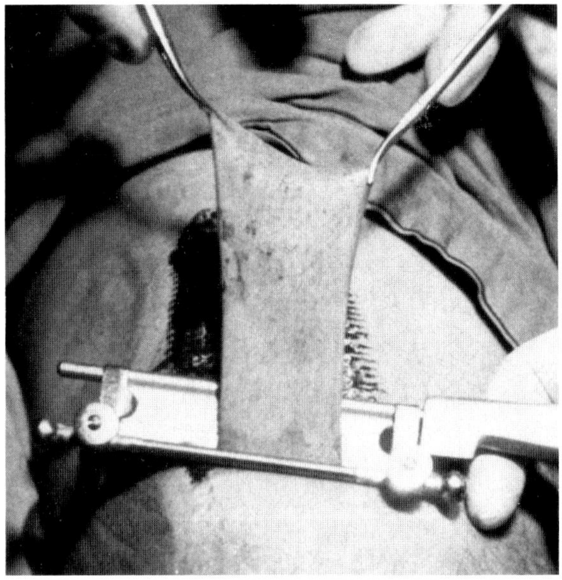

FIGURE 7
Cutting a split-thickness skin graft with a Humby knife.

superficial skin with sterile tapes. It is important to obtain a slight eversion of the margins of the wound and to remove the cutaneous sutures after a few days.

Skin Transplantation Skin transplantation is advisable in cases of massive tissue loss leading to wide scars and shrunken scars with distortion of neighboring regions. Skin grafts or flaps are employed. A systematic analysis of these techniques is beyond the scope of this chapter.[15–18]

Skin grafts consist of portions of skin, including the epidermis and the dermis, which are removed from a donor area of normal skin and transferred into the recipient area. They can be defined as split-thickness or full-thickness skin grafts according to the proportion of dermis they contain (Figs. 7 and 8), with the latter being preferred as more aes-

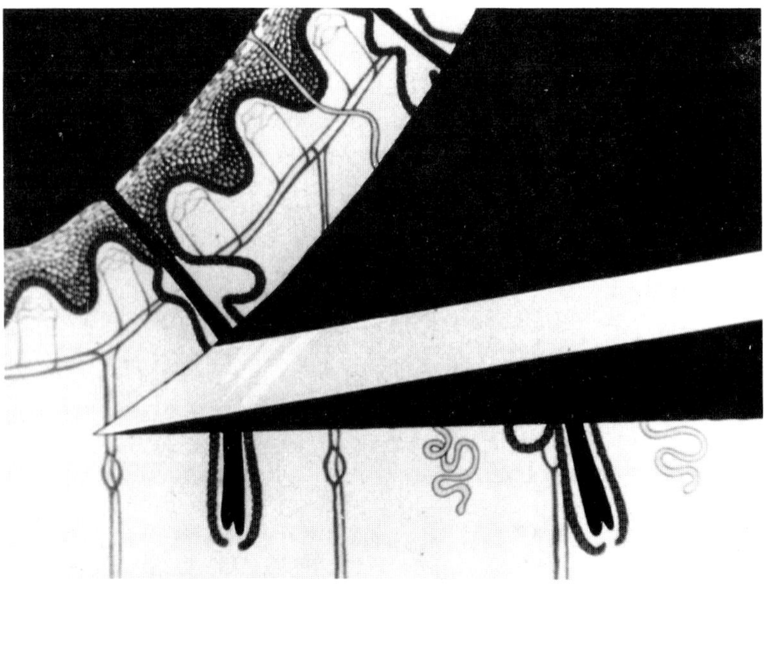

FIGURE 8
Cutting a split-thickness skin graft. The epidermis and the upper part of the dermis are removed from the donor area.

thetic although they are less easily adherent than the former. Skin grafts are recommended for wide and not very depressed scars and especially for reconstructing the skin surface of the eyelids (i.e., cicatricial ectropion) (Figs. 9 through 11). To obtain prompt and complete take of the graft, special care should be taken in establishing hemostasis, suturing, and compressing the graft. When working on the face, more aesthetic results can be achieved by using a graft that completely covers the entire anatomic region (*aesthetic units*) rather than only the scar area (Fig. 12).

Skin flaps are portions of skin that are transferred from the donor area to the recipient area, maintaining the original vascular connections either permanently (local flaps) or for a long enough period of time to allow the flap to adhere (distant flaps). Skin flaps are advisable for scars resulting from wide and deep tissue loss involving subcutaneous tissues. Local flaps are preferable since they

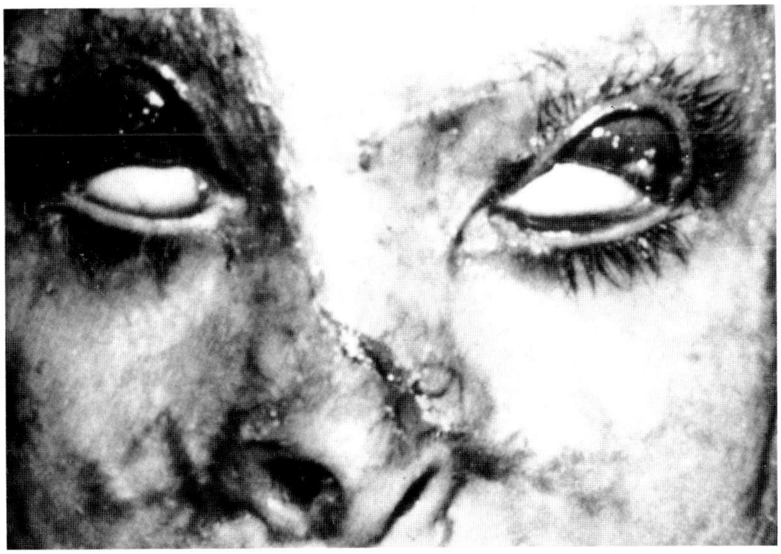

FIGURE 9
Burn scars causing ectropion of the upper eyelids.

FIGURE 10
A full-thickness skin graft is removed from the postauricular fold.

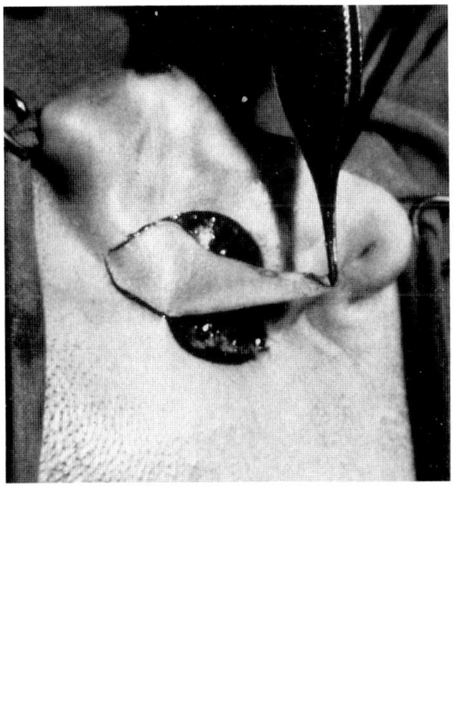

FIGURE 11
The patient seen in Fig. 9, 1-year postoperative view.

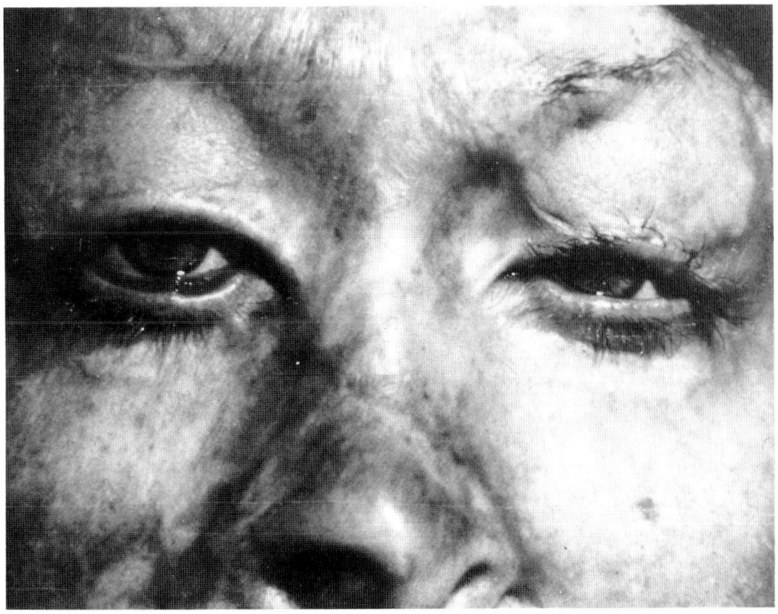

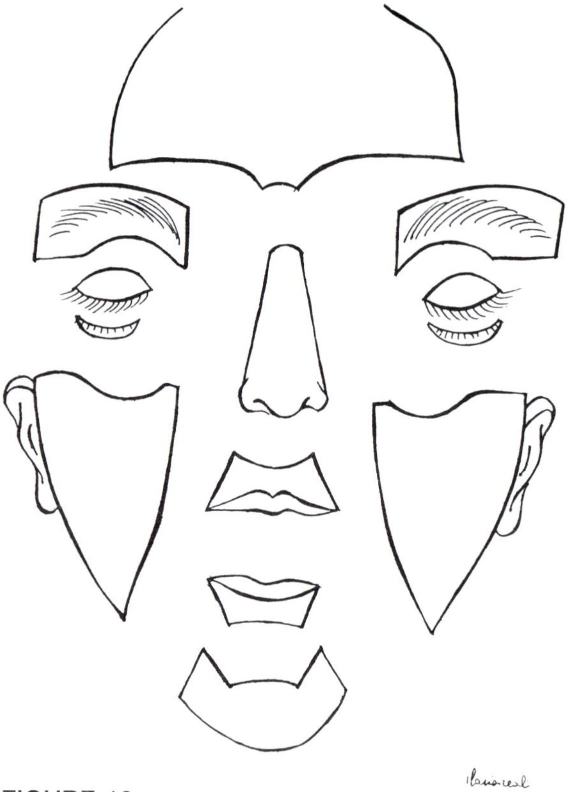

FIGURE 12
The aesthetic units of the face.

permit restoration of the defect definitively in a unique surgical step using tissues very like those which were lost (Figs. 13 and 14).

If possible, the surgeon should avoid making incisions across two contiguous aesthetic units or inside them in order to minimize the evidence of the surgical scars. The best results are achieved when the reconstruction is performed with a single skin flap for the entire aesthetic unit so that the surgical scars follow the contour of an aesthetic unit.

Many kinds of local flaps have been proposed for reconstruction of a large amount of lost tissue. Generally, one can distinguish advancement, rotation, and transposition flaps, depending on the movement of the major axes (Figs. 15 through 17). These flaps have specific indications which may be summarized as follows.

Advancement Flap This is a rectangular or square flap that moves forward to cover the defect without any lateral movement. These flaps are rarely used because the allowed movement is limited by re-

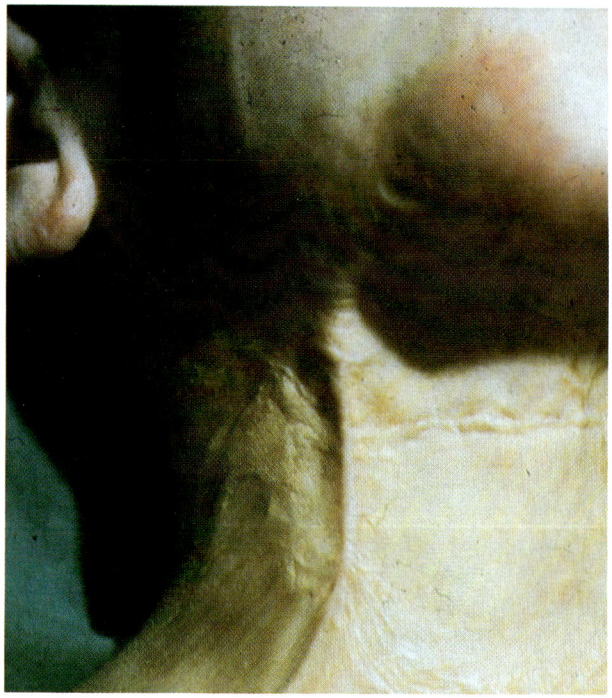

FIGURE 13
Burn scars and contracture of the neck.

FIGURE 14
Two-year postoperative view of the patient in Fig. 13. The cicatricial chorda was excised, and the skin flap, which is just visible in Fig. 13, was further advanced.

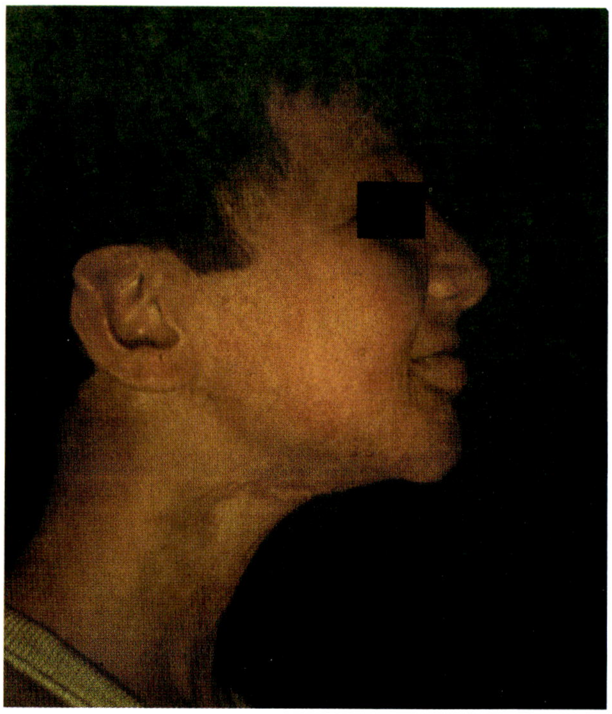

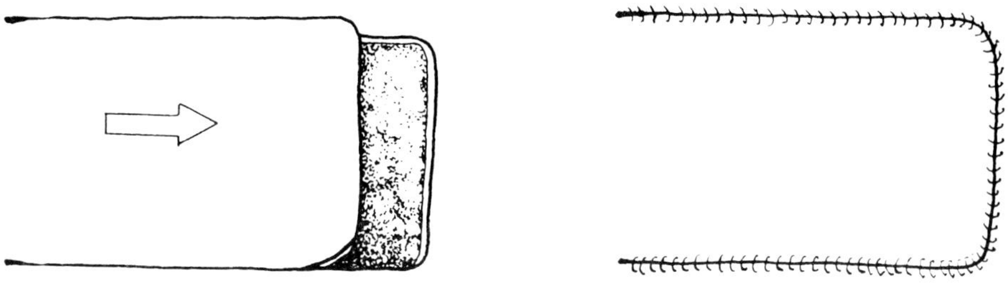

FIGURE 15
Advancement flap.

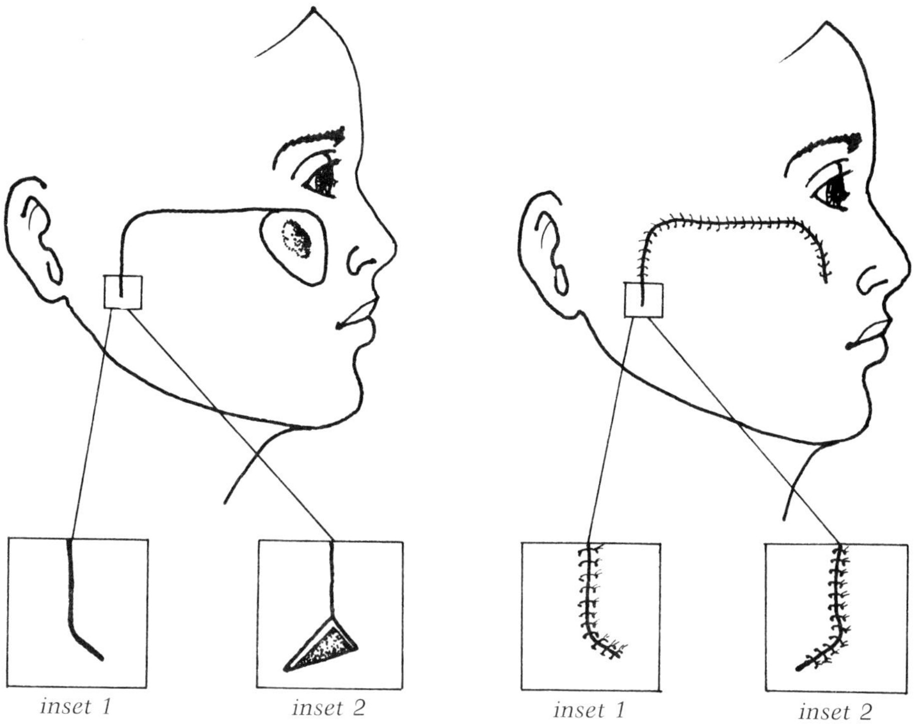

FIGURE 16
Rotation flap. *Insets:* 1. back cut; 2. Burow's triangle.

FIGURE 17
Transposition flap.

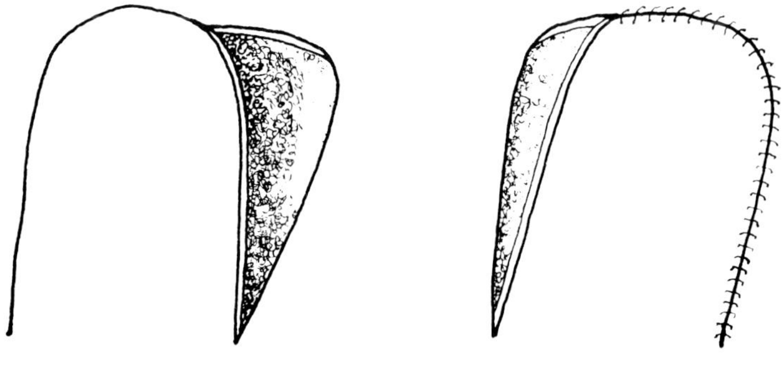

duced blood flow when the sutures are put in under tension. For this reason, only relatively small defects can be repaired; to minimize the hazard of necrosis, two opposite advancement flaps (Fig. 18) may be performed (H-plasty).

This technique is appropriate for round or square defects. Fusiform defects may be better repaired with another variant of this technique: the M-plasty. The procedure (Fig. 19) is performed as follows: Two opposite triangular flaps are raised at each corner of the wound and advanced toward each other; then the wound edges are undermined and approximated. The result is a minor length of scar without dog-ear deformities.

Minimal tissue displacement due to cicatricial contraction may be corrected with the V-Y advancement technique. After a V-shaped incision is made and the triangular flap is raised, the wound is sutured in a Y shape. In this manner, the tissue inside the V migrates toward the pedicle origin and tissue replacement is achieved (Fig. 20).

The Y-V advancement achieves the opposite effect. After undermining, the cutaneous area inside the oblique arms of the Y moves toward the apex of the final V.

Rotation Flap This is a semicircular flap that rotates about a pivot point toward the defect that is to be repaired; a back cut or the excision of an external triangular area (Burow's triangle) made at the pivot point may facilitate flap movement (Fig. 16, inset 2).

The rotation flap is best employed for reconstructing a defect that lies apart in an aesthetic unit, for example, in the cheek near the nasal region. In this case a flap raised from the uninvolved cheek rotates into the defect and at the same time resurfaces at the donor site so that other kinds of tissue are not needed. The incision, and therefore the future scar, lies around the aesthetic unit.

When the defect is close to an anatomic linear structure (lash line, alar cheek crease, etc.) that it is

FIGURE 18
H-plasty.

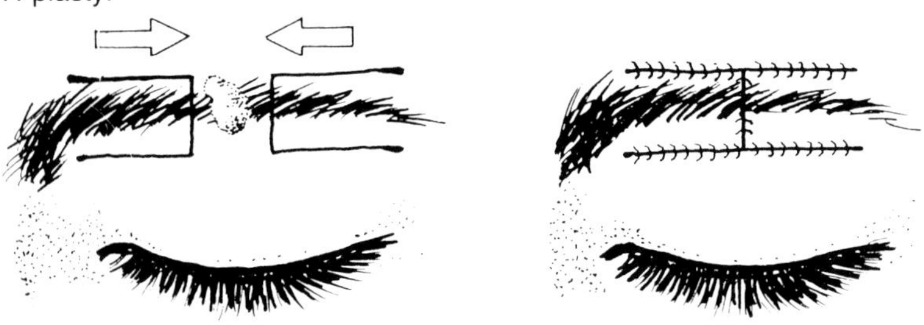

FIGURE 19
M-plasty.

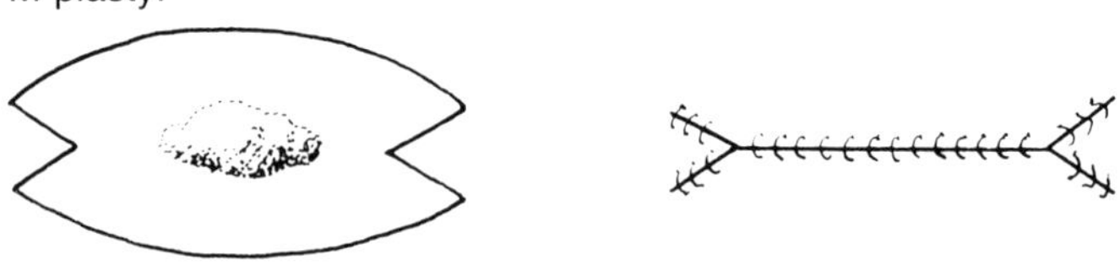

FIGURE 20
V-Y advancement flap.

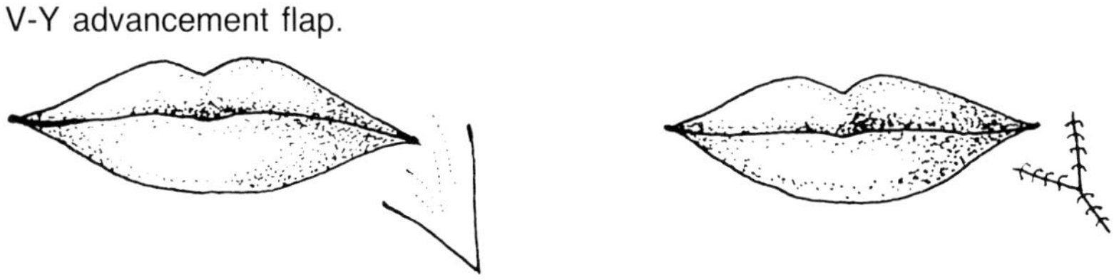

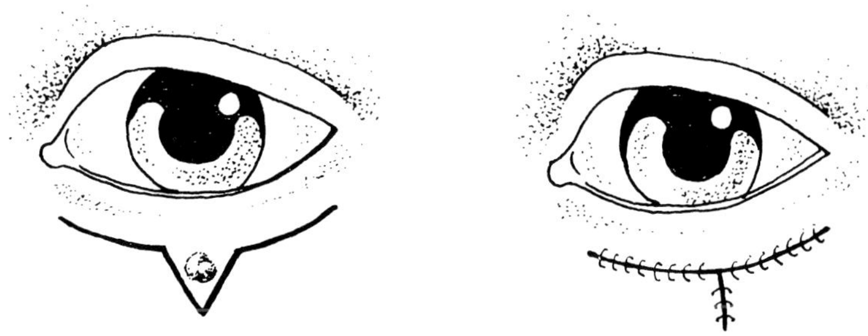

FIGURE 21
T-plasty.

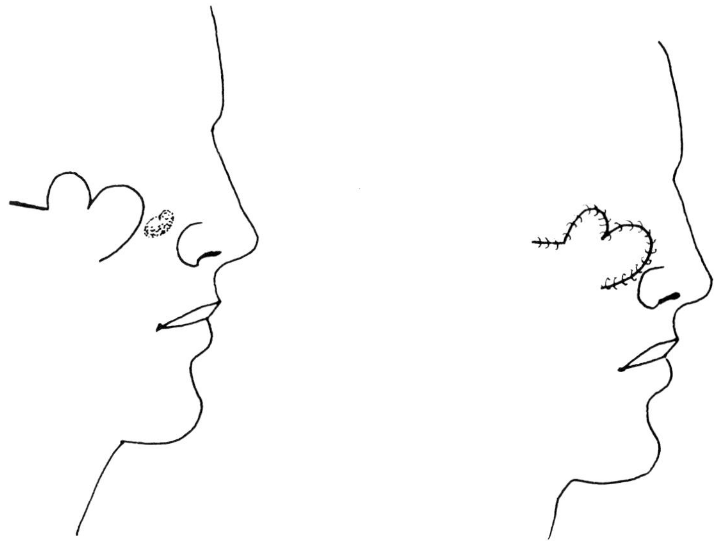

FIGURE 22
Bilobed flap.

preferable not to interrupt with a scar, two flaps raised in the opposite sides of the defect (Fig. 21) may be rotated toward it and sutured together (T-plasty).

Transposition Flap This technique is largely employed in reconstructive surgery. Many types of these flaps have been described.

The flap may be rectangular (Fig. 17), quadrangular, or triangular. Its major axis is turned laterally about a pivot point so that the flap will cover the defect. The donor area can be directly sutured, grafted, or repaired with a secondary flap (bilobed flap) (Fig. 22).

In the most typical use of this technique, two opposite triangular flaps are transposed into each other's donor areas so that they draw the letter Z (Z-plasty). Depending on the angle and width of the flaps, a progressive increase in length in a desired direction may theoretically be reached; however, 60-degree flaps are more commonly used.

Z-plasty joints with Y-V advancement flaps may be used. When wide flaps cannot be planned, multiple opposite flaps (Figs. 23 through 25) may be consecutively raised and then transposed (multiple Z-plasty). The Z-plasty is particularly useful in correcting cicatricial webs and contractures.

The method of geometric *broken-line* incisions, which is to modify the direction of a scar, gives a final cicatricial pattern resembling that of a Z-plasty (Fig. 26). It is in effect a direct suture method or, if the wound edges have been undermined, an advancement flap technique.

The use of the local flap technique may be precluded when an adequate amount of tissue is not available for transfer. If skin expanders (Chap. 29) cannot be employed to increase the donor area of local flap, the use of distant flaps is required. In this case, multiple surgical steps may be necessary and a less aesthetic result may occur.

More complex kinds of flaps, such as fasciocutaneous, myocutaneous, and free flaps, are seldom used in the surgical management of aesthetic dermatologic procedures.

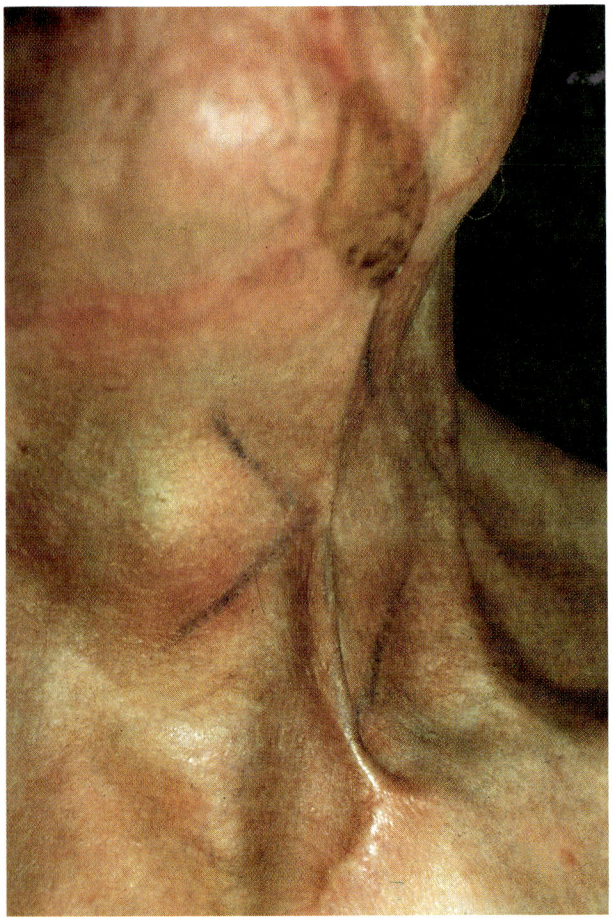

FIGURE 23
Burn scars causing a web on the left side of the neck. A multiple Z-plasty is planned.

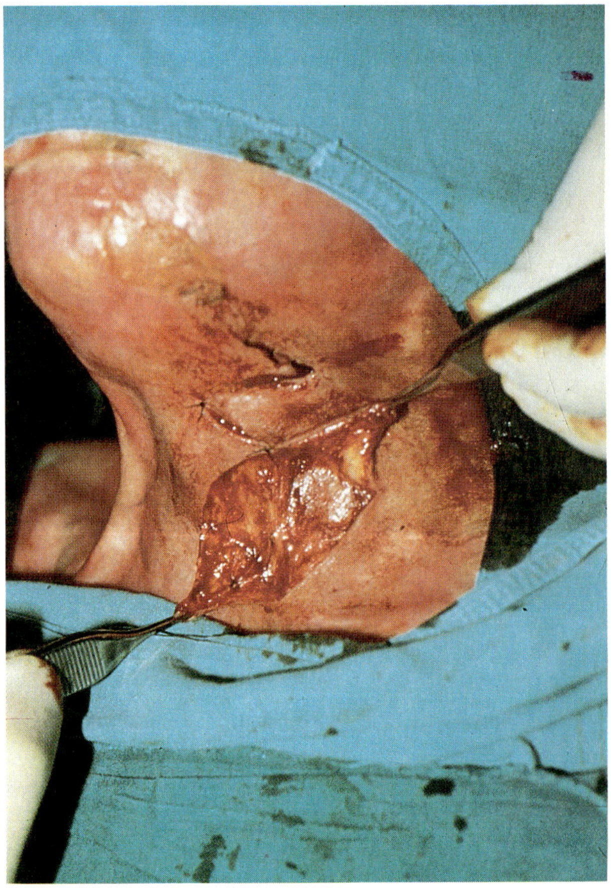

FIGURE 24
Intraoperative view of the patient in Fig. 23. Two flaps have just been transposed, while two are elevated before transposition.

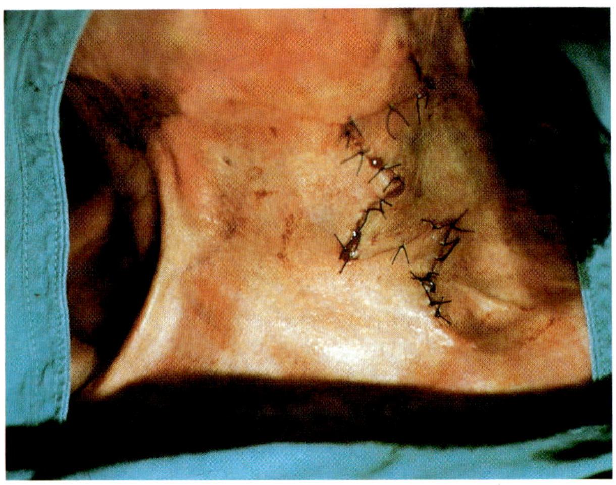

FIGURE 25
The patient in Figs. 23 and 24, postoperative view. The procedure has been completed. Note the complete recovery; an analogous cicatricial web is still uncorrected on the opposite side.

CONCLUSIONS

A scar can be considered an aesthetic deviation in wound healing, and several procedures can help minimize or possibly eliminate it. Intralesional steroids, pressure bandages, dermabrasion, excision, grafts, and flaps are just some of the possibilities for improving a situation of concern to a patient.

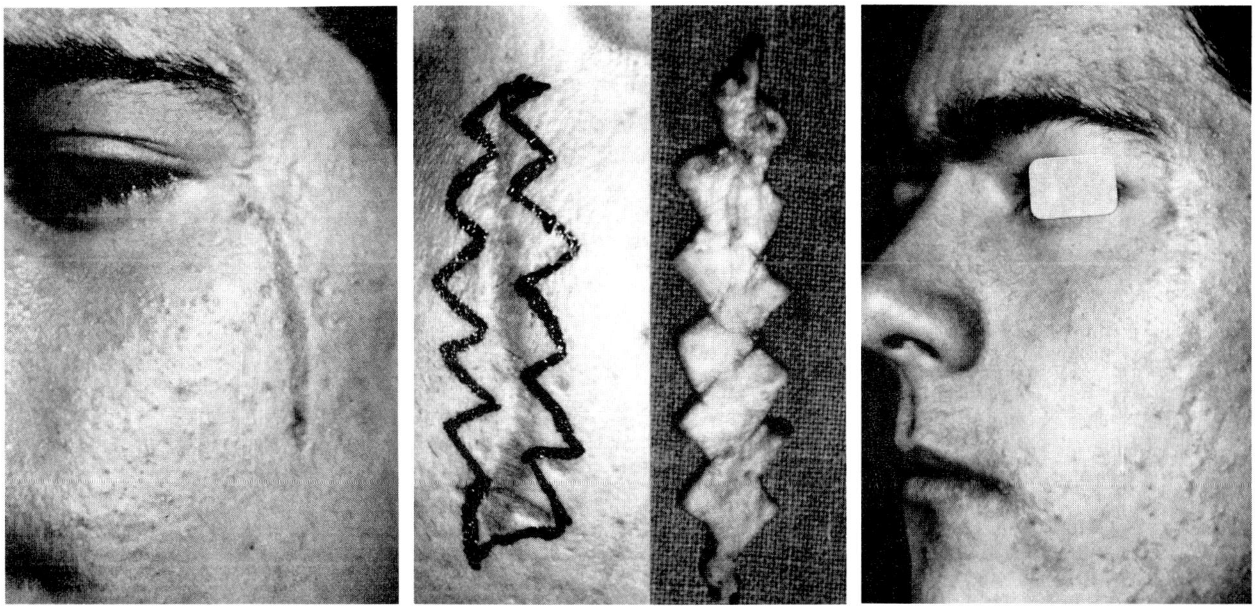

(a) (b) (c) (d)

FIGURE 26
Straight, enlarged scar due to a direct suture after the excision of a large congenital nevus. (*b*) "Broken-line" excision of the scar is planned. (*c*) The excised specimen. (*d*) Two-year postoperative view.

REFERENCES

1. Harris DR. Healing of the surgical wound: I. Basic considerations. J Am Acad Dermatol. 1979; 3:197–207.
2. Harris DR. Healing of the surgical wound: II. Factors influencing repair and regeneration. J Am Acad Dermatol. 1979; 3:208–215.
3. Wiegel PH, Fuller GM, LeBoeuf RD. A model for the role of the hyaluronic acid and fibrin in the early events during the inflammatory response and wound healing. J Theor Biol. 1986; 119:219–234.
4. Lisby G, Avnstorp C, Wantzin GL. Interleukin-1: A new mediator in dermatology. Int J Dermatol. 1987; 26:8–13.
5. Lacoure JP, Ortonne JP. La cicatrisation. Ann Dermatol Venereol. 1983; 110:159–173.
6. Grotendorst GR, Martin GR, Pewcev D, et al. Stimulation of granulation tissue formation by platelet-derived growth factor in normal and diabetic rats. J Clin Invest. 1985; 76:2323–2329.
7. Tengrup I, Ahonen J, Rank F, et al. Cytochemical study of granulation tissue in zinc treated rats. Acta Chir Scand. 1980; 146:243–246.
8. Stewart RJ, Duley JA, Rosman I, et al. The wound fibroblast and macrophage: I. Wound cell population changes observed in tissue culture. Br J Surg. 1981; 68:125–128.
9. Stewart RJ, Duley JA, Dewdney J, et al. The wound fibroblast and macrophage: II. Their origin studied in a human after bone marrow transplantation. Br J Surg. 1981; 68: 129–131.
10. Clark RAF, Della Pewe P, Dvorak KHF, et al. Fibronectin: A tissue matrix protein associated with fibroblast, epithelial cell and endothelial cell migration wound healing. J Invest Dermatol. 1981; 76:335–339.
11. West DC, Hampson IN, Arnold F, et al. Angiogenesis induced by degradation products of hyaluronic acid. Science. 1985; 228:1324–1329.
12. Beerens EGJ, Scott JW, Wander Leun JC. Rapid regeneration of dermal-epidermal junction after partial separation by vacuum: An electron microscopic study. J Invest Dermatol. 1975; 65:513–521.
13. Rudolph R. Location of the force of wound contraction. Surg Gynecol Obstet. 1979; 148:547–553.
14. Cossidente A, Sarti MG. Psychiatric syndromes with dermatologic expression. Clin Dermatol. 1984; 2:201–220.
15. Grabb WC, Myers MB. Skin Flaps. Boston: Little, Brown, 1975.
16. Grabb WC, Smith JW. Plastic Surgery, 3d ed. Boston: Little, Brown, 1979.
17. Cormack GC, Lamberty BGH. The Arterial Anatomy of Skin Flaps. London: Churchill Livingstone, 1986.
18. Thomas JR, Holt GR. Facial Scars: Incision, Revision and Camouflage. St. Louis: Mosby, 1989.

CHAPTER

12

Telangiectasia

LAWRENCE CHARLES PARISH
JOSEPH A. WITKOWSKI

Telangiectasia, or the condition of having *telangiectases,* is a permanent dilatation of preexisting blood vessels on the skin or mucous membranes. Telangiectases present as fine or coarse discrete red lines, erythematous macules, or patches. They may also appear as red puncta with lines radiating outward. These vascular dilatations may be divided into *primary* and *secondary* lesions (Table 1). The primary lesions may be idiopathic, as in familial essential telangiectasia or any number of genodermatoses. The secondary lesions may be due to physical trauma following radiation or sunburn, overuse of topical steroids, or an underlying systemic disease. Telangiectasia on the upper portions of the chest can even be a sign of AIDS.[1]

The telangiectases which appear on the legs appear to be hereditary. Many times the location will be nearly identical among family members; the extent of the condition can be the same in identical

TABLE 1
CLASSIFICATION OF TELANGIECTASIAS

Primary or idiopathic	
	Ataxia telangiectasia
	Familial essential telangiectasia
	Hereditary hemorrhagic telangiectasia
	Osler-Weber-Rendu disease
Secondary	
	Actinic damage
	AIDS
	Basal cell cancer
	Chemical burn
	Dermatomyositis
	Estrogen therapy
	Lupus erythematosus
	Pregnancy
	Radiation injury
	Scleroderma
	Steroid therapy
	Trauma
	Xeroderma pigmentosum

The interested physician may wish to join the North American Society of Phlebology, 3960 Park Boulevard, Suite E, San Diego, CA 92103 for up-to-date information on sclerotherapy.

twins.[2] While they occur in both men and women, there is a predominance in women, because estrogens seem to play a role in their development. The lesions usually appear after puberty, increase during pregnancy, and become noticeable with the use of estrogens or oral progestational agents with a high estrogen content.[3] Increased venous pressure can produce telangiectases and can be created by an enlarged pregnant uterus, tight garments, or excessive standing. Finally, telangiectases can follow trauma to the legs. Because of their morphology, they have been called spider veins, shooting stars, sunburst varicosities, and venous blemishes. They are most disfiguring in women approaching middle age[4] (Fig. 1, *a* and *b*).

The telangiectases found on the face often are located on the paranasal areas and the cheeks. Although these lesions measuring a few to several

FIGURE 1
(*a* and *b*) A 33-year-old woman noticed an increase in telangiectasia after taking oral progestational agents for 2 years.

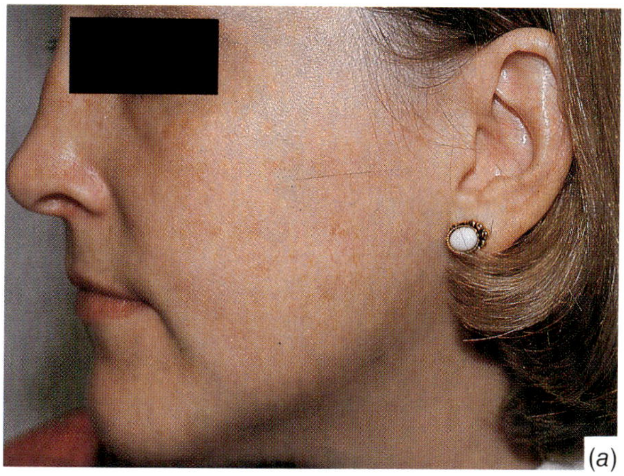

(*a*)

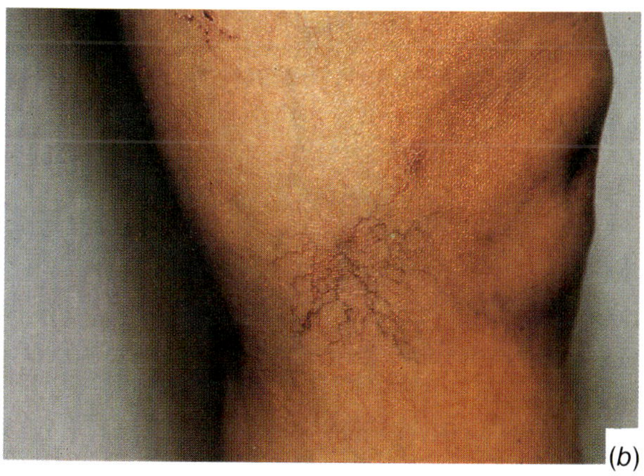

(*b*)

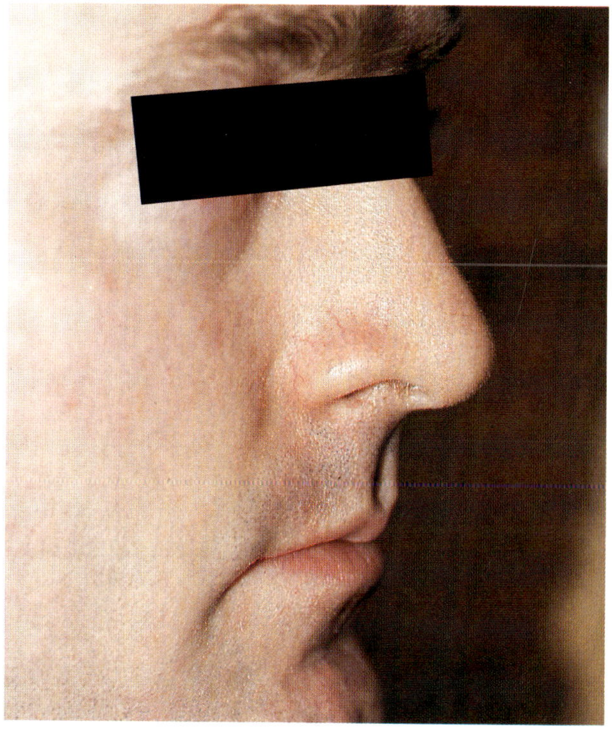

FIGURE 2
This 30-year-old man had many broken blood vessels appear on the paranasal area 2 weeks after a common cold.

millimeters can be due to hereditary factors, they more often result from actinic and aging processes or from the increased pressure of vigorous nose blowing (Fig. 2). Sometimes estrogens seem to play a role.

MANAGEMENT

At least four modalities of treatment exist: electrosurgery, sclerotherapy, dermabrasion, and laser surgery. Although high doses of vitamin C or even tetracycline were recommended in the past, no oral panacea exists.

With any form of treatment, the patient must be warned that scarring, most often minimal, can occur. Pain or discomfort should be minor but can be a problem with some patients. Generally, all telangiectases cannot be removed in one session. Frequently, when larger vascular spiders are eliminated, smaller ones tend to become more noticeable. In addition, new vascular spiders can develop for the same reasons that caused the recently destroyed ones to become visible in the first place.

With regard to lesions on the legs, patients with a history of thrombophlebitis, progressive thromboembolic disease, or pulmonary embolism are usually not good candidates for this treatment. Moreover, patients receiving anticoagulant therapy, patients with uncontrolled diabetes, and patients with severe renal disease should be discouraged from embarking on one of these procedures, as should pregnant or lactating women. Patients with large varicose veins should have the veins treated first.

Electrosurgery

This procedure involves the use of low-current electricity to desiccate the blood vessel. Electrosurgery is most often used on the face, but some workers use it to destroy vascular spiders on the legs. The advantages are the ease and quickness; the disadvantages are the electric type of pain created and the possibility of minor white atrophic scars being created. Rarely, keloids or hypertrophic scars have been produced.[5]

Any electrosurgical unit which has a high frequency and low amperage can be employed. With the Hyfercator, the procedure is monopolar. With the Bovie, it is possible to use bipolar reverse current by grounding the patient. An epilating or 30-gauge needle can be used with either unit.

The area is cleansed with alcohol, but treatment should not begin until the area is dry. Intradermal anesthesia cannot be used, as it can distort or obliterate the vessels.

The needle is inserted into the vessel, and a short burst of low power is given. If the procedure is successful, the vessel will blanch for many millimeters as the blood is pushed out. The collapsed vascular walls then stick together.[6]

During the next 24 h the treated area may appear urticarial. Some redness will be evident, and this may last for several days. Sometimes crusting can appear and remain for 1 to 3 weeks. Generally, within 1 to 3 months, the site shows no evidence of the procedure or of the broken blood vessel, but small atrophic scars can appear unpredictably and last indefinitely.

Sclerotherapy

This method involves the injection of sclerosing chemicals into the vascular spider. Sclerotherapy is most often used on the legs. Despite the variable pain on injection and the discomfort that occurs during the next several hours, there is infrequent scarring or hyperpigmentation. On the face, there is a possibility of telangiectatic mats occurring. The patient may be allergic to the selected sclerosing agent.[9]

Several agents can be used (Table 2), but hypertonic saline is selected most often in the United States.

When the patient is told about the procedure, warning is given that the sclerosing agent may burn when it is injected. The patient should also be informed that muscle cramps can occur in any part of the leg and generally disappear in 3 to 10 min. To prepare for the procedure, the patient is asked not to shave or use moisturizers on the day of sclerotherapy and to bring an elastic bandage to the office.

To prepare for sclerotherapy, assemble the mate-

TABLE 2
SCLEROSING AGENTS AND THEIR COMPOSITION

Hypertonic saline	23.4% saline
Sodium morrhuate*	Sodium salt of saturated and unsaturated fatty acids derived from cod liver oil
Sotradecol*	Sodium tetradecyl sulfate and benzyl alcohol
Polidocanol (Aetoxisclerol)	Polidocanol (Hydroxypoly-ethoxydodecane) (related to lidocaine)
Sclerodex	25% dextrose, 10% saline, with phenyl alcohol

* Approved by the U.S. Food and Drug Administration for sclerotherapy.
Source: Ramelet and Monti.[7]

TABLE 3
MATERIALS FOR SCLEROTHERAPY

Vial of sclerosing material
Disposable 3.0-ml Luer-lock syringe or 1.0-ml syringe
Needles: 30-gauge, 1/2-in, and 31- or 33-gauge, 1/4-in (after use, needle must be rinsed and wire inserted before sterilizing to prevent clogging)
70% isopropyl alcohol

rials suggested in Table 3. Two types of syringes are recommended, depending on whether air is to be used in the syringe. If the 3.0-ml Luer-lock variety is used, it is filled with 2.5 ml of sclerosant and 0.5 ml of air, using a large needle. If the 1.0-ml syringe is selected, it can be filled with the sclerosant. In either case, the small needle is placed on the syringe and bent at the hub 15 to 30 degrees.

The therapist should sit and rest the forearms on the table to minimize unsteady movement. Venules may be injected proximally to distally or distally to proximally because of the numerous anastomoses of these vascular complexes.

The patient is placed in a recumbent position, and the leg is positioned so that when the vessel is injected, the air precedes the sclerosant. The injection is made in an upward direction.

Liberal and frequent use of 70% isopropyl alcohol not only disinfects the skin but makes it much more translucent. This improves visualization of the vessels.

The thumb and index finger of the nondominant hand are used to exert tension on the skin, thus stabilizing the vessel. The bent needle is placed on the skin in the direction of the vessel about 1/8 to 1/4 in from the vessel to be treated. The needle is then pushed through the skin and into the vessel by slightly raising the syringe. For most telangiectasias, the tip of the needle can be seen through the skin and the vessel wall when properly positioned (Fig. 3).

Air injected before the sclerosant permits confirmation of the placement of the needle in the lumen. When the needle is correctly placed, the air displaces the blood. The vascular plexus or vein will blanch in a distinctive pattern. A diffuse urticarial blanch indicates that the needle is outside the lumen. The needle should then be withdrawn, and the air should be replaced in the syringe.

The air is used to ensure that the sclerosant will be injected within the vessel walls. This prevents additional pain and possible necrosis of adjacent tissue. Up to 250 ml of air can be injected intravenously before dire results occur.[8] When no air is

FIGURE 3
A small-gauge needle penetrating a vessel during sclerotherapy.

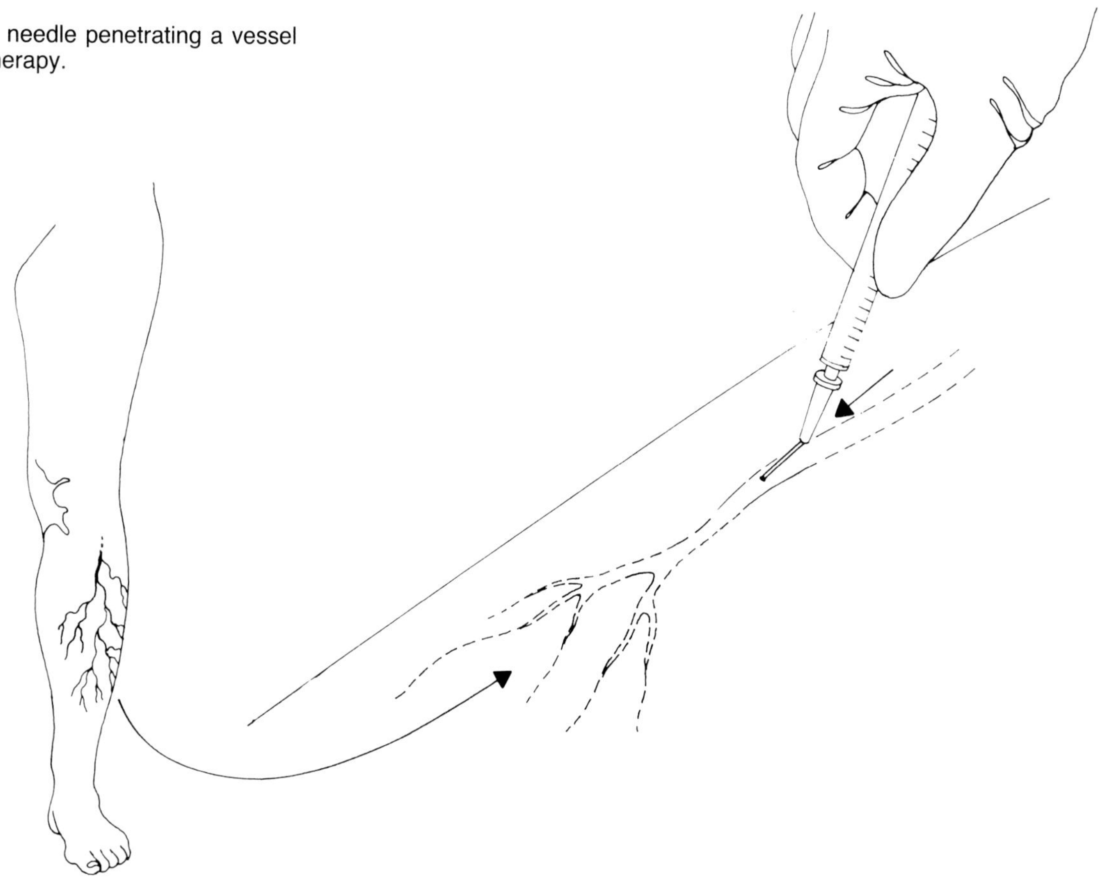

used, the operator may check that the needle is in the vein by moving the syringe. Slight injection of the material should disperse some blood.

Once the needle is in the desired position, 0.5 to 1.0 ml of sclerosant is injected until the vessel is fully injected. The needle is carefully withdrawn. Pressure is applied to the site to prevent extravasation of the sclerosant.

If the injection is successful, the vessel will fill with blood as the needle is being withdrawn. Within several seconds, the entire area will become red and the vein will become more prominent.

If the agent extravasates into surrounding tissue, lidocaine or sterile water, approximately 10 times the volume of the previously injected fluid, should be injected into the area. This reduces the pain and helps prevent a slough.

Some operators like to bandage the leg for 24 h after covering the sites with cotton balls and tape. The leg is then wrapped with the elastic bandage provided by the patient. Others prefer to apply Band-Aids when needed.

If vessels larger than 2 mm are treated, there is a possibility of thrombosis arising in 1 or 2 weeks. The affected vessel may appear blue and not blanch on pressure. The clot can then be expressed by making a small excision with a No. 11 blade.

Dermabrasion

When the physician is confronted with many telangiectases on the face due to such diseases as rosacea and familial essential telangiectasia, dermabrasion is a useful procedure. The postoperative discomfort may be a deterrent, but this should be balanced against the tedium of electrodessicating a large number of vessels.[10] Details of dermabrasion can be found in Chap. 14.

Laser Therapy

Argon Laser This is a very useful and effective modality for the treatment of facial telangiectasias. With parameters of 3.3 to 4.0 W, a 0.05-s pulse duration, and a 2-mm spot size, the entire vessel is traced. Minimal scarring and pigmentary changes can occur.

The argon laser is not recommended for use on the leg because the results are inconsistent. Moreover, noticeable scarring and both hyperpigmentation and hypopigmentation can occur.[11]

585 Pulsed Dye Laser This laser is recommended for use above the waist. Parameters are a 3- to 5-mm spot size with an energy density of 5.75 to 7.0 J/cm^2. The treatment can result in grayish spots lasting 5 to 14 days before an acceptable cosmetic appearance is achieved. Hyperpigmentation can appear and last for several weeks to months. This is seldom seen on the face when the power density is kept below 6.5 J/cm^2.

Some physicians also use this modality on the legs. The results have been disappointing because of scarring and hyperpigmentation.[12]

REFERENCES

1. Fisher BK, Warner LC. Cutaneous manifestations of acquired immunodeficiency syndrome. Int J Dermatol 1987; 26:615–630.
2. Duffy DM. Small vessel sclerotherapy: An overview, in Callen JP, Dahl MV, Golitz LE, et al. (eds). Advances in Dermatology. Chicago: Year Book, 1988:221–241.
3. Sire DJ. The vascular spider. Cutis. 1972; 9:619–622.
4. Bean W. Vascular Spiders and Related Lesions of the Skin. Springfield, IL: Charles C Thomas, 1958:1–372.
5. Otto JF. Principles of Minor Electrosurgery. Rochester, NY: Liebel Flarsheim, 1957;42.
6. Kobayashi T. Electrosurgery using insulated needles: Treatment of telangiectasias. J Dermatol Surg Oncol. 1986; 12:936–942.
7. Ramelet AA, Monti M. Phlébologie. Fribourg, Switzerland: Masson, 1988:223–230.
8. Goldman MP, Bennett RG. Treatment of telangiectasia: A review. J Am Acad Dermatol. 1987; 17:167–182.
9. Bodian EL. Sclerotherapy: A personal appraisal. J Dermatol Surg Oncol. 1989; 15:156–161.
10. Lapins NA. Dermabrasion for telangiectasia. J Dermatol Surg Oncol. 1983; 9:470–472.
11. Apfelberg DB, Maser MR, Lash H. Treatment of nevi aranei by means of an argon laser. J Dermatol Surg Oncol. 1978; 4:172–174.
12. Glassberg E, Lask GP, Tan E, et al. D-flashlamp pumped 577-nm pulsed tunable dye laser: Clinical efficacy and in vitro studies. J Dermatol Surg Oncol. 1988; 14:1200–1208.

CHAPTER 13

Micropigmentation Surgery: Cosmetic Tattooing and Removal

NORMAN GOLDSTEIN

Tattoos have both fascinated and repelled generations of people all over the world. Body art has been practiced since ancient times and was thought to have mystical or religious meaning.[1] While we in the west often tend to think of tattoos as something bizarre or perhaps unsightly, the result of a male bonding initiation of the night before, other cultures and people view tattooing as an extraordinary artform. See Figs. 1 and 2.

The medical practitioner will often become involved with tattoos at both ends of the spectrum: with micropigmentation*—or the cosmetic uses of tattooing—and with the removal of unwanted tattoos.

*The interested physician may wish to join the American Society of Micropigmentation Surgery, Inc. (C.S. Zwerling, M.D., 2709 Medical Office Place, Goldsboro, NC 27530), for up-to-the-minute information on cosmetic tattooing.

MICROPIGMENTATION SURGERY OR COSMETIC TATTOOING

Increasing numbers of people are interested in the expanding area of cosmetic tattooing.[2] See Fig. 3. While the major interest in micropigmentation thusfar has been with eyelid tattoos, the potential for other uses is limited only by the knowledge and skill of the dermatologist. Tattoos can help deemphasize a pigmentation defect or a scar. They can also be used to add cosmetic detail for the patient who wants a permanent change—for example, augmenting a thin eyebrow or aiding in breast reconstruction after a mastectomy. See Table 1.

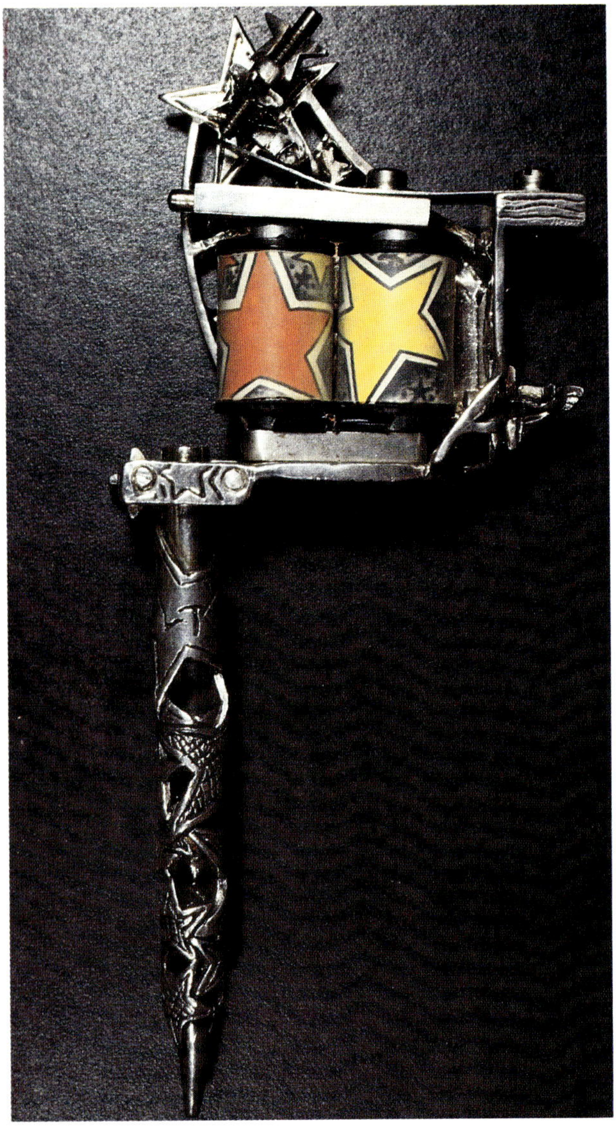

FIGURE 1
Close-up of a Lyle Tuttle instrument from the Tattoo Art Museum, San Francisco.

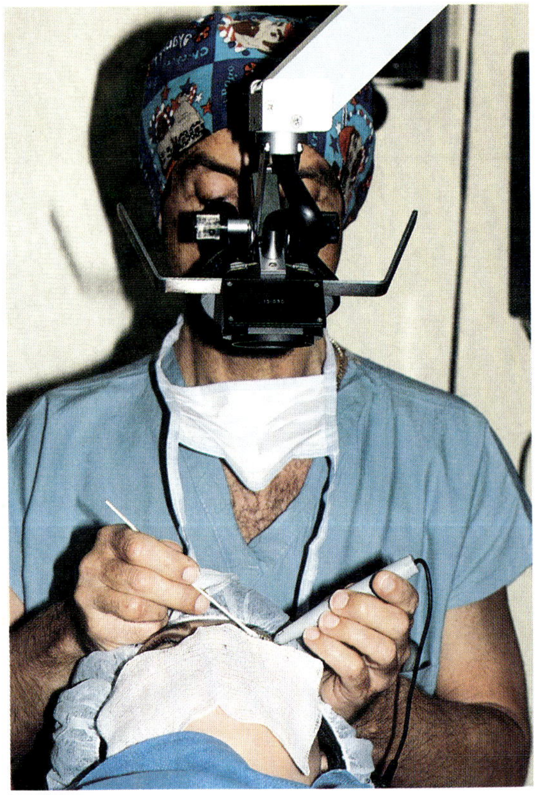

FIGURE 3
Cosmetic tattooing: John Corboy, M.D., using an operating microscope.

TABLE 1
USES OF COSMETIC TATTOOING

Eyelid tattoos
1. Permanent eyelining (see Fig. 4)
2. Eyelid pigmentation after cryosurgery
3. Eyelash enhancement for sparse lashes
4. Lid contour improvement after trauma or surgery

Eyebrows
1. Eyebrow enhancement or replacement (see Fig. 5)
2. Improved scarred areas

FIGURE 2
(a, b, and c) "MOM" and friends; (d and e) "MOM" stayed, but "KIM" and "TONY" were removed with argon laser techniques.

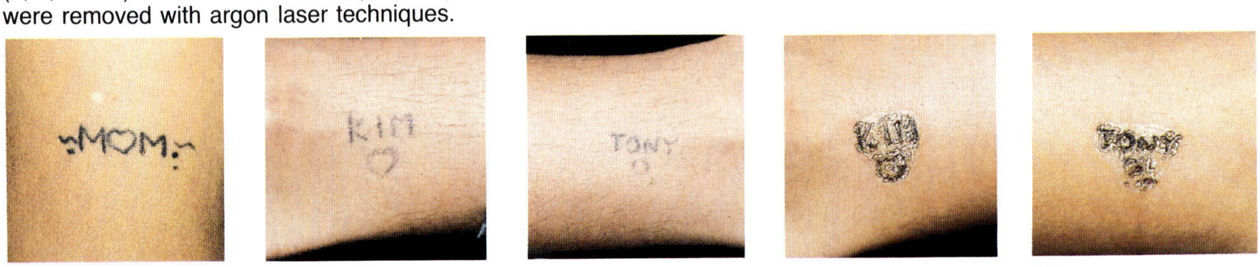

(a) (b) (c) (d) (e)

TABLE 1 *(Continued)*
USES OF COSMETIC TATTOOING

Lips
1. Contour repair/improvement (see Fig. 6)

Other general body uses
1. Countertattooing (covering or changing an existing tattoo)
2. Improvement of scars, skin grafts, or flaps after trauma or surgery
3. Nipple and areola reconstruction after trauma or mastectomy
4. Alopecia areata
5. Pinta
6. Vitiligo (see Fig. 7)
7. Cryosurgery hypopigmentation
8. "Filling-in" spaces between transplant plugs
9. Camouflaging drug users' needle tracks

Corneal and other tattoos (ophthalmologic surgeons only)
1. Congential corneal opacity
2. Heterochromia
3. Polychromia
4. Congential colobomas
5. Traumatic scars
6. Postinfection scars
7. Unilateral microphthalmus
8. Conversion for optical iridectomy
9. Postoperative conjunctival flaps
10. Operative defects of the iris

FIGURE 4
Eyeliner tattoo of the lower lids; (a) before and (b) after.

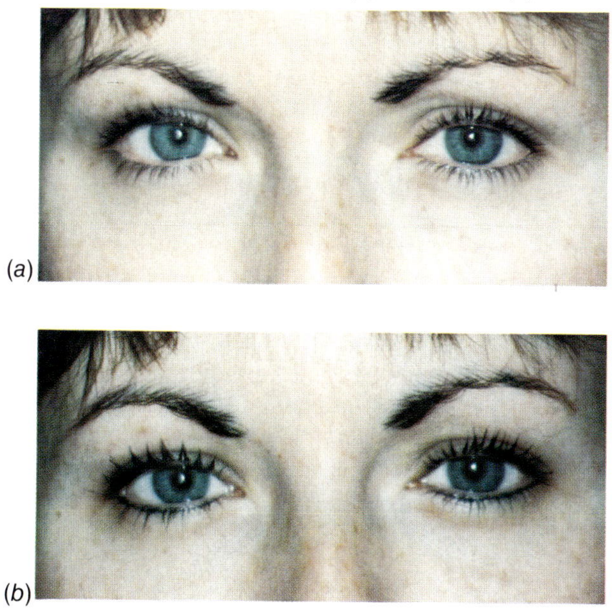

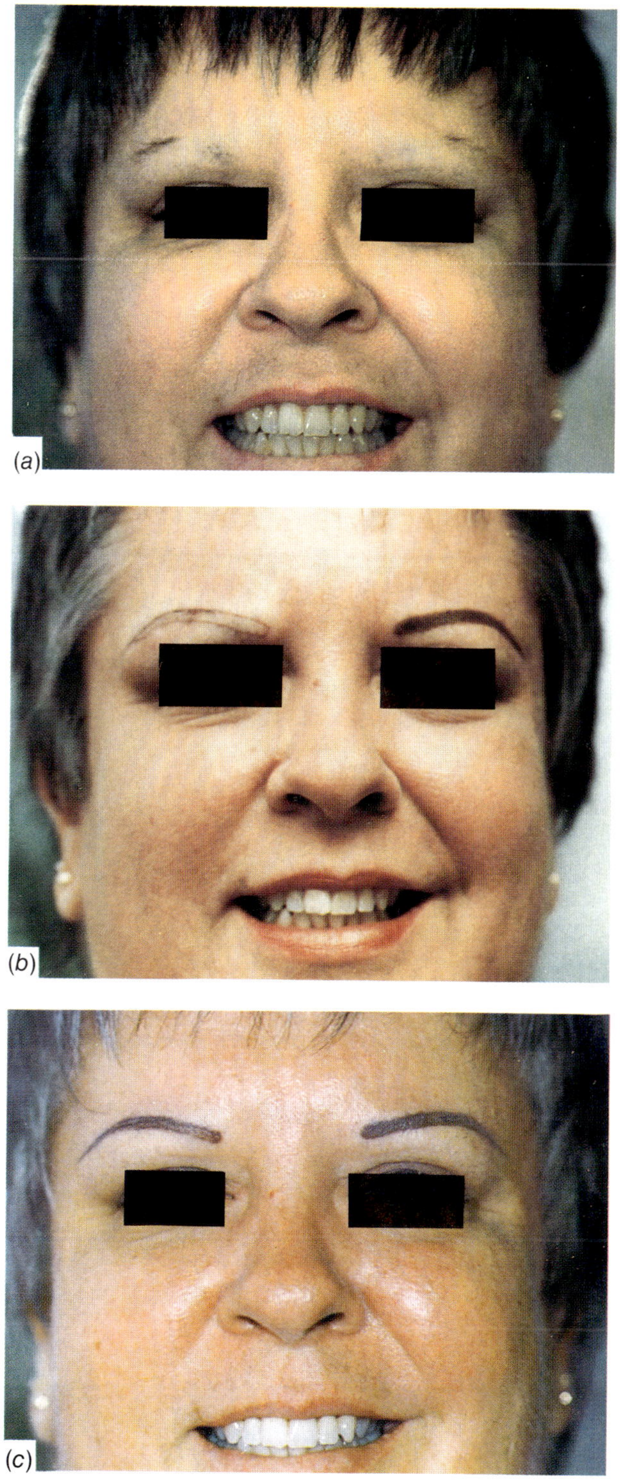

FIGURE 5
(a) Sparse eyebrows (hypothroidism); (b) eyebrow tattooing: right eyebrow is outlined, left eyebrow has been completed; (c) both eyebrows and eyelids have been completed.

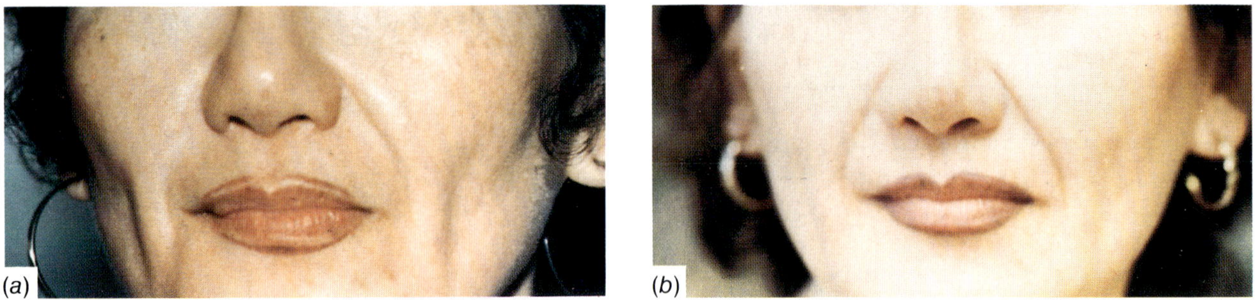

FIGURE 6
(a) Lip lining—note line on upper lip—and (b) full lip tattoo.

FIGURE 7
(a) Vitiligo of the hand and (b) after partial cosmetic tattooing.

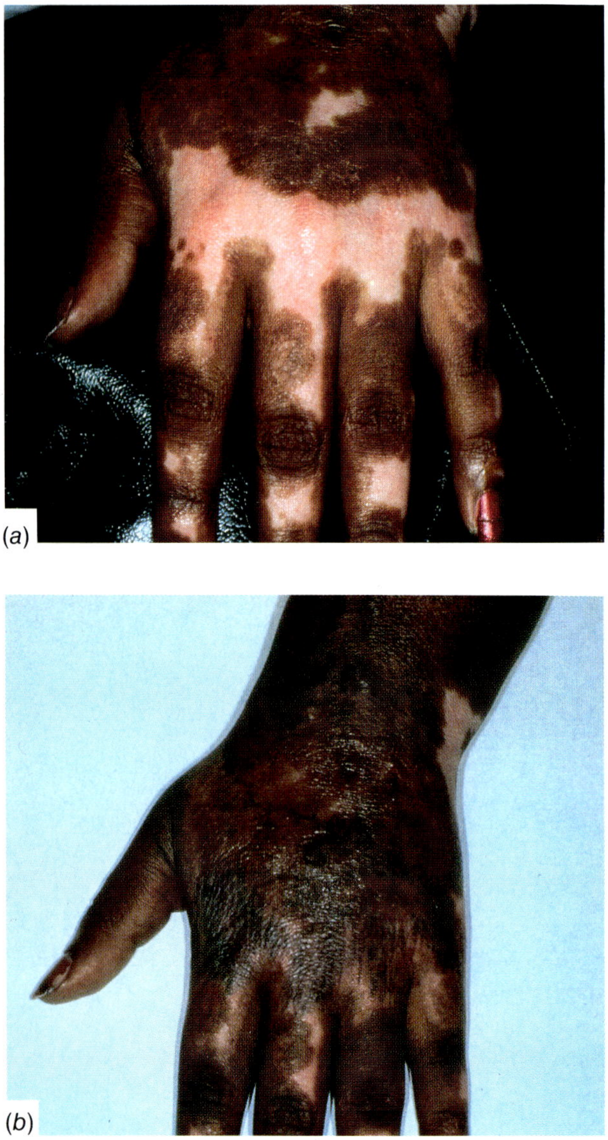

TATTOO EQUIPMENT

When physicians began to perform cosmetic tattooing, they had to use the types of instruments originally employed by tattoo artists, as shown in Fig. 8. As enthusiasm for eyelining tattoos increased, several manufacturers began to produce equipment specifically for the medical community. These include Cooper Vision (Natural Eyes), Penmark, Dioptics (Accents), Vision Concepts (Glamour Eyes), Cosmedyne, Alltek, and Eyelite.

It is recommended that aesthetic dermatologists take a course in micropigmentation surgery in order to learn and understand the techniques and problems of tattooing.

FIGURE 8
Cosmetic tattooing using a standard tattoo artist's instrument.

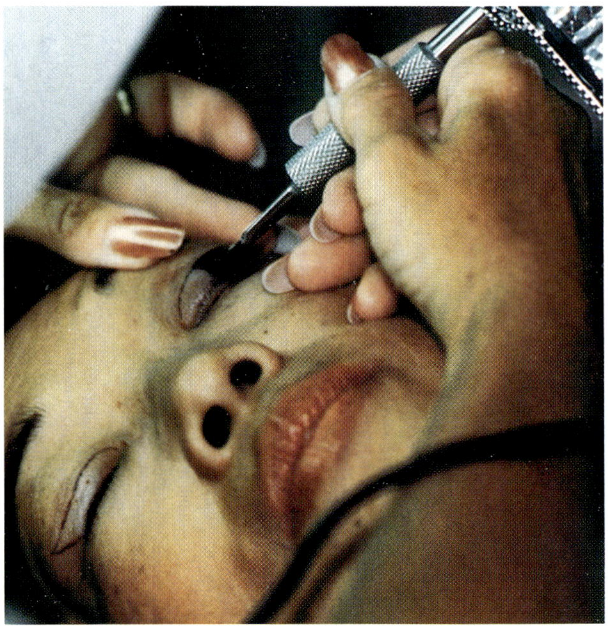

TATTOO TECHNIQUE

Modern cosmetic tattooing performed in a physician's office or surgical center is fairly simple technically, but there are caveats and complications.

Be conservative Do only as much micropigmentation surgery as necessary to obtain the desired results. The physician can always go back and add more pigment. Removal is not perfect, is usually difficult, and may be impossible. The patient must be made absolutely aware of the permanent nature of these procedures. Under no circumstances should cosmetic tattooing be performed at the initial consultation.

Be steady As with all cutaneous surgical procedures, a firm but gentle hand is mandatory. The pigment installed is permanent, although some superficially placed pigment may desquamate during the healing process.

Have good vision Binocular vision for full depth perception is helpful, if not mandatory. In addition, good color perception and sense can be important for matching the tattoo pigment to the skin color. This is less significant in eyeliner tattooing but could be problematic if judgment is impaired when performing this surgery for breast reconstruction, scar improvement, and the treatment of vitiligo.

Preoperative photographs should always be obtained for medical documentation as well as legal reasons. Pigments vary depending on the supply company and the instrument. The pigments can be premixed or mixed and matched. The colors used should be slightly darker than the shade desired in general, because the final color is usually lighter than anticipated.

After the skin is cleaned with benzalkonium chloride or alcohol, a small amount of local anesthetic is injected into the site to be tattooed. Some cosmetic surgeons and tattoo artists apply a thin layer of antibiotic ointment or petroleum jelly to the site before beginning. When an electric or battery-operated instrument and either a single-needle or a three-needle setup are used, the needles are dipped into the pigment and brought to the site, usually holding the needles at a 45-degree angle (some hold it at 90 degrees). Then the current is turned on. The tattoo pigment is inserted, the area is wiped, examined for any missed spots, and retouched if necessary. *Remember that pigment is permanent.* Tattoo less rather than more.

INFECTIONS AND OTHER COMPLICATIONS

Medical complications used to be fairly routine after being tattooed. Fortunately, side effects or adverse reactions tend to be minor and self-limiting bacterial infections these days. (And no case of acquired immunodeficiency syndrome has been reported to date of transmission by tattooing techniques.[3,4] A rare case of necrosis required amputation; even more rare were deaths reported in 1869[5] and in 1972.[6] Among the millions of people with tattooed arms, buttocks, and other sites, remarkably few have suffered any medical complications (personal communication, Michael Patipa, M.D., May 1988). Psychological problems are another consideration. With the surge in cosmetic tattooing, including lip lining and lip coloring, two recently observed complications have been noted. Within a 1-month period, I examined two women who presented with exacerbations of herpes simplex infections of the lips after having their lips tattooed with red pigment, as in Fig. 9. Another developed verruca vulgaris subsequent to lip coloring, as in Fig. 10. While herpes simplex infection probably represents latent herpes with photosensitization from cadmium in the red pigment, this has not been confirmed. Similar cases have been reported after red tattoos had been applied to some military personnel.[7] Because other cases have been

FIGURE 9
Herpes simplex infection after red full lip tattoo (sun sensitivity?).

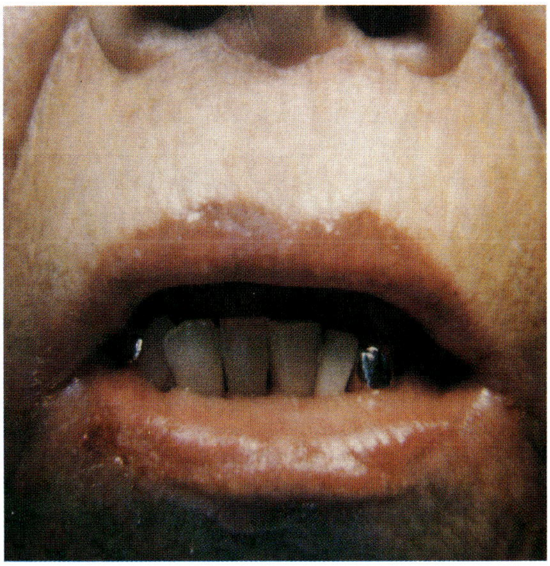

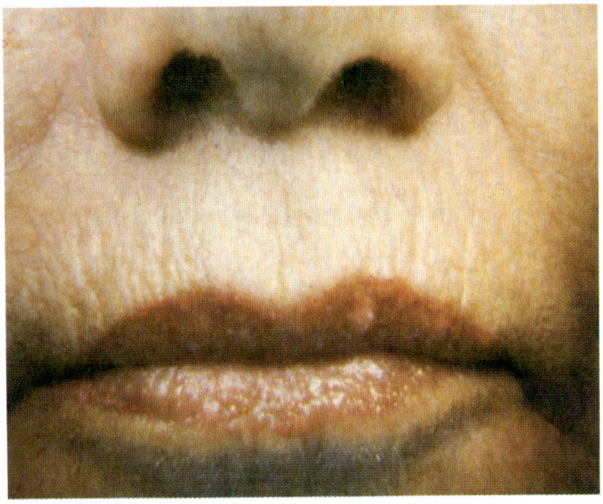

FIGURE 10
A wart appeared after a full lip tattoo. This patient also had a herpes simplex infection (sun sensitivity?).

TABLE 2
CAVEATS RELATED TO MEDICAL TATTOOING

1. Legal considerations
   a. State laws pertaining to tattooing (cities, counties, and states may have specific rules and regulations[8])
   b. Potential and real malpractice suits from dissatisfied patients[9]
2. Medical contraindications
   a. *Absolute:*
      Psoriasis
      Lichen planus
      Warts
      Molluscum contagiosum
      Active herpes simplex or herpes zoster
      Allergy to mercury or cadmium
      Active tuberculosis
      Darier's disease
      Keloid formation
      Anticoagulant therapy
      Hemophilia
   b. *Possible:*
      Chronic pyoderma
      Dermatographism
      Atopic dermatitis
      Alopecia areata
3. Psychological contraindications: mentally unstable patients; if in doubt, don't tattoo, or at least get a psychiatric consultation.

reported of reactions to lip coloring, tattoo artists and cosmetic surgeons no longer seem to be performing this procedure. See Table 2 which lists caveats to tattooing.

Blepharopigmentation—or eyelash tattooing—is another common form of cosmetic tattooing. See also Chap. 19. One potential hazard of this procedure has been reported by researchers who tattooed human cadaveric and rabbit globes in an attempt to show that accidental tattooing of the cornea or sclera may cause eyeball damage. However, in 48 corneal and 48 scleral tattoo wounds, no penetration of the globe was seen. Aqueous and vitreous leakage and only superficial tattoo pigments were seen in the cornea and sclera. The authors stated that "the risk of occular penetration is real."[10] To date, this has not been confirmed.

TATTOO REMOVAL

Patients as well as dermatologists must be aware that some form of scar or pigment abnormality usually results from any technique employed to remove dermal pigment.

Why Are Tattoos Removed?

The majority of tattooed individuals do not want their tattoos removed; however, a commonly cited reason for desiring removal is literally a "change of heart"—a new relationship or spouse. Another reason often involves the patient's occupation, e.g., a bank clerk who is required to wear short-sleeved shirts and has a large tattoo on the forearm, a momento from military days. And often a tattoo now occupies a site that is more visible than it was when it was first applied, for example, as necklines plunge or shorts and bikinis get smaller (see Fig. 11).

Methods of Tattoo Removal

The most common methods of tattoo removal are listed in Table 3.

Before undertaking a tattoo removal, remind the patient that *pigment placed in the skin should be thought of as permanent.* In addition, several preoperative factors must be considered before attempting to remove a tattoo:

1. Was the tattoo performed by an amateur or a professional?
2. How old is the tattoo?
3. Where is the tattoo situated on the body?
4. How many and of what size are the tattoos?
5. How motivated and how old is the patient?
6. What are the artistic and surgical skills of the physician?

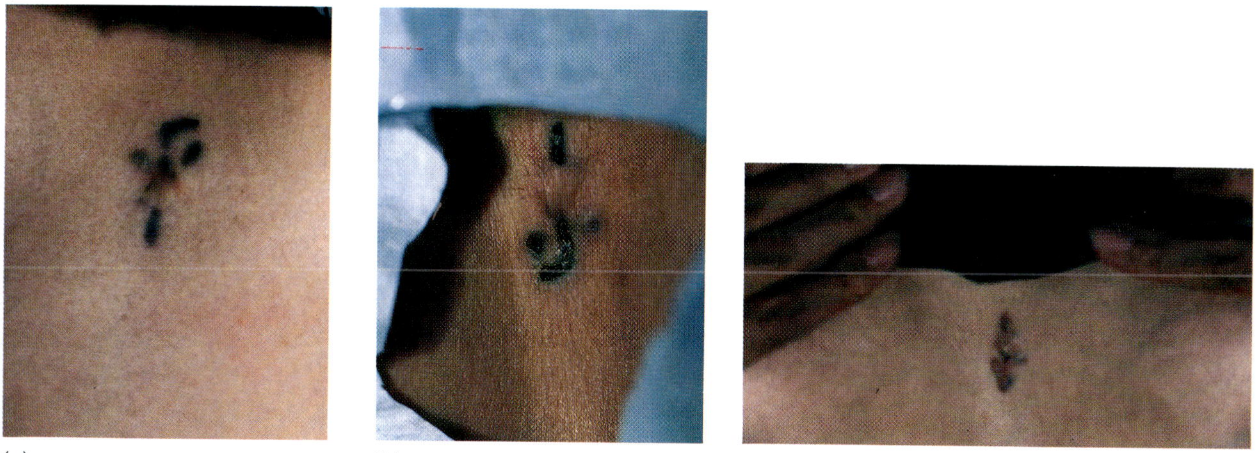

(a) (b) (c)

FIGURE 11
(a) Patient attempted to remove an amateur tattoo at home, which left a residual scar in the center. (b) Patient requested tattoo pigment and hypertrophic scar removal; argon laser treatment was used. (c) Six weeks after treatment.

TABLE 3
MEDICAL METHODS OF TATTOO REMOVAL

1. EXCISION
   With closure
   Tangential
   Punch
2. SALABRASION
   Table salt
   Hawaiian salt
   Kosher salt
3. DERMABRASION
   Standard or deep
   Superficial
   French method (modified by Penoff)
   Toothbrush
   Curettage after dermabrasion
4. LASERS
   Argon
   Carbon dioxide
   Ultraviolet
   Neodymium-yttrium-aluminum-garnet (Nd:YAG)
   Q-Switched ruby lasers
   Frequency-doubled YAG
   Tunable dye lasers
   Lasers and acids (e.g., urea)
   Chemolaser combinations
5. OTHER METHODS
   Cryosurgery
   Electrofulguration
   Grafting
   Mohs' chemosurgery
   Infrared coagulation
   Tissue expansion

In general, amateur tattoos cannot be as successfully removed as those done by professional artists. The depth of tattoo pigment varies greatly in amateur tattooing. Since professional tattoos are performed by electric tattoo equipment or by hand with multiple puncture methods, the same depth into the dermis is achieved, making removal easier.

Newer tattoos (weeks or months) are usually more successfully removed because the macrophages have not yet dispersed the pigment. Older or faded tattoos tend to be deeper and have spread out under the skin surface.

The site of the tattoo greatly influences the outcome of removal. Deltoid and art tattoos (Fig. 12) are notorious for poor results irrespective of size, age, or method of removal. More keloids and hypertrophic tattoos occur on the deltoid than on all other sites combined, and they are frequently the subject of litigation. The anterior chest is another common site for postremoval keloids. Tattoos in sun-exposed sites have a higher incidence of photosensitive reactions in allergic individuals.[7]

The size and number of tattoos must be carefully evaluated by the surgeon. A single small tattoo can be removed by any of the methods listed in Table 3. Multiple small tattoos compel the surgeon to consider the possibility that the patient will go back for additional tattoos.

Patient motivation is also a consideration in removal procedures. A young person brought in by a parent may not be very cooperative and may in-

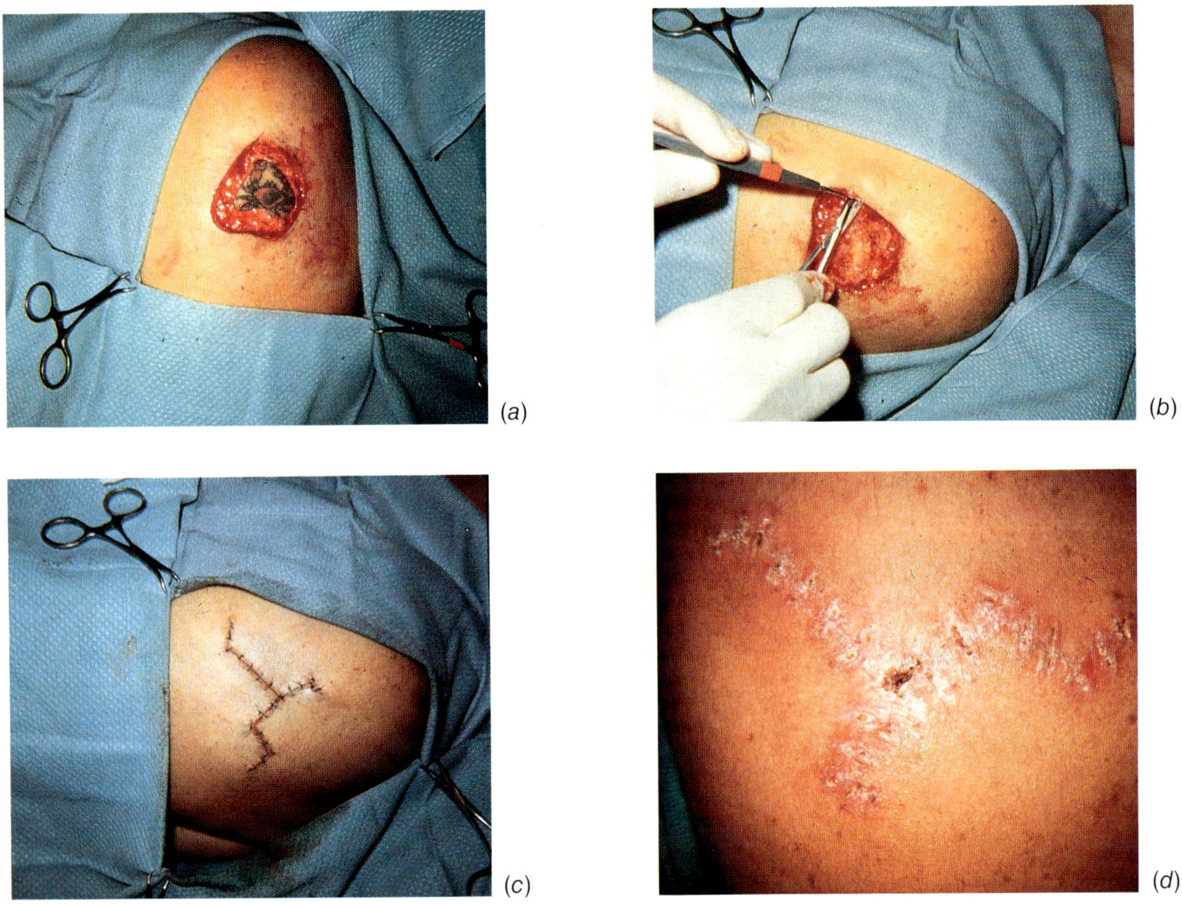

FIGURE 12
(a) Excision of a deltoid tattoo. (b) Undermining of surrounding skin. (c) Closure with a Hawaiian petroglyph-like technique. (d) Site healing nicely 2 months postoperatively. No keloids have developed, although this is a common area for keloids and hypertrophic

... get another tattoo soon after the removal of the first. As in any elective cosmetic procedure, the psychological status of the patient must be considered.

The surgical technique and skill of the dermatologist obviously will affect the outcome of the removal. Although there are many removal methods, most physicians have tried only a few and usually limit their procedures to the one or two that they feel most proficient in and that will give the best results.

REMOVAL TECHNIQUES

Excision

Excision and closure Small tattoos are probably best removed by excision if the anatomy of the area permits simple closure. Larger tattoos may be removed in stages: removing a central part, closing the site, and returning for excision of the remainder of the tattoo. (In my experience, the patient often does not return for the follow-up procedures.)

Technique A standard operating tray with scissors, scalpel, forceps, needle and suture material, local anesthetic, and syringe is prepared. Using a skin dye, the physician marks the ends of the excision site. The area does not have to be shaved, but hair removal allows better dressing adhesion. The area is infiltrated using a local anesthetic with epinephrine and a Luer-Lok type of syringe with a 30-gauge needle. Using scalpel and scissors, the entire tattoo is removed, with bleeding controlled by fine electrocautery. The site is closed in two layers, the first a deep dermal or subcuticular stitch just approximating the deeper dermal layers. The skin is then closed with an over-and-over continuous suture knotted at both ends.

A variant of this procedure is the punch biopsy excision, which is used for small (i.e., dotted) tattoos.

Split-thickness tangential excision With this method, a Brown, Davol, or similar oscillating dermatome is used. This method is frequently employed by plastic and reconstructive surgeons. It is preferred for many large professional tattoos, because most of the pigment is found at the same dermal level.

Technique Using local infiltration with epinephrine, the physician actually lifts up a portion of the tattoo. The dermatome, set at 0.15 in, removes the elevated tattoo, similar to the removal of a split-thickness skin graft. The operation site is managed like a graft donor site. Fine-mesh cotton gauze cut to conform to the site is applied. Some surgeons apply a slightly occlusive wet dressing and remove it the next day. A crust forms in the mesh gauze and usually separates in 7 to 10 days, with a good to excellent result seen in several months.

Tissue expansion One of the most recent methods for tattoo removal, reported by Agris[11], is tissue expansion. Plastic and reconstructive surgeons have used these techniques for breast reconstruction after mastectomy, for scalp replacement, and for head and neck cancer surgery. While there may be a limited use for it, this method is currently too time-consuming, inconvenient, and expensive to be used for ordinary tattoo removal.

Salabrasion

In 543 AD, the Byzantine Greek physician Aetius suggested the use of salt to remove tattoos.[9] His technique consisted of applying an irritating substance to the tattoo for several days and then rubbing salt into the site—a method that has been modified over the centuries but which remains essentially the same.

Klovekorn[12] revived the technique in 1935, suggesting daily salt rubbings until the skin became red. The term *salabrasion* was coined by Frank Crittenden in 1971.[13,14] The histologic changes were later found to show no granulomatous formation.[15] Better results were found with three separate abrasions rather than a single procedure,[16] although increased wrinkling of the skin may occur with repeated salabrasions.[17] A power-driven, cotton-tipped wooden applicator may be used for small or linear tattoos after dermabrasion with a dental burr.[18] Another modification of the salabrasion technique is the addition of heat treatments.[19]

Techniques Hair is shaved and the skin is prepared with povidone-iodine. A local anesthetic may be used but is not necessary. The tattoo site is rubbed with a slightly moistened sterile gauze and dipped in salt until the skin surface is removed and a uniform glistening erosion can be seen. Fine table salt or a coarse grade of salt, such as Hawaiian crude or kosher salt, can be used. Try different kinds of salt to see the results.

Some physicians use wooden or plastic doorknob-like devices to hold the salt and gauze and improve the abrasion. The treated area can be left uncovered, or an occlusive dressing with or without an antibiotic ointment may be applied. Dressings should be changed daily; pigment comes out with the dressing removals.

Dermabrasion

Before the advent of laser technology, derm[illegible]a-sion was the preferred method of tattoo re[illegible]al among most dermatologists and it still has [illegible]-ponents. The term was coined by Saul B[illegible] perfected the dermabrasion wheel for acn[illegible] and tattoo removal.[20] Accidental or gunsh[illegible] toos have been removed with a toothbrush or hand brush.[21,22] While most dermatologists [illegible]-ploy a fraise for dermabrasion procedures, a pow[illegible]-driven rotary brush can be used because of its "speed and reduced friction."[23]

Standard or deep dermabrasion technique[21,24,25] With this technique, the physician attempts to remove as much pigment as possible. Because of the depth of abrasion, the process is usually quite bloody. Sterile technique is not necessary; a clean operating room and office routine are sufficient. To guard against the possibility of HIV transmission as well as the requisite messiness, protective operating garments, gloves, and face shields are mandatory.

The tattoo site can be marked with gentian violet using 4-in by 4-in gauze pads. A small area of the tattoo is then exposed and frozen with dichlorotetrafluoroether (Frigiderm) or a similar spray or with a liquid nitrogen cryospray unit. The frozen area is then physically scraped with the fraise or brush, although care should be taken as brushes can get caught on the gauze. An adaptic or similar dressing is applied and removed in a day or two. Serum, epidermal cells, and pigment are seen lodged in the dressings.

As with any removal method, if the outline of tattoo is followed too closely, a ghost will remain. Blending the entire tattoo and fanning out the edges will improve the result.

Superficial dermabrasion technique With this method, the physician does not attempt to remove all tattoo pigment.[26] Frequently the residual tattoo is covered by reepithelialization. The most superficial dermabrasions do not require repeat procedures.[26]

After a preparation similar to that used for standard dermabrasion, the tattoo site is abraded very superficially. Only the epidermis and part of the papillary dermis are removed. When the tattoo pigment appears in the skin scrapings, the abrasion is stopped. This is a fast procedure even for an average-sized tattoo. The abraded site is painted with 2% gentian violet solution, and an adaptic dressing is applied and covered with gauze and tape. Dressings are change daily for 7 to 10 days.

Dermabrasion with tannic acid, or the French method technique Tattoo artists have relied on a method first described by Variot in 1888 to remove their handiwork.[27] Variot removed tattoos by making linear incisions, scratches, or punctures and then applying tannic acid and a silver nitrate solution. Penoff[28] reported his results, using a modified technique, on 85 patients with 207 tattoos over an 11-year period.

After the tattoo is anesthetized, the area is very superficially dermabraded (as above). The tattoo actually becomes more prominent since the dermis is exposed. When oozing occurs, the tattoo is painted with a tannic acid solution using a cotton swab. Penoff's solution is composed of two parts tannic acid, one part glycerin, and one part distilled water. It is thick and syruplike and goes over the abraded area easily.

A second superficial dermabrasion is done, with the wheel turned very slowly so as to rub the tannic acid gently into the dermis. Tannic acid painting is then performed using a hand-held tattoo needle or a cluster of three 18- or 21-gauge needles. The tannic acid solution is actually embedded into the dermis with the needles. The site is washed with saline, followed by silver nitrate stick rubbings. A black dry eschar forms in 2 to 3 min, and it separates in 2 to 3 weeks. Showers and baths are permitted and analgesics may be required for 2 to 3 days. Any residual pigment usually disappears over the ensuing 1 to 3 months.

LASERS

Carbon Dioxide Laser

Currently the CO_2 laser is considered the best to use for tattoo removal. The tattoo is infiltrated with 1% lidocaine with or without epinephrine. Carbon dioxide laser parimeters are 5 to 10 watts, defocused beam, and a continuous wave mode. The entire tattoo is vaporized, and the eschar is removed with saline solution or hydrogen peroxide. Repeated passes with the CO_2 laser are performed until the desired depth is obtained. Some operators recommend removing the entire tattoo pigment; however, with very deep tattoos this may result in a disfiguring scar. Thus, the removal of the pigment to the mid-dermis with the laser and further removal with urea may give a better aesthetic result. See Fig. 13.

Technique Several reviews[32–35] on laser technique for tattoo removal have been published and there are textbooks on laser therapy which offer additional information. The laser therapy course offered by the American Academy of Dermatology is highly recommended. The following factors should also be considered:

1. **Patient education, information, and instruction:** As with any cosmetic procedure, these are vital. Brochures, printed instructions, slides, or video presentations can help to alleviate fear or uncertainty; they are, however, no substitute for careful informed consent procedures. Patients must understand the process fully and be made aware of any possible complications, such as pigment problems (hyper- or hypopigmentation), incomplete removal of tattoo pigment, keloid formation, hypertrophic scars, and ghosting.
2. **Patient selection:** Patients must be highly motivated, especially if serial treatments are neces-

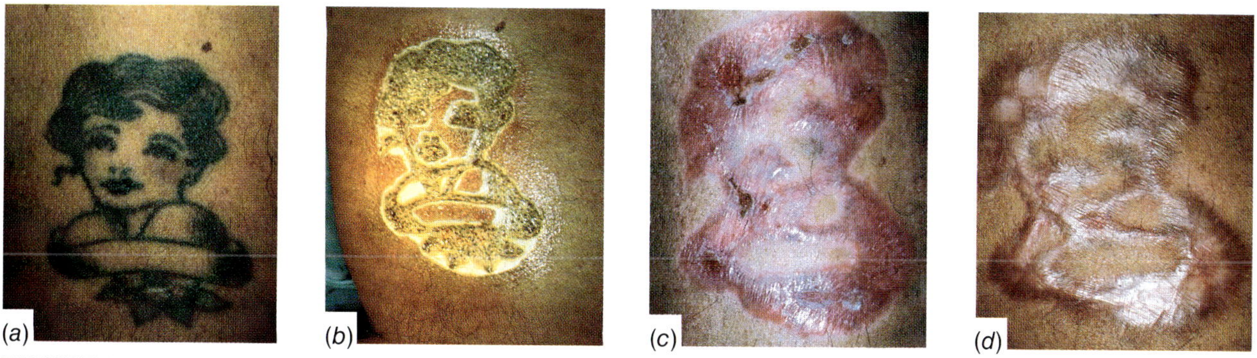

(a) (b) (c) (d)

FIGURE 13
(a) A 30-year-old tattoo on the arm of a 50-year-old man. (b) One month after carbon dioxide laser treatment. (c) Six months after treatment. (d) Nine months after treatment, showing keloids. Subsequent treatment with intralesional steroids reduced the keloids. (*Courtesy of Paul Takiuchi, M.D.*)

sary. Those who only want the procedure in order to please others are not likely to cooperate in follow-up.

3. Anesthesia: Preoperative sedation may be needed for younger or apprehensive patients. With a cooperative patient, even a local anesthetic may be unnecessary for the removal of a small tattoo. For a larger one, a local is needed.
4. Smoke evacuation: Smoke evacuation is mandatory. The nozzle of the vacuum cleaner-like device[36] is held 2 to 3 cm away from the laser site. Since the evacuator is noisy, some physicians provide their patients with earphones during the procedure so they can be distracted by music.
5. Laser safety: Lock the door to the laser surgery room and/or use a flashing sign to indicate the room is in use and prevent others from entering while the procedure is taking place. Also, test a small area of the tattoo with both the argon and CO_2 lasers before engaging in extensive treatment. After 4 weeks the patient should return for evaluation and further treatment as needed.
6. Laser beam: The beam is used to trace the outline of the tattoo and to obliterate an entire small tattoo or a portion of a large one. No site larger than 3 in by 3 in should be treated at one sitting.
7. Postoperative care: An antibiotic ointment is applied and a Telfa dressing is taped into place. The patient is instructed to avoid exposing the treated area to sunlight for a minimum of 6 weeks. Give patients a sunscreen with a sun protection factor (SPF) of 15 or higher and tell them to apply it to the site once the crust has fallen off, usually in 7 to 10 days. Patient acceptance of and follow-up for tattoo removal by laser have been excellent.

Lasers in Combination with Other Methods

There is not yet, and perhaps never will be, a perfect method for tattoo removal. Combination therapies involving lasers and other modalities have therefore become more common. Chemolaser methods[37] have been tried, and work is also being done with a modification of Dismuke's technique using CO_2 lasers and urea.

OTHER METHODS OF TATTOO REMOVAL

Cryosurgery

Cryosurgery with liquid nitrogen cotton-tipped applicators or spray units have not been very successful with tattoo removal. Too many repeated treatments are necessary for equivocal, if not poor, results.[35] Although one of my nontattoo patients suffered a cardiac arrest during liquid nitrogen treatment in the office,[38] I continue to use it for other procedures. Several practitioners[39,40] have reported their experiences with cryosurgery and cryospray.

Electrofulguration

Thermocautery was once considered "as crude as daubing with powerful chemical caustics and about as effective."[41] Shen and Mehlmauer,[42] on the other hand, treated eight patients with 12 tattoos using a ball-tipped needle on a Surgitome FFPF machine. They found electrofulguration to be a reasonable method, easy to perform, effective in removing pigment at various levels in an amateur tattoo, and less costly than other methods.

Grafting

Grafting is still performed by many plastic and reconstruction surgeons. Depending on the site and size of the tattoo, this procedure can be useful; however, most dermatologic surgeons elect not to graft tattoos since faster, less expensive methods exist that produce better results.

Infrared Coagulation

Infrared coagulation was developed recently for tattoo ablation and was used to treat 21 patients.[43] This technique has been compared with the CO_2 laser and it was found that infrared coagulation had a faster healing time and easier postoperative care but was not as effective in pigment removal as the laser.[44] Doses using the infrared coagulator have not been compared with other methods.[45]

Mohs Chemosurgery

Several of my associates have indicated interest in Mohs chemosurgery for tattoos, but I am not aware of any reports of anyone actually using this technique for removal.

CONCLUSION

As we have seen, tattoos can be removed, more often than not, by a number of methods. In general, some kind of scar will remain, but patients should know that something can be attempted and the overall effect of having the tattoo removed may be more felicitous than having it remain.

My thanks to John Corboy, M.D., Michael Patita, M.D., Gerald Faulkner, M.D., Norman Algiers, Marjorie King-Star, R.N., Raven McMurrin, and Deanna King who contributed photographs.

REFERENCES

1. Goldstein N, Sewell M. Tattoos in different cultures. J Dermatol Surg Oncol. 1979; 5:857–864.
2. Zwerling CS, Christensen FH, Goldstein N. Micropigmentation. Thorofare, NJ: Slack, 1986.
3. Goldstein N. Tattoos today—From eyelashes to ankles and some in "3-D." Arch Dermatol. 1985; 121:604–605.
4. Fish P. More about plague prevention. Tattoo Life. 1988; May:8.
5. Berchon E. Histoire Medicale du Tatouages. Paris: JB Bailliere et fils, 1869.
6. International comments. Death after tattooing. JAMA. 1972; 22:1194.
7. Goldstein N. Mercury-cadmium sensitivity in tattoos: A photo-allergic reaction in red pigment. Ann Intern Med. 1967; 67:984–989.
8. Goldstein N. Laws and regulations relating to tattoos—An updated survey. To be published.
9. Zimmerman M. Suit for malpractice based on alleged unsightly scars resulting from removal of tattoos. J Dermatol Surg Oncol. 1979; 5:911–912.
10. Kreter JK, Sall KN, Keates RH. Potential hazards of blepharopigmentation. Ophthalmic Surg. 1985; 16:693–695.
11. Argis J. Tissue expansion—A new vista in reconstruction. Am J Plas Reconstr Surg. 1987; 4:301–308.
12. Klovekorn GH. Ein Einfache der Enterfernung von Tatowierung. Dermatol Wochenschr. 1935; 101:1271.
13. Crittenden FR Jr. Salabrasion: Removal of tattoos by superficial abrasion with table salt. Cutis. 1971; 7:295–300.
14. Crittenden FR Jr. Salabrasion: Removal of tattoos, in Epstein E, Epstein E Jr. (eds). Skin Surgery, 5th ed. Springfield, IL: Charles C Thomas, 1982.
15. Koerber WA Jr, Price NM. Salabrasion of tattoos: A correlation of clinical and histologic results. Arch Dermatol. 1978; 114:884–888.
16. Catterall MD. Removal of tattoos, letter. Lancet. 1980; i:981.
17. Horn W. Effects of tattoo removal and results after salabrasion. Z Hautkr. 1983; 58:336–342.
18. Shell WB, Shelley ED. Focal salabrasion for removal of linear tattoos. J Dermatol Surg Oncol. 1984; 10:216–218.
19. Johannesson A. A simplified method of focal salabrasion for removal of linear tattoos. J Dermatol Surg Oncol. 1985; 11:1004–1005.
20. Burchfield RW. The Compact Edition of the Oxford English Dictionary. New York: Oxford Univ. Press, 1971. Vol 1, 777.
21. Goldstein N. Tattoos: Cosmetic and therapeutic tattoos and removal techniques in, Epstein E, Epstein E Jr (eds). Skin Surgery, 6th ed. Philadelphia: Saunders, 1987, 625.
22. Notaro WA. Dermabrasion for the management of traumatic tattoos. J Dermatol Surg Oncol. 1983; 9:916–918.
23. Yarborough JM Jr. Dermabrasion by wire brush. J Dermatol Surg Oncol. 1987; 13:610–615.
24. Bunke HJ, Conway H. Surgery of decorative and traumatic tattoos. Plast Reconstr Surg. 1957; 20:67–77.

25. Chai KB. The decorative tattoo: Its removal by dermabrasion. Plast Reconstr Surg. 1963; 32:559.
26. Clabaugh W. Removal of tattoos by superficial dermabrasion. Arch Dermatol. 1968; 98:515–521.
27. Variot G. Nouveau procede de destruction des tatouages. Compte Rendu Soc Biol (Paris). 1888; 8:836–838.
28. Penoff JH. The office treatment of tattoos: A simple and effective method. Plast Reconstr Surg. 1987; 79:186–191.
29. Goldstein N, Hay-Roe V, Penoff JH. Tattoo Removal Methods (video tape). The World of Tattoos, Honolulu, 1979.
30. Goldstein N, Penoff JH, Price N. Techniques of removal of tattoos. J Dermatol Surg Oncol. 1979; 5:901–910.
31. Goldman L, Rockwell RJ, Meyer R. Laser treatment of tattoos: A preliminary survey of three years clinical experience. JAMA. 1967; 201:163–166.
32. Apfelberg DB, Manchester GH. Decorative tattoos: Biophysiology and removal. Clin Plast Surg. 1987; 14:243–251.
33. Eastern JS. Lasers in private practice. Cutis. 1986; 37: 293–299.
34. Bailin PL, Ratz JL, Wheeland RG. Laser therapy of the skin—A review of principles and applications. Advanced Dermatologic Surgery Dermatology Clinics. 1987; 5:259–285.
35. Goldstein N. Tattoo removal—Review article. Derm Clinic. 1987; 5:349–358.
36. Laser Institute Study. Raises concern over plume safety. Clin Laser Monthly. 1988; 6:61–65.
37. Dismukes DE. The chemo-laser technique for the treatment of decorative tattoos: A more complete dye removal procedure. Lasers Surg Med. 1986; 6:59–61.
38. Goldstein N. Cryo corner cardiac arrest following application of liquid nitrogen. J Dermatol Surg Oncol. 1979; 7:602.
39. Lembo G, Donofrio P, DeLuca F. Tattoo treatment with cryotherapy. G Ital Dermatol Venereol. 1983; 118:187–188.
40. Colver GB, Dawber RP. Tattoo removal using a liquid nitrogen cryospray. Clin Exp Dermatol. 1984; 9:364–366.
41. Goldman L. Thermal cautery by fulguration of lasers. J Dermatol Surg Oncol. 1979; 5:910.
42. Shen JY, Mehlmauer M. Tattoo removal with electrodessication. J Dermatol Surg Oncol. (to be published).
43. Colver GB, Cherry GW, Dawber RPR. Tattoo removal using infrared coagulation. Br J Dermatol. 1985; 12:481–485.
44. Groot DW, Arlett JP, Johnston PA. Comparison of the infrared coagulator and the CO_2 laser in the removal of decorative tattoos. J Am Acad Dermatol. 1986; 15:518–522.
45. Venning VA, Colver GB, Millard PR. Tattoo removal using infrared coagulation: A dose comparison. Br J Dermatol. 1987; 117:99–105.

PART III

TOPICAL CONSIDERATIONS

CHAPTER

14

Facial Scarring: Punch Grafting and Dermabrasion

WAINE C. JOHNSON

Scarring of the face is most commonly caused by acne, although varicella and other infections occasionally result in disfiguring marks. Acne can produce scarring which varies from narrow to wide and from shallow to deep and may be depressed or hypertrophic. *Dermabrasion* has been used for many years to remove superficial scars and improve deeper scars by beveling the edges of a scar and thus reducing shadows. Pitted or ice-pick-like bound-down scars cannot be improved significantly by dermabrasion. In the past, deep, pitted scars were treated with simple surgical excision prior to a dermabrasion procedure, but after the dermabrasion a linear scar with relatively little pigment remained. In my experience, full-thickness skin grafts using the punch graft technique represent the best way of treating pitted scars of the face.[1–3] After a dermabrasion procedure, the sites of the grafts in most instances look like normal skin and cannot be detected. Another technique known as *punch graft elevation* has been reported.[4] This technique consists of separating the scar from the surrounding skin by means of a surgical cutaneous punch and allowing the tissue to rise but still remain attached to the subcutaneous fat which serves as its source of blood supply. The disadvantages of this method are that most scars are not perfectly round with straight edges but are V-shaped (Fig. 1).

Pitted scars that are round and reasonably flat at the base often retract from the adjacent skin and

FIGURE 1
Most pitting scars are V-shaped. Excision and allow-to-rise techniques give an inadequate result.

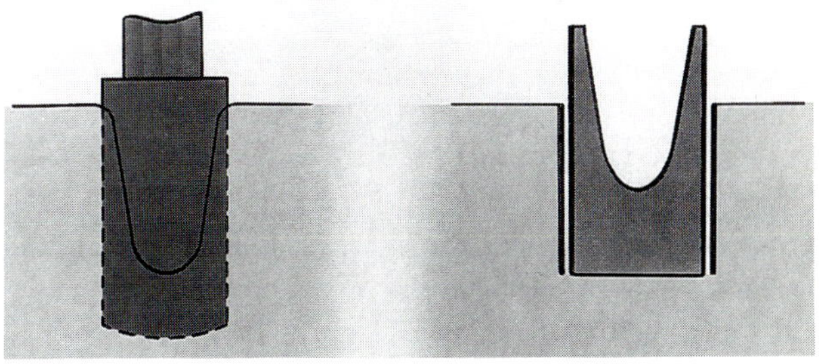

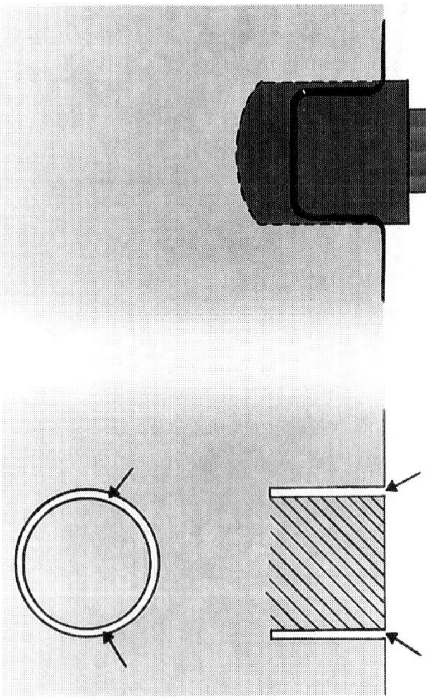

FIGURE 2
Even rounded scars leave a retraction space and do not always heal well.

fail to heal properly (Fig. 2). Even after technically successful treatment, the tissue remains scar tissue. This technique is best used in large, relatively round depressed scars 5 mm or more in diameter which might not take as free, full-thickness grafts.

A patient seeking treatment for scarring of the face must be examined carefully to determine the types of scars present and the best approach to treatment. The examination should be conducted with a unidirectional light source parallel to the plane of the skin surface; this technique emphasizes and allows close examination of the defect. Overhead diffuse lighting must be turned off because it tends to minimize defects. Many shallow and mildly to moderately atrophic soft scars are probably best treated with soft tissue augmentation (my preference usually is silicone). Deep, pitted scars, especially bound-down pitted scars, are best treated with the punch graft transplant technique. If patients have large (greater than 5 mm) atrophic scars, a simple excision can be performed, and the scar tissue can be replaced later with punch graft transplants prior to a dermabrasion procedure. When the scars are less than 1 mm deep, dermabrasion alone is usually adequate to correct or significantly improve the defects. Some physicians recommend dermabrasion for the treatment of telangiectasias, but I do not recommend this.

PUNCH GRAFT TRANSPLANTS

Prior to the procedure, the patient is advised to avoid aspirin and aspirin-containing preparations. Patients are placed on tretinoin (retinoic acid, Retin-A), which seems to improve healing and reduce the number of milia after dermabrasion. Prophylactic oral erythromycin or another antibiotic may be given the day before surgery and for 10 days after surgery. It is desirable to have someone accompany the patient. The supplies and instruments needed are listed in Table 1.

Procedure

The scars to be removed are marked with gentian violet or another dye, using a sharpened wooden applicator stick to prevent obliteration of the scar by the local anesthetic. Lidocaine or another local anesthetic with epinephrine is used to achieve appropriate nerve block and local infiltration into the donor and recipient sites. Injection into the subcutaneous tissue is less painful than dermal injection.

The surgical punch used to remove the pitted scar must be large enough to remove all the epidermis extending into the pit. If any epidermis remains, the transplant will not heal properly and

TABLE 1
INSTRUMENT AND SUPPLIES FOR PUNCH GRAFT TRANSPLANTS

1. Surgical punches 1.5 to 4 mm in 0.25-mm increments
2. Surgical punches 4.0 to 6.0 mm in 0.5-mm increments
3. Iris or other small scissors
4. Fine forceps
5. Flat surgical instrument
6. Needle holder and suture
7. Tissue glue and applicator [bucrylate (isobutyl cyanoacrylate)]
8. Liquid adhesive (mastic)
9. Adhesive remover (Detachol)
10. Steri-Strips, 1/8 in
11. Gauze sponges
12. Cotton-tipped applicators
13. Gentian violet
14. Lidocaine (Xylocaine) 1% with epinephrine
15. Syringe and 30-gauge needles
16. Petri dishes
17. Sterile, normal saline
18. Cold plate
19. Hydrogen peroxide
20. Alcohol swabs

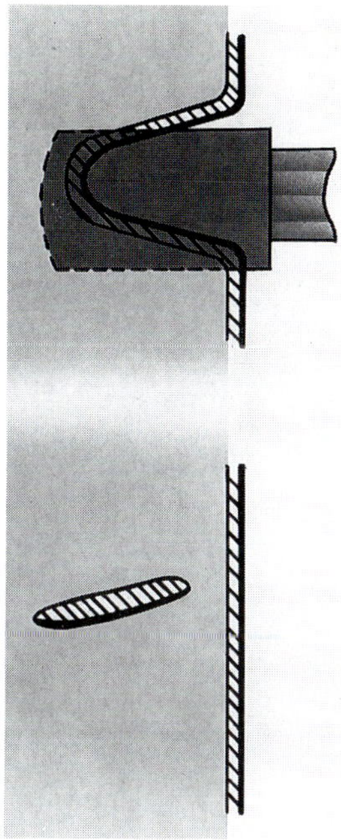

FIGURE 3
The entire thickness of the epithelial wall of the pit must be completely removed to avoid the formation of a sinus tract or cyst.

will form a sinus tract or a cyst (Fig. 3). All scars from a single area (up to one-half of the face) are removed, and the areas are covered with damp, cool gauze. The entire thickness of the dermis is removed. A fine-toothed forcep or a 30-gauge needle may be used to lift the graft for removal. The number and sizes of the grafts removed should be recorded.

The preferred donor site is the postauricular skin in the nonhairy area. If there is not enough donor skin in this site, the skin from the back of the ear is used. The skin from the back of the ear is usually thinner than that in the postauricular area. Donor grafts should be large enough to fill the recipient hole firmly on all its margins but not large enough to cause trouble in pushing the graft into the hole. When the graft is too large, it may later elevate to a greater extent than is desirable. If it is too small, it may retract from one margin and leave a sinus tract or depression. The ear should not be bent excessively or enough to significantly stretch the skin, since this may result in an oval graft rather than a round graft. The size of the donor graft varies from person to person but generally is 0.5 mm larger than the recipient site for grafts up to 2.25 mm, 0.75 larger for grafts from 2.25 to 3.25 mm, and 1 mm or more larger for grafts greater than 3.5 mm. A 1.5-mm punch is the smallest size recommended, since smaller grafts often do not take.

It is best to perform a few donor grafts for the various sizes needed to be sure of a proper fit and then do the remainder. The donor grafts are placed in a petri dish on top of gauze which is covered with sterile, cold normal saline; the dish is kept on a cold plate. When the grafts are cut from the donor site, a minimal amount of subcutaneous tissue is removed to prevent the subcutaneous fat from trailing up along the side of the graft and extending to the surface, causing a defect between the opposing skin margins. When one is treating a large number of scars, it is best to place the donor grafts into the holes by sections and secure them in place. Skin tissue glue should be used to secure the graft to the adjacent skin. The delivery method involves dropping the glue, using the plastic applicators which are included (Fig. 4 and 5). If one is particularly concerned about a graft or if the graft is large,

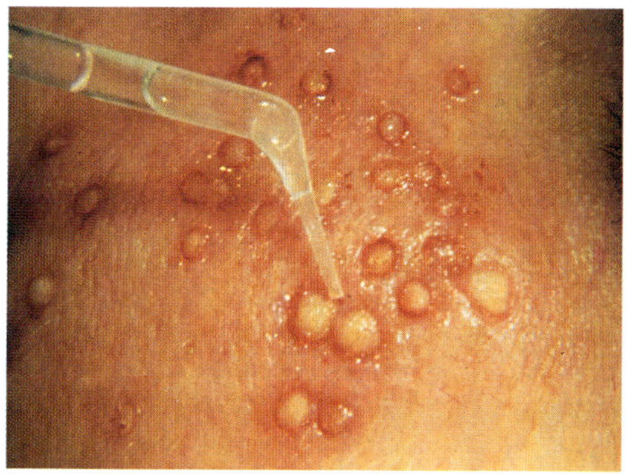

FIGURE 4
Tissue glue is applied by drop, using the applicator provided.

FIGURE 5
Appearance of tissue glue after application.

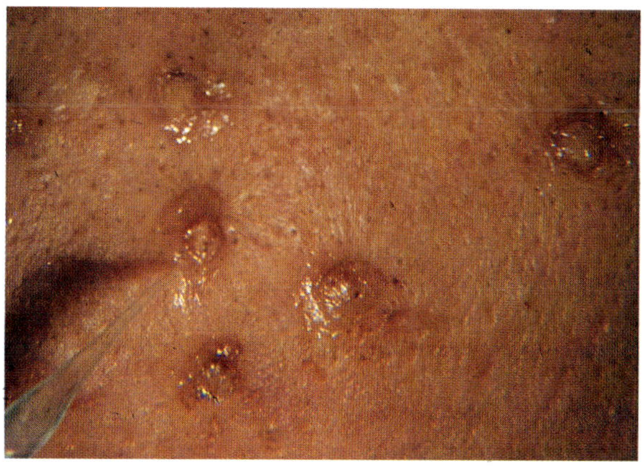

one can use tissue glue and then place a Steri-Strip over it. In previous years Steri-Strips were used for holding all grafts in place except in the case of large grafts. When Steri-Strips are used, the adhesive mastic (Mastisol) is used on the adjacent skin to hold the strips in place (Fig. 6). For transplants 4.5 to 5 mm, one can use sutures over the transplant (Fig. 7), a steel pin through the transplant, or sutures into the transplant itself.

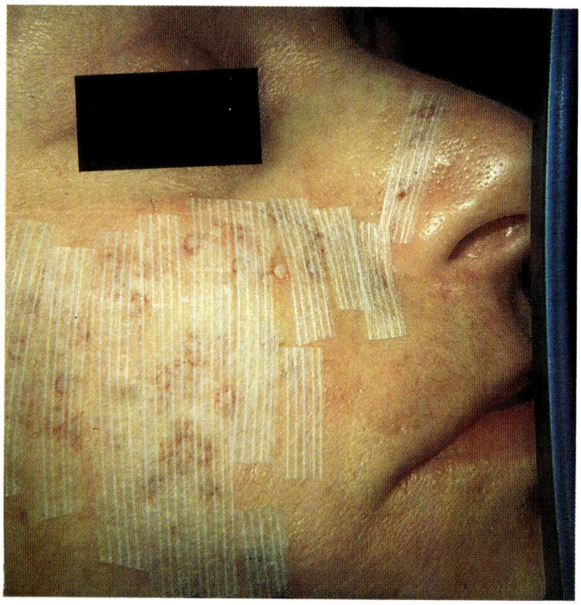

FIGURE 6
Steri-Strips can be used to hold grafts in place.

FIGURE 7
The dotted line indicates the suture beneath the skin surface. The suture lies above the graft and prevents it from rising.

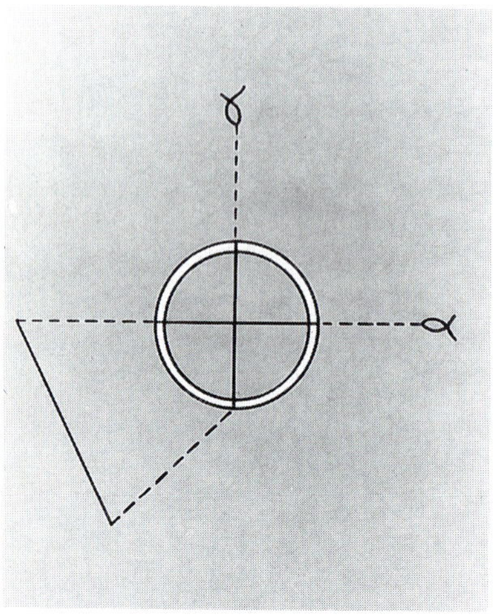

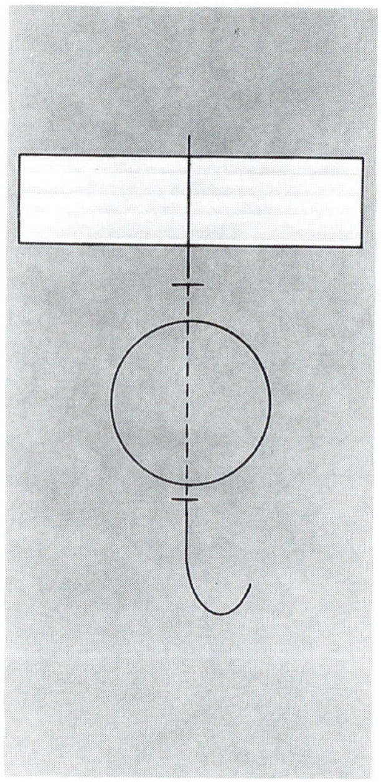

FIGURE 8
A stainless steel pin is placed through the graft and held in place with a Steri-Strip.

FIGURE 9
Transplants of 5 mm or more are best sutured. Tissue glue or Steri-Strips can also be used.

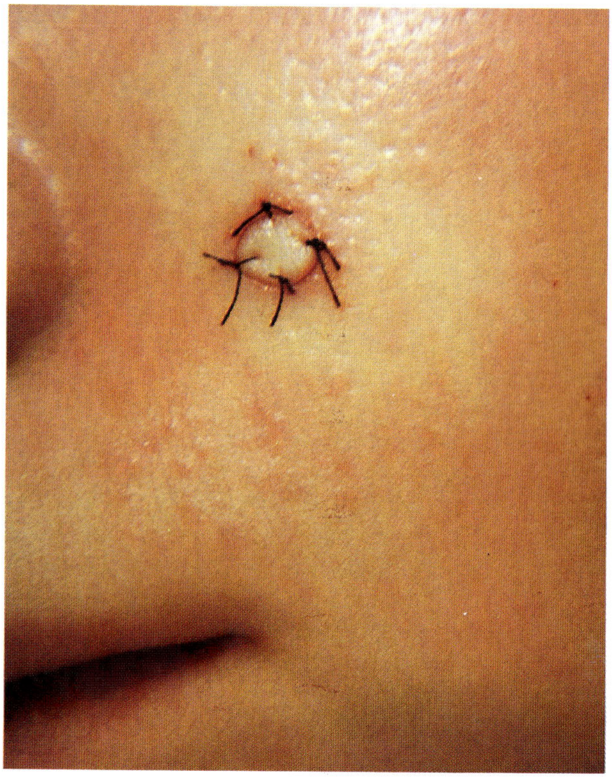

TABLE 2
OPERATIVE PROCEDURES FOR PUNCH GRAFT TRANSPLANTS

1. Mark scars with gentian violet.
2. Infiltrate recipient and donor sites
3. Remove scars using surgical punches
4. Remove donor grafts
5. Place grafts in a petri dish
6. Place grafts in recipient holes
7. Clean and dry recipient area
8. Secure grafts with tissue glue or Steri-Strips

The technique used for steel pins has been reported for hair transplants,[5] but when this procedure is done on the face, the pins are taped on one end or both ends with Steri-Strips (Fig. 8). Steel pins are not as effective on the face as they are on the scalp, because they tend to come loose as a result of the movement of the facial muscles. Transplants 5 mm or larger should be sutured using 7-0 simple sutures (4 or more) per transplant (Fig. 9). The plan of the procedure is to have the top of the transplant slightly elevated in relation to the adjacent skin. The operative procedure is summarized in Table 2.

Postoperative Care

Patients are instructed not to touch or attempt to wash the sites of the transplants for 4 days. They are told to take liquid or soft foods by mouth and avoid unnecessary facial expressions and unnecessary talking. An antibiotic (erythromycin 250 mg qid) is taken for 10 days. If Steri-Strips are used to secure the transplant, the patient returns to the office in 2 or 3 days and the crusts are soaked with hydrogen peroxide solution. Then the adhesive remover (Detachol) is liberally applied with a cotton-tipped applicator stick. A flat surgical instrument is inserted beneath the Steri-Strip and over the graft, and the Steri-Strip is gently removed with a forcep (Fig. 10). The patient is advised to use warm water compresses beginning 4 days after the procedure (15 minutes three times a day) until the crusts spontaneously separate. A hydrogen peroxide compress is used at the end of each period of warm water compresses. If it is convenient, the patient returns to the office in 5 to 7 days to have excess glue and debris cleaned off. The patient is usually seen 2 weeks after surgery to determine whether all the grafts have taken, and any necessary regrafting is usually done 3 weeks after the operation.

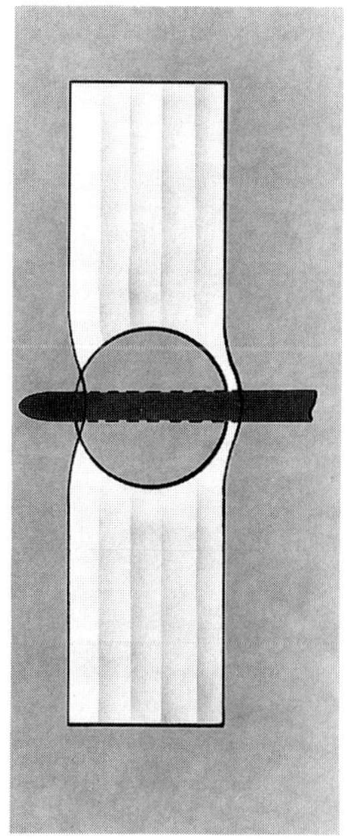

FIGURE 10
A flat surgical instrument is placed beneath the Steri-Strip and over the graft, and the Steri-Strip is gently removed.

Dermabrasion or another leveling procedure is usually done 3 to 4 weeks after the grafting is complete. If only a few grafts have been done, they may be leveled with either focal dermabrasion or surgical shaving at the skin level and light electrodesiccation of the graft and an area of normal skin 1 to 2 mm about the graft. The sites of the graft usually can be seen immediately after the dermabrasion or other leveling procedure, but as the skin heals, the sites of the grafts generally cannot be seen. Stages of treatment and results are shown in Fig. 11 through 13.

Complications

Failure of an entire graft to take, a depressed groove at the junction with normal skin, a depressed graft, and rarely a hypertrophic scar reaction are possible complications. When a large number of transplants are performed, some of the transplants often have to be redone. This may be due to excessive bleeding, lack of bleeding to seal the wound, or trauma to the graft. Regrafting is performed and sometimes requires a slightly larger graft. If a graft or a part of a

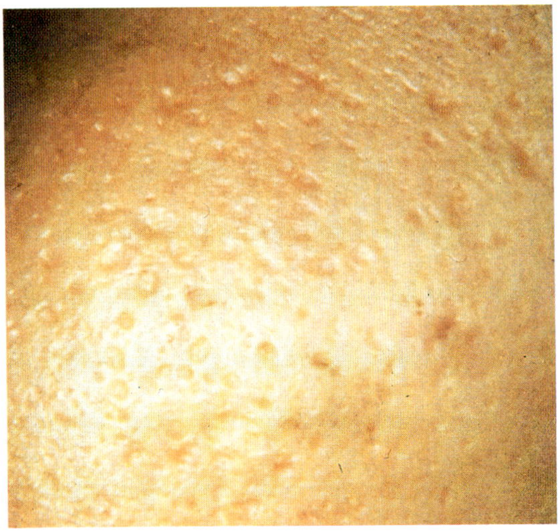

(a)

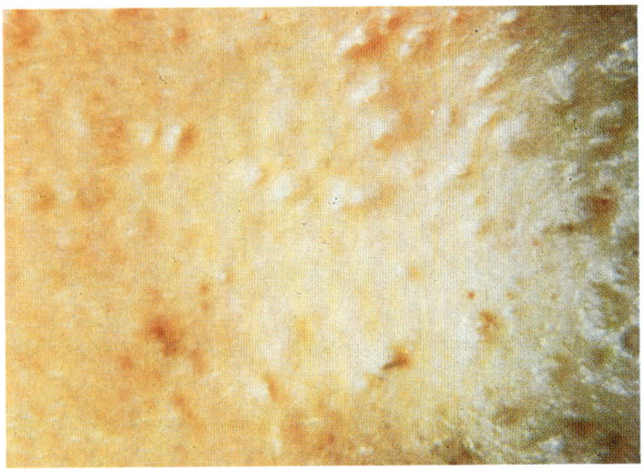

(b)

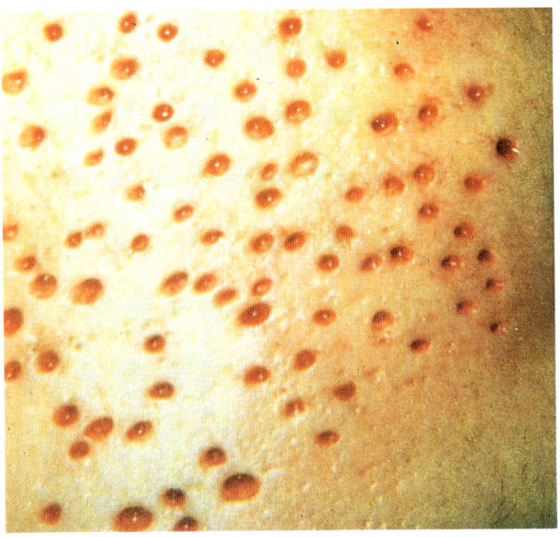

(c)

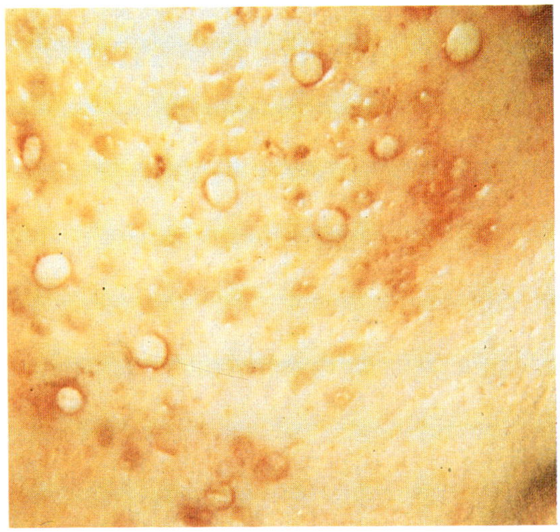

(d)

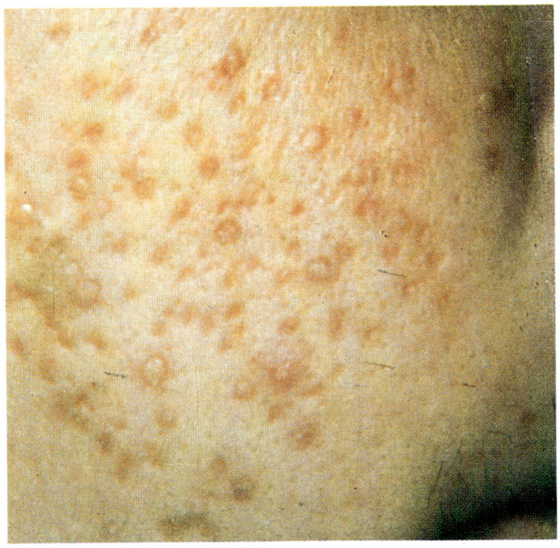

(e)

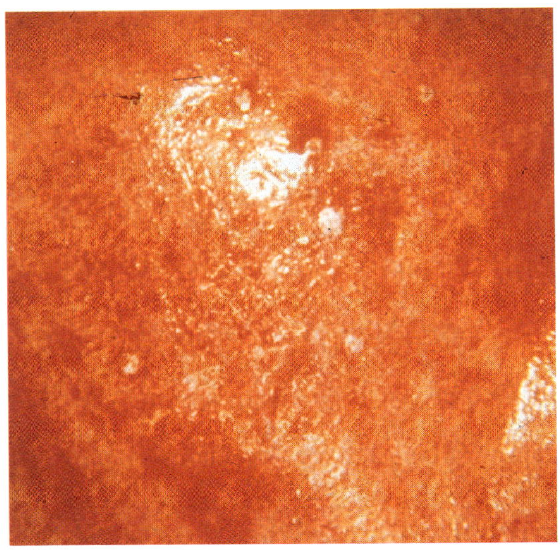

(f)

FIGURE 11
(*a*) Before treatment; (*b*) closer view; (*c*) after removal of scars; (*d*) grafts in place; (*e*) grafts before dermabrasion; (*f*) immediately after dermabrasion; (*g*) 4 months after dermabrasion.

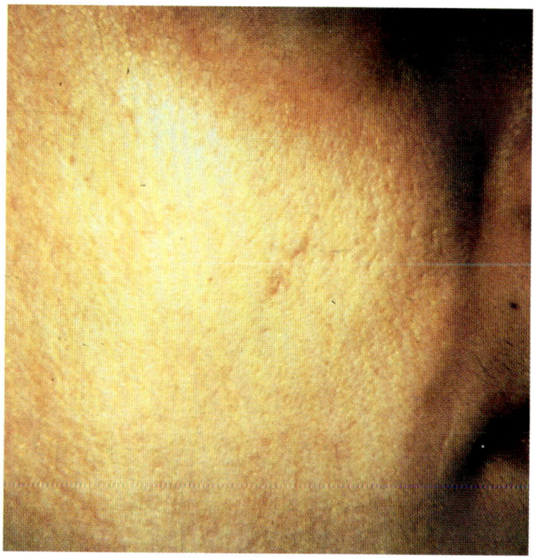

(g)

FIGURE 11 (*Concluded*)

FIGURE 12

(*a*) Before treatment; (*b*) after punch grafts; (*c*) 3 months after dermabrasion.

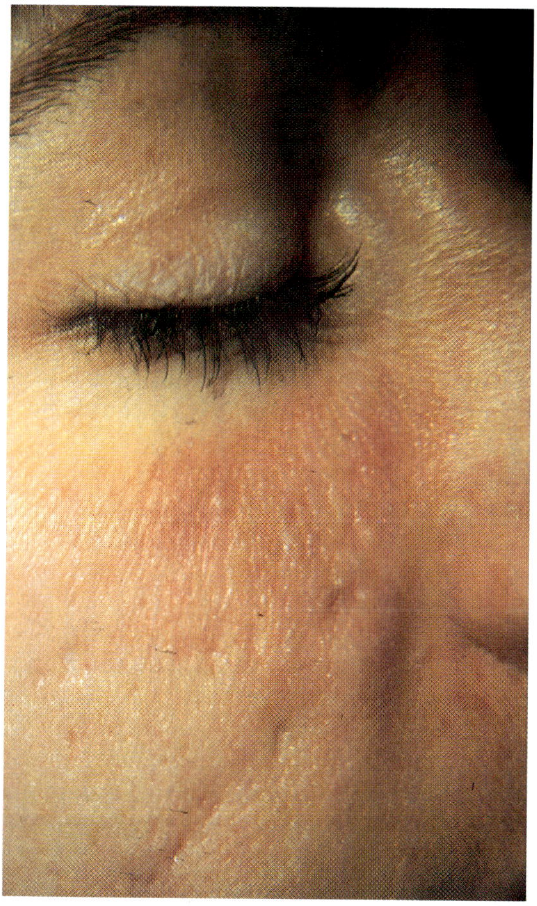

(*a*)

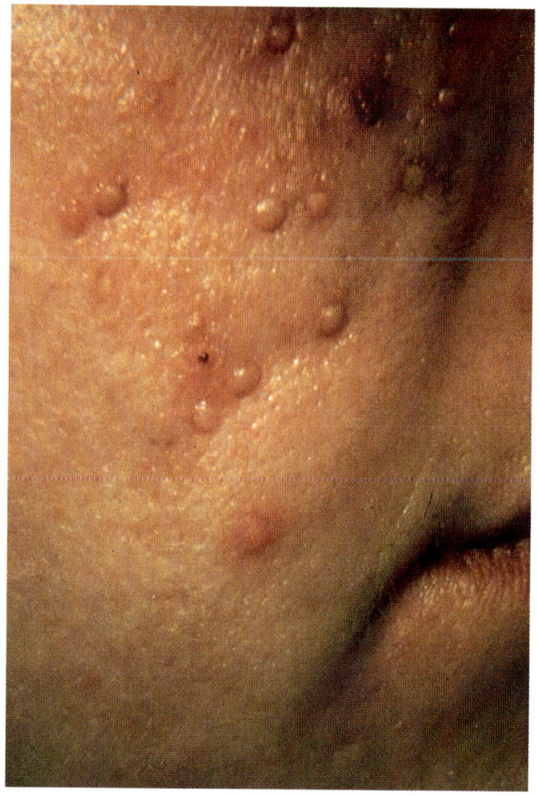

(*b*)

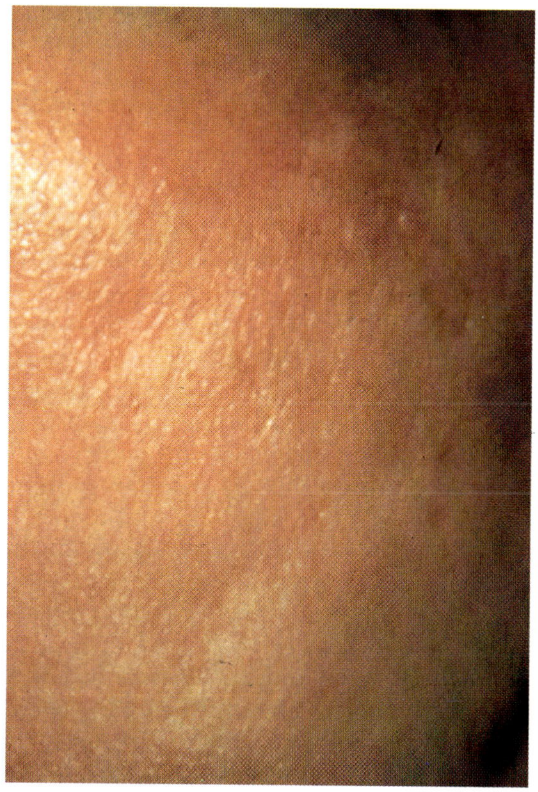

(*c*)

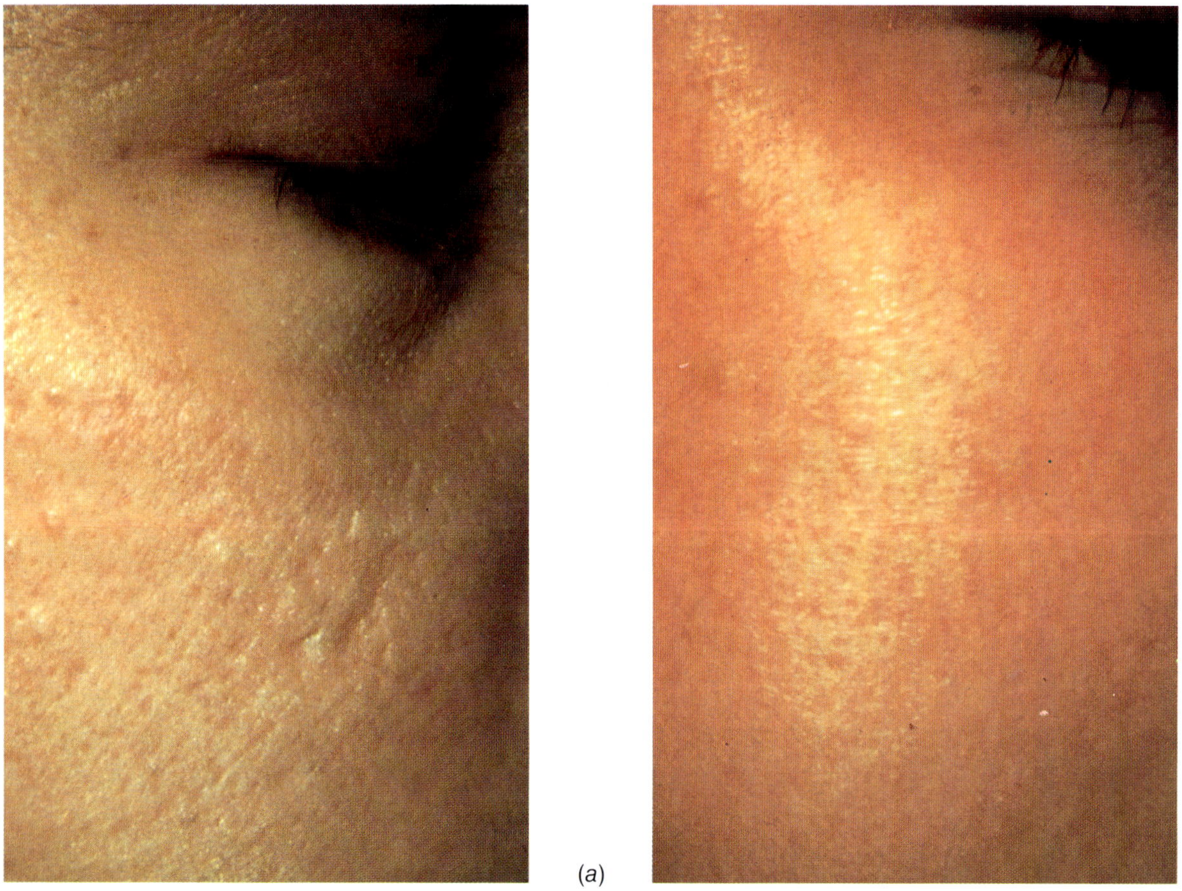

(a) (b)

FIGURE 13
(*a*) Before treatment; (*b*) after grafting and dermabrasion.

graft is depressed, it is probably best to regraft, although a slight depression can be corrected if a dermabrasion procedure is being performed. Soft tissue augmentation, such as a silicone injection, can also be used for slightly depressed grafts. A depressed groove may occur if the graft is too small or sustains trauma and pulls away from the adjacent skin. It is recommended that the physician regraft any defect as deep as 1 mm.

Problem areas for using the punch graft technique include the bearded area of men and the areas lateral to the angles of the mouth. In the bearded area of men, the initial punch excision must be parallel to the hair follicles to avoid the complication of ingrown hair or intracutaneous cysts secondary to the overgrowth of the epithelium surrounding the hair. The problem with areas at the angle of the mouth is related to the marked movement of the skin at these sites when the patient is talking or otherwise moving the facial muscles, making it difficult for the graft to take.

DERMABRASION

Abrasion of the skin has been used for the treatment of scars for many years. In the early 1950s, Abner Roenigk[6] used a wire brush motor-driven dermabrator and employed refrigeration to achieve anesthesia. He recommended this method for the improvement of acne scars, keratoses, wrinkles, and many other abnormalities. The extensive experience of James Burks' associates was published as a textbook in 1956.[7] As with any new procedure, this was very popular at first, but interest was lost to some extent when the degree of improvement was balanced against potential complications. In the past several years, this technique has again become popular because considerably greater improvement can be obtained when dermabrasion is used in association with other techniques, such as punch graft transplants and tissue augmentation. I began using the procedure in 1955 and have continued to use it.

Preoperative blood work on dermabrasion patients varies with each physician. Some prefer to obtain a complete blood count, Sequential Multiple Analyzer (SMA) panel, and bleeding and clotting panels. Some physicians test for hepatitis and human immunodeficiency virus infection.

Preoperative medication also varies greatly and includes secobarbital sodium, promethazine hydrochloride, prochlorperazine dimaleate, dimanhydrinate, diazepam, and midazolam Hcl (Versed). I usually prefer 10 mg of diazepam given orally and 75 to 100 mg of meperidine and 50 mg of dimenhydrinate given intramuscularly 30 min before the procedure. In addition, Versed may be given intravenously if needed at the start of the procedure.

Nerve block to the major facial nerves using xylocaine or bupivacaine hydrochloride is recommended. I sometimes use local infiltration to extend anesthesia away from the sites of the nerve blocks.

Equipment

The equipment developed and recommended by Roenigk[6] was a cable-driven dermabrator manufactured by the Robbins Instrument Company. The motor was connected to the hand piece by a flexible wire cable. In the past several years, advances in technology have led to the development of small electric engines that can be held by hand. This represents a considerable improvement in convenience to the operator. Some of the instruments available for use are listed in Table 3. Every operator has a personal preference. I use one of the older Dremel power tools, because the current models are larger than I like to hold. The operator and assistants should wear face shields.

It is absolutely necessary to have backup equipment available in case the instrument becomes defective while one is doing a dermabrasion procedure. It is often recommended that a grapefruit be used for practice or to develop the physician's technique prior to performing dermabrasion of human skin.

The endpieces or cutting tools include diamond fraises, wire brushes, and various types of serrated wheels.[8] In the 1950s and 1960s most operators used wire brushes, but diamond fraises are more popular today. Diamond fraises are less likely to cause grooves or gouges in the skin. I buy the coarsest grade of diamond fraise and select for a particular procedure a relatively new coarse or a used less coarse fraise.

TABLE 3
INSTRUMENTS AND SUPPLIES USED IN DERMABRASION

- Dermabrator
  - Motor driven
    - Bell International Hand Engine
    - Mill-Bilt Equipment Company
    - Robbins Instrument Company
    - Dremel Power Tool (hand-held unit)
  - Air-driven: Stryker Company
- End Piece
  - Fraises
  - Wire brush
- Gentian violet
- Syringe with 30-gauge needles
- Lidocaine 1% with epinephrine
- Pillow to position patient's head
- Sterile towels
- Hydrogen peroxide
- Bandaging materials

Procedure

The operating room should be relatively cool, and precooling of the patient's face may be done using cold packs. This probably is not necessary if adequate nerve blocks have been performed. Cotton should be used to prevent drainage into the patient's ears. A pillow should be placed under the head, neck, and shoulder areas so that the physician can position the patient differently when doing various parts of the face. It is desirable to keep the section of the face being operated on relatively flat and positioned so that liquid refrigerant will run away from the eyes. A number of spray refrigerants are available,[9] but I prefer diclorotetrafluoroethane (Frigiderm). Some of the newer and colder refrigerants are thought to have caused prolonged erythema, delayed healing, and scarring.[10] Sterile towels (dishcloth type) are used to protect adjacent areas and can be used to keep the skin firm during the abrading procedure. I prefer to do the freezing without stretch or pull on the skin and then maintain moderate pressure during the abrading procedure. I also use cotton gloves beneath the rubber gloves to provide insulation against the cold spray. The area to be dermabraded is painted with 1% gentian violet, which helps assure that dermabrasion is applied to all the designated areas.

Most operators visually or mentally mark the face into sections and approach the procedure in a uniform fashion. I prefer to begin in the preauricular area on the side of the face opposite the operator, proceed to the center of the face, do the forehead from the opposite side to the near side, do the near side beginning in the preauricular area, and finish with the nose and central areas of the face. Freezing of the forehead area tends to be painful and should be completed while the local anesthetic and sedation are still effective. Except for the peripheral areas, which are abraded lightly, I prefer to have the skin frozen "rock-like." The depth of the cut is determined by the degree of freezing, the speed of the cutting tool, and the downward pressure exerted by the operator. The plane of the section of the face being abraded should be relatively flat in relation to the operator's hand piece, although each operator develops a special technique. I prefer to do a full-face dermabrasion so that the "age appearance" of all areas of the face is similar, especially if there is significant damage from sunlight.

Postoperative Care

After the surgical procedure is completed, cold gauze is placed on the face for several minutes; a nonsticking surface (Telfa) dressing with a liberally applied topical antibiotic is placed over the abraded areas, and then a layer of gauze and an outer layer of conforming gauze bandage (Kling) are applied. A number of precut, preformed dressings are available for the outer dressings to make application simpler. A number of membrane materials are available to apply to the wound surface (Table 4).[11] These materials minimize postoperative pain and cause faster healing by keeping the skin surface moist. Disadvantages include the need for daily or frequent reapplication, and there is always a possibility of infection developing beneath the membrane. I prefer the older technique of applying an antibiotic and nonsticking surface dressing with regular bandaging and having the patient remove the bandage the following day. Cool compresses are recommended for 15 min four to six times a day after the dressings have been removed. Hexachlorophene (pHisohex) may be added to the compress solution to achieve detergent and antibacterial action. As the drainage diminishes, the patient uses a topical antibiotic to prevent drying and cracking of the crust. Liquids or soft foods are recommended. After the swelling has decreased (2 to 4 days), the cool compress is replaced by a warm compress.

Analgesics and antipruritic preparations are used as needed. Patients are usually seen in the office for examination at 1- and 2-week intervals. After the crusts have separated, topical steroids may be used to achieve antipruritic effects and to reduce the redness more rapidly.

TABLE 4
WOUND SURFACE DRESSINGS

1. Perforated plastic films with absorptive pad backing (Band-Aid, Telfa)
2. Hydrogel dressings (Vigilon, Second Skin)
3. Hydrocolloid dressings (Duoderm)
4. Adhesive polyurethane dressings (Op-Site, Tegaderm)

Source: Zitelli.[11]

Complications

Hypertrophic scar formation is the most common serious complication of a dermabrasion procedure. The cause is unknown, but the patient's genetic background (which may be related to darker pigmentation), the depth of the dermabrasion procedure, the depth of the freezing, and the anatomic site (over the jaw line) are possible causes. The first clue to a hypertrophic scar reaction is that the crust does not separate as quickly as the crusts on the rest of the face do. Another sign is increased redness in the involved areas, when palpation may reveal thickness. The reddened areas should be treated with a potent topical steroid, and as soon as evidence of increased thickness is noted intralesional steroids should be used. It is important to assure the patient that the increased thickness will become level after a variable period of time. The skin markings may be lost as a result of the scar formation, but the elevations will respond to intralesional steroids, topical steroids, and the passage of time. This may take up to 1 to 2 years and rarely longer, and the patient must be assured that the condition will continue to improve. In addition to the possible causes of hypertrophic scars mentioned above, a hypertrophic scar may occur even in very light-skinned individuals after a very superficial dermabrasion.

The second most important complication is pigmentation problems. *Hyperpigmentation* routinely occurs if a patient is exposed to sunlight during the first 2 to 4 months after dermabrasion. This almost always clears spontaneously over a period of several months. A more significant problem is *hypopigmentation*, which may remain as a permanent residual. This is more likely to be a problem in people with darker complexions. Patients should be advised to avoid sunlight as much as possible for the first few months after the dermabrasion procedure and to use sunscreens appropriately.

The most common complication is *milia* formation, but this may be treated by surgical removal, topical retinoic acid, or a peeling agent. The use of topical retinoic acid for 3 to 6 weeks before dermabrasion will reduce milia formation.

Contour defects such as grooving of the skin may occur if the operator does not use the proper technique. Such grooves may be prevented by appropriate steady strokes, strokes perpendicular to the initial strokes, or circular strokes.

An uncommon complication is fine telangiectasia, which usually regresses spontaneously but may require treatment. Telangiectasia almost always occurs in association with hypertrophic scar formation.

Rare complications may include various bacterial and viral infections of the skin.

CONCLUSION

The use of dermabrasion for the treatment of facial scarring has been greatly extended during the past few years in combination with other surgical techniques. Most commonly, these other techniques are removal of pitted scars by the punch graft transplant method and soft tissue augmentation for depressed or atrophic scars. Patients with large areas of atrophic depressed scars may require surgical excision of the scars and then punch graft transplants to remove the linear scars created. This is done in two procedures to remove the scar tissue completely and create overlapping grafts of normal skin. The use of these special techniques greatly extends the benefits which can be obtained from dermabrasion alone.

REFERENCES

1. Johnson WC. Treatment of pitted scars: Punch transplant techniques. J Dermatol Surg Oncol. 1986; 12:260–265.
2. Solotoff SA. Treatment for pitted acne scarring: Postauricular punch grafts followed by dermabrasion. J Dermatol Surg Oncol. 1986;12:1079–1084.
3. Johnson WC. Treatment of pitted scars: Punch-graft transplant technique. Am J Cosmet Surg. 1988;5:73–77.
4. Orentreich N, Durr NP. Rehabilitation of acne scarring. Dermatol Clin. 1983;1:405–413.
5. Johnson WC, Baker GK. Use of steel pins in hair transplantation. J Dermatol Surg Oncol. 1977;3:220–221.
6. Roenigk HH Jr. Dermabrasion, in Roenigk RK, Roenigk HH Jr. (eds) Dermatologic Surgery, New York: Marcel Dekker, 1989:959–978.
7. Burks JW. Wire Brush Surgery. Springfield, IL: Charles C Thomas, 1956.
8. Koranda FC. Dermabrasion, in Thomas JR, Holt GR (eds) Facial Scars: Incision, Revision & Camouflage, St. Louis: CV Mosby, 1989:123–136.
9. Hanke CW, O'Brian JJ, Solow EB. Laboratory evaluation of skin refrigerants used in dermabrasion. J Dermatol Surg Oncol. 1985;11:45–49.
10. Dzubow LM. Histologic and temperature alterations induced by skin refrigerants. J Am Acad Dermatol. 1985; 12:796–809.
11. Zitelli JA. Wound healing and wound dressings, in Roenigk RK, Roenigk HH Jr. (eds) Dermatologic Surgery. New York: Marcel Dekker, 1989:97–138.

CHAPTER

15

Facial Peeling: Phenol

ROBERT KOTLER

Chemical skin peeling (chemexfoliation) is an established technique for improving or erasing wrinkles, reducing superficial acne scarring, removing keratoses, and correcting pigment problems. When it is properly performed on well-selected patients, the results are very gratifying to both patient and physician.

The procedure relies on penetration of an escharotic agent into the skin. This results in sloughing of the superficial skin layers and evokes a nonspecific tissue regeneration, creating a smooth, more youthful-appearing skin. Sir Harold Gillies is recognized as the first physician-practitioner to employ the acid painting and taping techniques. He published the results of his work in 1957.[1] Further investigation followed including histologic studies by Kaplan and Brown (1960),[2] Litton (1962),[3] and Baker (1962).[4] By the mid-1960s, the procedure became an accepted treatment modality.[5]

The author's technique is based on principles taught by Richard Ariagno, M.D., Chicago, IL, and Jack P. Startz, M.D. (deceased), Beverly Hills, CA.

This chapter concentrates on the use of phenol, the peeling agent I have used extensively. (For an alternative method of facial peeling, see Chap. 16, which concentrates on tricholoracetic acid.)

INDICATIONS AND PATIENT SELECTION

Chemical skin peeling is indicated for any and all fine lines, wrinkles, keratoses, and pigmentary problems on any or all parts of the face. The areas most commonly demonstrating the more profound wrinkles are the upper and lower lips, forehead, and periorbital and glabellar regions.

Some patients are better candidates than others. The best candidate is of fair complexion with thin, dry skin and with no or minimal pigmentation. Generally, blond and red-haired women with green or blue eyes are considered more favorable candidates because of their intrinsically lighter pigmentation. Men, because of the potential for an end color difference between treated and untreated areas, are rarely ideal candidates. While chemical skin peeling is not a substitute for surgery of redundant tissue about the eyelids, neck, and jawline, frequently some improvement in such sagging tissues may be realized.

Patients who are not suitable candidates for the procedure have thick oily skin, with dark complexion. Those with a history of reactive pigmentation to previous surgical procedures, including dermabrasion, should be approached with caution. Proceed more cautiously with those who have a history of very large doses of radiation to the face or long-term topical steroid treatment that resulted in dermal atrophy. Thinning of the dermis may follow chemexfoliation, and this, superimposed on a preexisting thinned dermis, may give an unacceptably thin and shiny appearance to the skin. This is often a telltale sign of the chemical skin peel. The potential for increased pigmentation after the administration of oral contraceptives or postmenopausal supplementation hormones must always be considered.

A hedge against uncertainty of pigmentary response can be provided by a "patch" or sample test of phenol, at a concealed site such as the frontal hairline. This test area should be observed for 10 to 12 weeks.

Patients may be disqualified for medical reasons. For example, because phenol, the most frequently employed major agent, requires conjugation by the kidneys, patients with borderline or poor kidney function are not candidates. Likewise, patients with cardiac and hepatic insufficiency are not candidates, in deference to the recognized potential cardiotoxic effect of phenol and detoxification of anesthetic agents by the liver. Because phenol is an irritant, allergic reactions do occur.

A person with thick and porous skin who expects some improvement in the general skin texture from the chemexfoliative procedure may be disappointed. In my experience, this result has been unpredictable; even when the procedure is done aggressively, the pores are often still visible and the patient may not be satisfied. The procedure should not be performed on skin involved in eyelid or face and neck lifting within 10 to 12 weeks after surgery; tissue edema and wound immaturity often persist for this period. While some practitioners advocate peeling the skin that has been undermined in a face and neck lift, I see this as unwise, having witnessed several unfortunate consequences of this practice. It is illogical to assume that the skin will heal ideally after being undermined and thus deprived of its blood supply and concomitantly undergoing an assault to its surface by the chemexfoliative agents. The dictum so frequently employed by wise cosmetic surgeons should be heeded: "When you are not sure, don't" (Kazanjian).

TISSUE CHANGES INDUCED BY CHEMICAL SKIN PEELING

Numerous investigators have vividly documented the histologic changes in the skin following application of chemexfoliative agents.[4,5,7,12] Phenol has been the most frequently employed agent, with concentrations ranging from 30 to 90 percent. Additives have included croton oil, cresol, olive oil, sesame oil, sodium salicylate, camphor, anhydrous glycerin, and ethanol with or without a saponifying agent. Likewise, techniques have employed both occlusive taping and lack of it for specific treatments. Seemingly paradoxically, a more dilute concentration of phenol is a stronger chemexfoliative agent. Spira et al.,[6] in their study in which varying concentrations of phenol were used, concluded that "phenol concentrations of 50% or more all had a similar effect on the . . . skin." At this concentration, maximum coagulation usually occurred with no further penetration by any higher concentration. The use of the soap or detergent as a wetting agent and the use of occlusive dressings seem to have a bearing on the penetration and clinical effect of the peeling agent. Mullins and Lettiere[7] contended that waterproof tape prevents evaporation of the phenol and macerates the underlying skin, thereby increasing penetration. This may also, of course, increase systemic absorption.

Chemical cauterization induces a limited destruction of the corium, not dissimilar to the injury produced by a thermal burn, hastening formation of new collagen beneath the basal layer of the epidermis.[18] It is accepted that the gross changes in the appearance of the epidermal surface result from replacements in the papillary layer of the corium with young collagen and from an increased vascularity.[18]

ANESTHESIA

Until 3 years ago, in our practice, chemical face peels were performed with the patient under intravenous sedation. A small number of arrhythmias occurred, none of which proved difficult to control. Since converting to general endotracheal anesthesia with full monitoring devices, such as electrocardiograph, pulse oxymetry, and end-tidal CO_2 monitoring, we have seen a marked decrease in the incidence of arrhythmias. We attribute this to the more efficient exchange of oxygen and carbon dioxide as well as less dependency on narcotic analgesics in general endotracheal anesthesia. We have hypothesized that cardiac arrhythmia is more likely to occur under intravenous sedation than under general endotracheal anesthesia with assisted ventilation for the following reasons:

1. Sedatives, particularly barbiturates and benzodiazepines, tend to depress respiration, leading to hypoxia and hypercarbia, both of which predispose to arrhythmia.
2. Narcotic analgesics likewise depress respiration with the same potential ventilatory and cardiac consequences.
3. A sedated, but not unconscious, patient, made uncomfortable by the application of the chemicals, particularly under the influence of sedative agents, may become restless, agitated, and uninhibited—behavior which will overlap with the ensuing hypoxic restlessness. Such a scenario can occur with subsequent increased cardiac irritability, arrhythmias, and hypertension.
4. The combination of increased endogenous catecholamines causing cardiac sensitization and hypercapnia and hypoxia secondary to respiratory depression portends a dangerous trend of circumstances.

Therefore, a well-ventilated patient under general endotracheal anesthesia is less likely to develop arrhythmias during the application of the phenol peeling solution.

OPERATIVE TECHNIQUE

Preoperative Counseling: 2 Weeks Prior to Procedure

Patients are routinely seen 2 weeks prior to the scheduled date of procedure. Prior to this preoperative visit, they will have had a preoperative medical consultation and clearance by their personal physician. That examination should minimally include basic history and physical examination, complete blood count, urinalysis, and determination of creatinine level. An electrocardiogram or chest x-ray is needed at the discretion of the consulting physician. Our office provides a checklist form for the consultant to complete.

At the preoperative visit, the sequence of events on the day of the procedure is explained in detail to the patient. Consent forms are signed. The patient is given a prescription for a hexachlorophene detergent cleanser (pHisoHex) to be used as facial soap and shampoo for the 5 days prior to the procedure. The patient is advised to eat or drink nothing after midnight the day before the procedure and that the anesthesiologist will call the patient the evening prior to the procedure to obtain another history and discuss the anesthetic.

Preoperative Preparation: Day of Procedure

The surgical nurse reviews the history and results of the physical examination. Careful examination is performed for any signs of infection. The patient is then taken to the preoperative holding area, where the hair is restrained. An intravenous line of a 5% dextrose and balanced salt solution is started by the surgical nurse or anesthesiologist. The patient is then placed in the sitting position on the operating room table. The operator, using a surgical marking pen, delineates the inferior limit of the procedure (Fig. 1), while the patient is sitting;

FIGURE 1
Deepest wrinkling about eyes and mouth. Note blue marking line to delineate inferior limit of application.

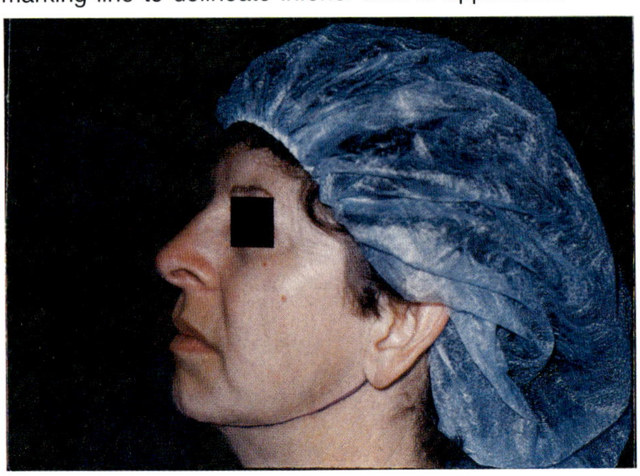

otherwise, normal anatomic landmarks may be misconstrued. Ideally, the line should be placed beneath the visible inferior mandibular margin; if a color demarcation between the treated face and the untreated neck develops, it should be concealed in the "shadow" of the mandible. Patients of lean habitus with prominent mandibles afford the ideal circumstance for concealing this "zone of transition."

Next the patient is placed in the supine position. All electrocardiographic leads, pulse oxymeter, and CO_2 monitor are attached; the anesthesiologist induces general endotracheal anesthesia. The surgical nurse then washes the face with surgical soap and uses acetone or other skin degreaser to remove residual oils from the skin.

Technique of Chemical Application

For extremely deep, craggy lines of the glabella, nasolabial creases of cheeks or forehead, a pretreatment with 50% trichloracetic acid (TCA) to these specific lines is performed (Fig. 2). Extreme caution

FIGURE 2
First application is 50% trichloracetic acid to deep glabellar creases, periorbital wrinkles, and upper lip.

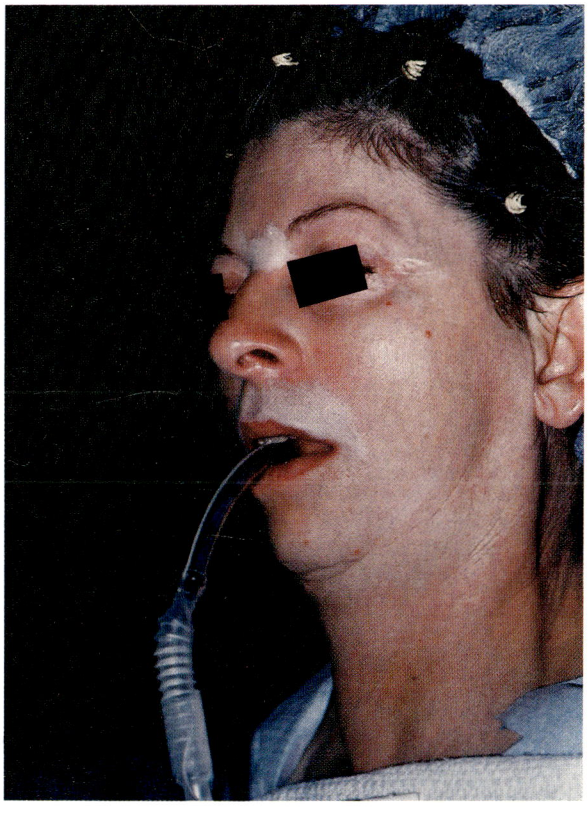

TABLE 1
BAKER'S FORMULA FOR PHENOL SOLUTION

Phenol, liquid USP	3 cc
Water, distilled	2 cc
Croton oil	3 drops
Soap, liquid	8 drops

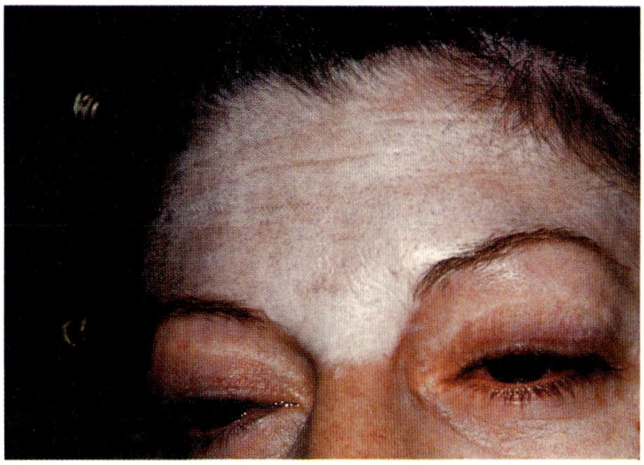

FIGURE 3
Glabellar and forehead areas treated with phenol solution. Frost appears in a few minutes.

against overapplication is advised. In the very thick-skinned patient, overapplication of TCA can result in overthinning of the stratum corneum in those areas pretreated with TCA. This could manifest as a contour discrepancy that cannot be concealed.

The phenol solution, prepared in the manner of Baker,[5,14] and shown in Table 1, is applied with a cotton-tipped swab (Fig. 3). I prefer to perform the procedure in a staged manner, with given aesthetic zones being treated sequentially. The forehead zone is treated first, beginning with the glabella and inferior forehead. The application continues in a cephalic direction until the hairline is reached. Great care must be taken to apply the solution well beyond the first rows of hair, to avoid a visible area of untreated scalp at the hairline. As classically described, the endpoint of chemical application occurs when the skin develops a chalk-white color, the so-called frost. A lesser number of applications or applications using a less moist applicator will result in a less profound white frost, indicating less dense penetration and a "weaker" peel. Strive for uniformity of application as judged by the consistency of the white color. The white color gradually

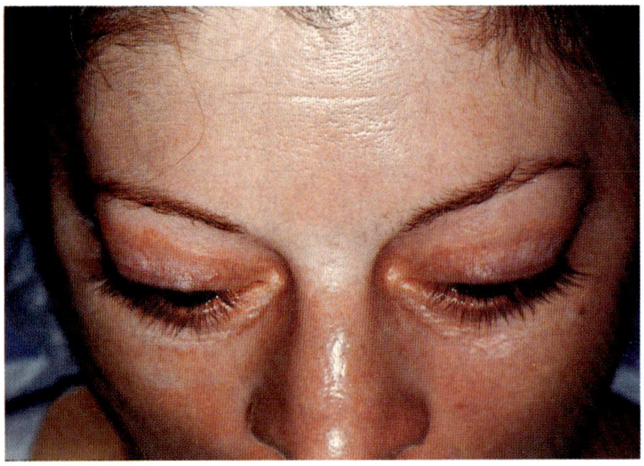

FIGURE 4
After frost disappears, edema of treated forehead skin gives a waxen appearance.

disappears over 5 to 10 min; the skin appears pinker, shows signs of early edema, and has a waxen appearance, as in Fig. 4. Schedule a rest break for 10 min or more. This diminishes the clearance load to the excretory organs. Phenol toxicity is related to blood level, the latter being a function of application dose and time.

Treat the nose and orbital areas next, beginning with the eyebrow and infrabrow skin. (There is no untoward effect on hair follicles.) The application is carried inferiorly from the brow to the supratarsal crease. The eyelid skin below the crease is usually not peeled, because this tissue is almost never wrinkled. Applications to the lower eyelid skin must avoid inadvertently touching the globe. To minimize such occurrence, the operator or assistant should retract the cheek downward, allowing the lower lid to detract from the globe. Simultaneous elevation of the upper lid by an assistant gains additional exposure for the operator. The identical procedure is then performed on the opposite side. To ensure against "skip" on untreated areas, the chemical solution application onto a given zone should overlap the adjacent, previously treated zone.

Following treatment of the nose and both periorbital areas, the forehead will have lost its whitish color. An efficient use of the break time between chemical application is to apply dressings to a previously treated zone, if needed. Dressing application will be discussed separately.

Now treat the left cheek, extending medially to the nasolabial crease. After a 10-min pause, the right cheek zone receives the peel solution; the tragus and earlobe are treated next, and the final zone is the upper and lower lip and chin areas.

Allow a minimum of 1 hr for application to the entire face. Because faces come in various sizes, of course, you can expect to take longer and to apply more solution to the patient with the larger facial surface area. Total operative time, including anesthesia induction and emergence and dressing application, may be 2 hr. The anesthesiologist administers 1 liter of fluid over a 2- to 3-hr period for an average 60- to 70-kg patient.

Technique of Occlusive Dressing Application

It is an axiom in chemical skin peeling that if you want deeper penetration in areas of more profound wrinkling, such areas mandate occlusion.

The concept of occlusion has been modified recently to include occlusion with adhesive tapes. Some experienced practitioners have been satisfied with petrolatum coating instead of tape.[9] Such a technique obviates the need for a separate dressing removal session. We are currently comparing this nontaping technique with taping those areas where the "extra-strength" medicated plaster occlusive dressing (below) is not indicated. Traditionally, we have used white waterproof tape in a minimum of four layers to all areas that seem to need moderately aggressive peeling. Often, significant portions of the face may not require such an aggressive technique. Therefore, the dressing is customized for each patient. In our experience with a quite sun-damaged population, 20 percent of patients will require dressings to the entire face.

For patients who have profoundly deep wrinkles, particularly in the glabellar, periorbital, or perioral areas, it has been our experience that a very aggressive taping technique is needed to produce a superior result. The use of a medicated plaster tape containing methyl salicylate, menthol, camphor, and glycol salicylate apparently yields better results by causing additional irritation and maceration of the skin. This becomes the "first layer" of tape and is then covered by the standard white waterproof tape mask. It must be emphasized that as the reward and satisfaction of removing nearly all the wrinkles become greater, the attendant potential risks of delayed healing and of scarring also increase. However, this remains a proven technique for eliminating the deepest wrinkles that are otherwise not removable. This medicated plaster tape, marketed as Salonpas, is made in Japan and is generally available through Oriental food stores, where it is sold for "temporary relief of minor muscular aches and pains."

Tapes may be applied in the same "zone" manner used for the application of the chemical peeling solution. If one chooses to use an adhesive, various adhesives are appropriate including the aerosol spray adhesives frequently used to apply Elastoplast dressings or commercial-grade rubber cement (see Fig. 5). After the application of the waterproof tape layers (Figs. 6 and 7), two additional layers of pink Hy-Tape may be applied (see Fig. 8). This plastic tape is an excellent outer layer since it resists staining and may be washed.

To achieve maximum chemexfoliation, the skin surface should not be allowed to dry out; taping

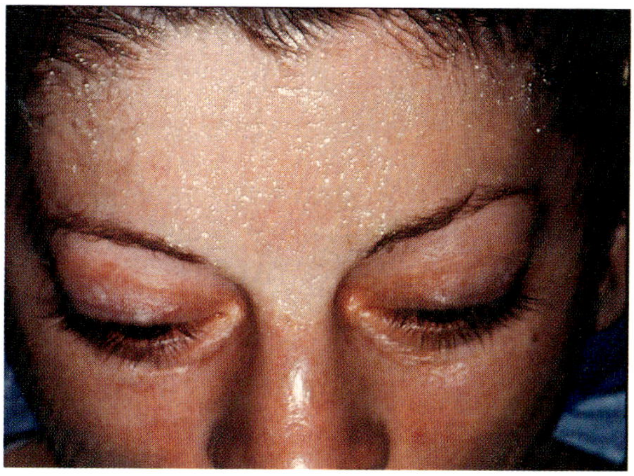

FIGURE 5
Adhesive is applied to forehead zone.

FIGURE 6
Waterproof adhesive tape is applied to forehead zone, in four layers with overlapping edges.

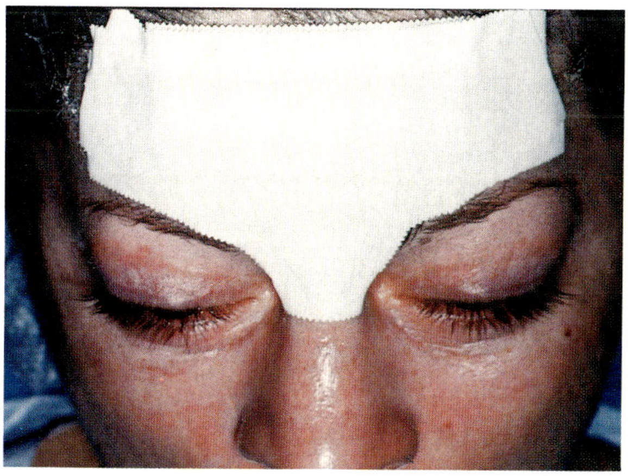

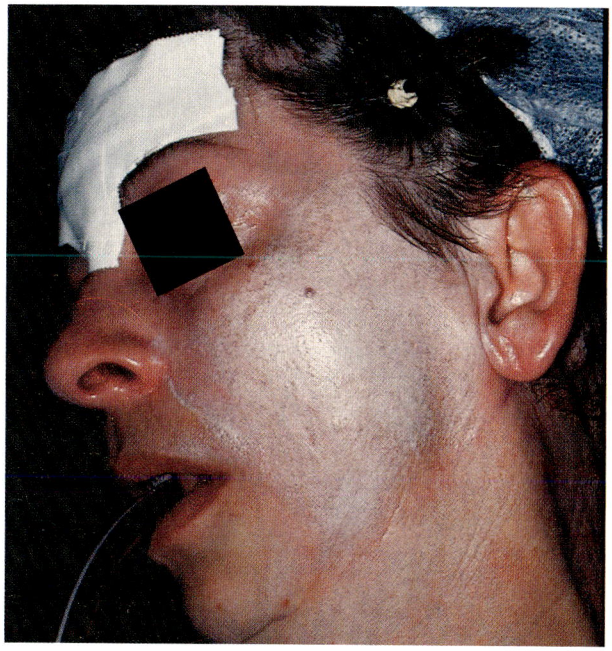

FIGURE 7
Forehead zone has been occluded. Periorbital zone has been treated, and frost has disappeared. Now the cheek zone receives application. Note that application is carried into hairline.

FIGURE 8
After solution applied to cheek has been absorbed, occlusive dressing is applied to crow's feet area. Then final area to receive application is lip/mouth zone. Note that final layer of plastic coated tape has been applied to forehead zone.

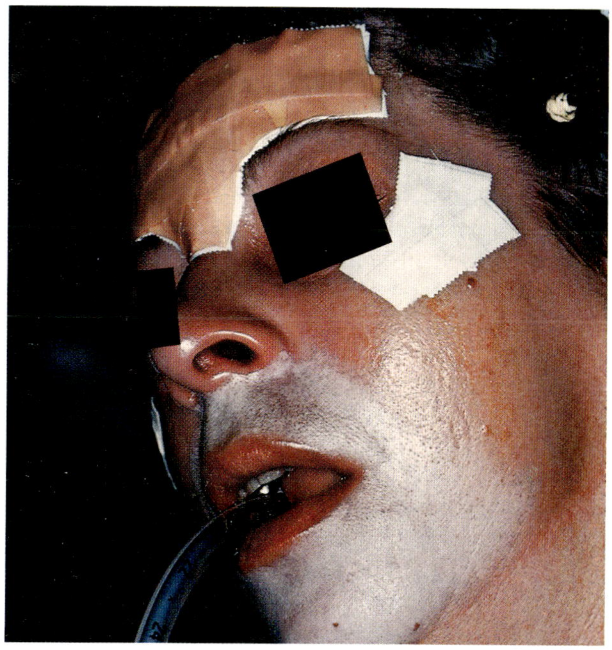

TABLE 2
FACIAL REJUVENATION POSTTREATMENT INSTRUCTIONS

Days 1 and 2:	The dressings, if placed, stay on the skin. Liquids per straw only. No chewing. Skin not covered by dressings turns dark and becomes dry. The face and neck are normally swollen.
Day 3:	If your face has any dressings on it, you will have them removed in the office, usually under a brief anesthetic; *do not* eat or drink anything after 11 p.m. the evening before coming to the office. Some areas may be redressed for another 24 hours. Today we begin covering the entire face with the triple antibiotic ointment. Swelling begins to subside. "Weeping" may still be present.
Day 4:	Continue to apply the antibiotic ointment to the entire face. Ointment should be applied as often as necessary to keep entire treated area covered at all times. This ointment helps to soften and remove the old skin.
Day 5:	Begin to wash off remaining crust with Ivory soap and water. If some crust remains, keep applying ointment to soften. Wash several times during the day and apply ointment to keep skin from being dry. Continue this process until all the "crust" is off. This may take another day or so.
After day 5:	We shall set an appointment for you to be seen.

must be meticulously done. Careful overlapping of the edges provides the most effective airtight seal. Patients are given posttreatment instructions, as in Table 2.

Dressing Change

I usually remove the dressings 48 hr after application. It may be appropriate to remove the dressings after 24 hr; previously peeled skin and very thin atrophic skin require greater caution and hence a more conservative taping approach. Certainly, it is technically easier to remove the dressing at 48 hr, by which time there has been liquefaction of the chemexfoliated skin which allows the dressing to spontaneously loosen from the face.

I treat the patient with intravenous sedation for the 5 to 10 min that it takes to remove the dressing, cleanse the skin of the desquamated and necrotic epithelium, and perform general tidying about the face and neck. We are currently evaluating the efficacy of a light abrasion of the denuded skin and using gauze sponges to further enhance the chemexfoliation (see Fig. 9). This can be an alternative to retaping or even lightly repeeling and retaping of those areas requiring the most radical treatment, for example, deep glabellar or transverse forehead furrows. The weeping is stopped by using a hair dryer. Triple antibiotic ointment is then applied. Our practice is to have the anesthesiologist perform the intravenous sedation, although with proper monitoring equipment and experience the

FIGURE 9
After mask removal, skin is given light abrasion and is dried. Triple antibiotic ointment is being applied here.

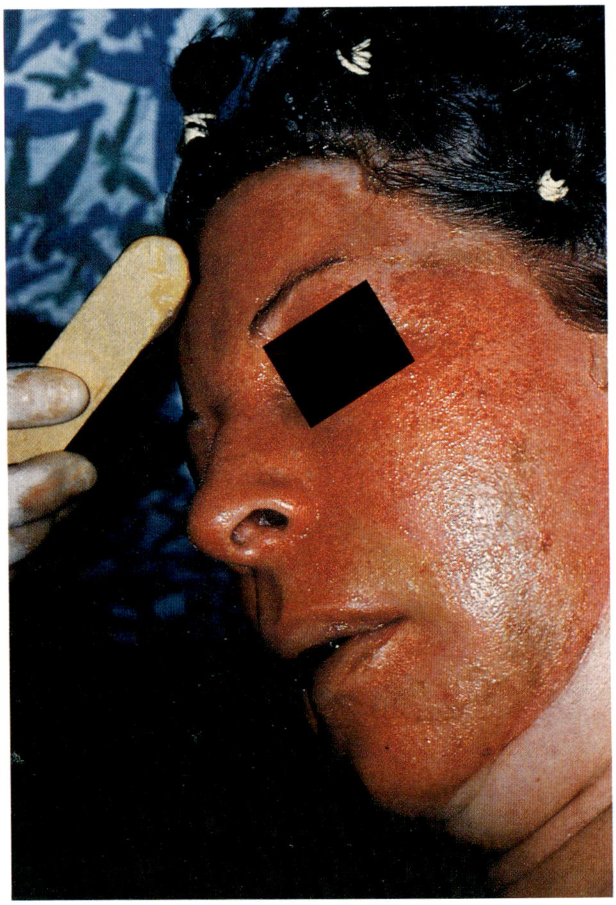

operator may choose to perform the procedure independently. Patients recover for an appropriate time and are then discharged to home, with appropriate supplies and instructions.

Aftercare for the Next 4 Days

We do not routinely use thymol iodide powder, preferring to coat the skin with triple antibiotic ointment. This shortens the time between dressing removal and erasure of the crust that forms on the skin surface. Our timetable calls for 2 days' continuous application of triple antibiotic ointment, followed by 2 days of several showers a day and using Ivory soap to remove the crust from the face. What crusting remains after these washings is treated again with the triple antibiotic ointment. Generally within 48 hr of beginning the washing, over 95 percent of the face is free of crust. Those areas most apt to remain crusted are the crow's feet, forehead, and mouth. Generally these areas will have been treated more aggressively, evoking a deeper peel process, hence development of a thicker crust. The patients are comfortable, do not require pain medication, and complain only of a sunburn-like sensation. This may be relieved with a mild anti-inflammatory medication such as aspirin, acetaminophen, or a nonsteroidal anti-inflammatory agent.

The 1-Week Visit

An appointment is always made to see the patient 6 or 7 days after the application day. By this time the entire face is clear of the crust and appears bright pink and dry. The patient is asked to begin a program of skin care after rejuvenation. You may want to deliver a single intramuscular dose of long-acting steroid, particularly if the patient is beginning to itch. Our center's pharmacy compounds 2.5% hydrocortisone in Aquaphor ointment. There are no additional ingredients such as alcohols or propylene glycol, which are frequently found in commercial preparations. The patient is advised to use this at least once a day. Those who will not be returning to work or venturing forth into the world may use the hydrocortisone ointment preparation continuously. This provides moisturization and some degree of anti-inflammatory effect. Patients often complain of itching, beginning 10 to 14 days after the procedure is performed. A prescription is given for trimeprazine (Temaril) 2.5 mg 4 times a day. We have recently added nonsteroidal anti-inflammatory agents to the regimen and are currently evaluating the efficacy of this additional treatment. For those patients for whom itching becomes intolerable and who complain of the tightness and soreness of the skin, we have frequently resorted to a 6-day course of methylprednisolone (Medrol Dose Pak) for excellent relief of symptoms. Generally the most trying time for patients will be in the second and third weeks of the process when the skin is quite red, often itchy, and dry and when patients think they will be destined to endure this forever (Fig. 10). They must be reassured that the pink color will fade, the skin will become less sensitive, and the itching will disappear. Often I have asked patients who are veterans of the experience to talk with the new patient, which provides a sense of support and rejuvenates morale.

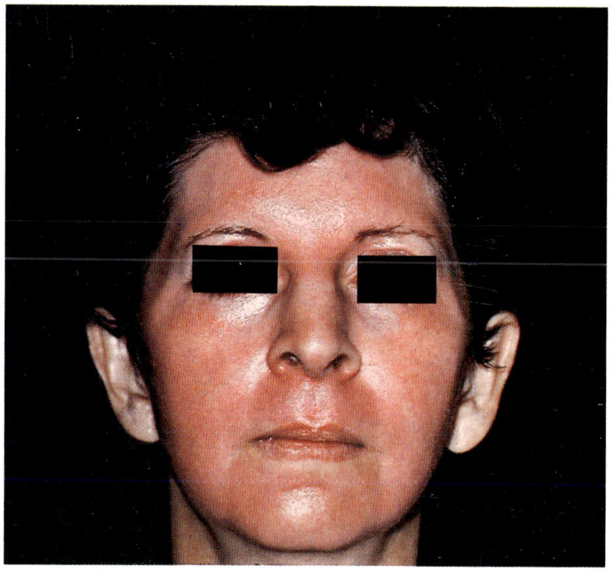

FIGURE 10
The patient 2 weeks after rejuvenation.

Skin Care after Rejuvenation—Long-Term Management

I believe that patients need education concerning the long-term optimal management of the skin following the procedure. For this reason, we provide them with a starter kit of products that have proved reliable and are not apt to cause sensitivity. This includes a sunscreen that does not contain PABA, a hypoallergenic moisturizer, and an emollient oil for those for whom dry skin has always been a problem. I advise against using soap, preferring lipophilic cleansing lotions (Cetaphil, CAM).

Patients are urged to apply the moisturizer during the day as an integral part of their makeup technique. Pamphlets concerning skin care are included in our starter kit. Also, the office staff gives advice on cosmetic techniques, particularly those needed to obscure the red hue of the skin.

We see the patient at least twice in the first month. This gives us a chance to be aware of any problems, complications, or dissatisfactions. Our instruction sheet provides a list of the most common side effects or possible complications, for example, milia or pigment formation. Generally, the peak incidence for milia is in the sixth to eighth week after the process. Pigmentary problems have been observed as early as 2 to 3 weeks after the process, particularly in those who were obviously predisposed to such. The management of these problems is discussed in the following section. The patients are told to expect 8 to 12 weeks to elapse before the redness will disappear and that ultimately the skin color of their face may be lighter than that of their neck. I show photographs of patients with an obvious demarcation between the face and the neck, both with and without makeup, so they can understand that this is not necessarily an insurmountable or unacceptable result of the procedure.

COMPLICATIONS

Atrophy

Depending on the aggressiveness of the procedure, that is, the strength of solution, application of occlusive dressings, and so forth, there may be atrophy of the skin. Thus, repeat skin peels are to be avoided or performed in a very conservative manner. Obviously, a thicker-skinned patient will have greater latitude and will tolerate more procedures.

Scarring

Scarring remains the most feared complication of chemical skin peeling. Unquestionably, its development is related to the depth of dermal injury produced by the chemexfoliative process. Therefore, it is most likely to occur in areas where more potent solutions have been generously applied and where the skin has been occluded. Intercurrent infection, which deepens the level of tissue injury, will predispose to such scarring.

Several experienced practitioners have observed that scarring almost always occurs on the lower third of the face. Perhaps this is related to the greater amount of tissue movement during eating and speaking. My personal observation has been that those patients whose mouths habitually widen greatly during speaking, who gesticulate with very broad lip and mouth movements, have more prolonged posttreatment perioral stiffness and edema.

The incidence of hypertrophic scarring can be reduced nearly to zero if early warning signs such as persistent induration and edema of tissues are aggressively treated, particularly with topical steroids. A high-potency topical steroid is extremely effective in reversal of that persistent induration and edema which may predispose to scarring. The medication must be used twice daily for 2 weeks, at which time the patient is reevaluated. I have used it "prophylactically" in those patients who appeared to be at higher risk for scarring, as manifested by persistent redness and induration of the tissues. Whether any of these patients would have necessarily gone on to develop hypertrophic scars is uncertain, but the treatment has been successful in early resolution of those prognostically unfavorable findings. Should such scarring actually manifest, intralesional steroids should immediately be injected and reinjected until the scar disappears. Surgical excision and repair are less favorable modalities and should be reserved for those cases that fail to respond to more conservative treatment.

The two patients in my experience who developed perioral hypertrophic scars both failed to report for routine posttreatment evaluations. Had they been seen, perhaps early intervention could have prevented frank scar formation.

Color Change, Demarcation Line, and Depigmentation

It must be accepted that with more aggressive peel procedures, there will be some change in the skin color, with hypopigmentation being most uncommon. Less commonly, some patients, thought to be ideal candidates with no evidence of predisposition to increased pigmentation, may develop focal or diffuse hyperpigmentation. It has been well said that "the only thing which can be stated with certainty about color changes in chemical skin peeling is that there will be some."[21]

Hyperpigmentation can manifest extremely early, even within the first 2 weeks after the procedure has been performed. Unquestionably the gradation in color change is related to the aggressiveness of the procedure.

At the first signs of increased pigment formation in the skin, the areas may be treated with topical steroids, topical bleaching agents such as hydroquinone, or both. The Kligman bleach cream compound,[11] which includes topical steroid, retinoic acid, and a hydroquinone, may be used for those cases that defy more conservative treatment. Obviously, sun exposure may precipitate the development of hyperpigmentation, and therefore a nonsensitizing sunscreen or sun block should be an essential ingredient in postpeel skin care. It is of the utmost importance that patients be aware of the hazards of sun exposure in the early posttreatment period, particularly during the summer months when sun intensity is strongest.

Those patients whose skin has been particularly darkened and weathered by sun exposure will most often demonstrate a significant line of demarcation between the treated areas of the face and the untreated area of the neck. This disparity in color will be most noticeable if the patient's habitus is such that there is no strong cervicomental angle whose shadow will conceal the line of demarcation. We are currently evaluating the efficacy of retinoic acid (Retin-A) to "soften" the zone of transition.

I am unaware of a specific technique of chemical application which can completely "feather," and hence make invisible to the eye, this line of demarcation. It is generally best concealed by satisfactory makeup techniques.

Should one choose to peel the neck, the same dilemma of a line of demarcation at the cervicothoracic junction exists. This line of demarcation may be even more difficult to conceal than that between the face and the neck. Therefore, patients who usually cannot (such as men) or will not consider applying cosmetics should be strongly advised against having the procedure performed.

Persistent Redness

Some patients will endure prolonged redness of the treated areas. This is generally related to the aggressiveness of the procedure. Nonetheless, even in some patients on whom the procedure may be more conservatively performed, there is persistent redness which is a source of great consternation. Sun exposure and applications of photosensitizing agents including cosmetics may be responsible for the prolonged erythema. Whether topical steroids hasten resolution is uncertain. Those patients who have the fairest skin are less likely to have prolonged redness; conversely, those who are quite ruddy can anticipate such prolonged redness. In my experience, 6 to 8 weeks is our minimum "fade time" prediction. A minority of patients will take up to 3 or 4 months.

Infection

Prior to the availability of oral acyclovir (Zovirax), the incidence of herpes simplex was not insignificant and a cause of great consternation to both patient and physician. Currently many practitioners prescribe prophylactic acyclovir 200 mg 5 times daily, beginning the day prior to the procedure and continuing for up to 7 to 10 days after the procedure. This has nearly eliminated the threat.

Pyogenic infections remain quite rare because of the inherent resistance of the facial skin to infection, particularly with the increased vascular supply attendant to the procedure. Should there be any signs of incipient infection, aggressive treatment with topical or systemic antibiotics is indicated.

Pore Size Change

Peeling less than the entire face is often not satisfactory because of resultant regional texture differences. Patients requesting regional skin peels fail to appreciate that while the treated skin will be satisfactory, the adjacent untreated areas will offer a texture contrast to the eye. For this reason, patients with large pores must be advised that pore size may increase as a result of the "planing" effect of the process or that the pores may become more obvious as the other unsatisfactory elements of the skin, including the wrinkling and keratoses, are no longer present to distract the eye.

Itching and Burning

A significant number of patients develop annoying itching, usually in the first 2 weeks after treatment. Antihistamines may be effective. Topical steroids may reduce this postinflammatory reaction. Aspirin and nonsteroidal anti-inflammatory agents may also be helpful in relieving the symptom. Most patients are reassured to know that it is a temporary phenomenon that generally peaks at 2 to 3 weeks after the procedure. Low-level pain medication is also advisable, and in some patients one must combine all or several of the above drug modalities to relieve this itching, which distracts from the pleasure of the result.

Milia

Milia, or small inclusion cysts, occur with unpredictable incidence. The peak incidence seems to be between 6 and 8 weeks after the process has been performed. In some patients there may be 50 to 100 or more of these, if the entire face has been treated. Although most will disappear spontaneously after several months, for those patients who find the situation unacceptable, each cyst may be "shucked" from its bed. The skin is then treated with topical antibiotics until reepithelialization has taken place.

CONCLUSION

Chemical skin peeling is a reliable, effective modality for the treatment of wrinkles and other signs of aging. With proper patient selection and appropriate technique, the level of satisfaction for both patient and physician can be extremely high.

REFERENCES

1. Gillies HD, Millard DR. The Principles and Art of Plastic Surgery. Boston: Little, Brown, 1957;403.
2. Brown AM, Kaplan LM, Brown MG. Phenol-induced histological skin changes: Hazards, technique and uses. Br J Plast Surg. 1960;13:158–169.
3. Litton C. Chemical face lifting. Plast Reconstr Surg. 1962;92:371–380.
4. Baker TJ. Chemical face peeling and rhitidectomy. Plast Reconstr Surg. 1962;29:199–207.
5. Baker TJ, Gordon HL, Seckinger D. A second look at chemical face peeling. Plast Reconstr Surg. 1966;37:47–48.
6. Spira M, Dahl C, Freeman R, et al. Chemosurgery: A histological study. Plast Reconstr Surg. 1970;45:247–253.
7. Mullens JF, Lettiere MD. Chemosurgery of facial wrinkles. Texas Med J. 1963;59:488–495.
8. Baker TJ, Gordon HL. Chemical face peeling and dermabrasion. Surg Clin N Am. 1971;1:387–401.
9. Collins P. Personal communication.
10. Stegman S. Personal communication.
11. Kligman AM, Willis I. A new formula for depigmenting skin. Arch Dermatol. 1975;111:40–48.
12. Aronsohn RB. Complications of chemosurgery. Eye, Ear, Nose and Throat Month. 1972;51:48–56.
13. Aronsohn RB. Facial chemosurgery. Eye, Ear, Nose and Throat Month. 1971;50:20–28.
14. Baker T, Gordon H. Chemical face peeling, in Surgical Rejuvenation of the Face. St. Louis: CV Mosby, 1986: Chap. 3.
15. Coopman CF Jr. Phenol toxicity during face peels. Otolaryngol, Head, Neck Surg. 1982;90:383–388.
16. Litton C. Observations after chemosurgery of the face. Plast Reconstr Surg. 1963;32:554–556.
17. Litton C, Fournier P, Capinpin A. A survey of chemical peeling of the face. Plast Reconstr Surg. 1973;51:645–647.
18. McCollough EG, Beeson WH. Chemical peel, in McCollough E (ed), Aesthetic Surgery of the Aging Face. St. Louis: CV Mosby, 1986:182–212.
19. McCollough EG, Hillman, RA. Chemical face peel. Otolaryngol Clin N Am. 1980;13:353–365.
20. Spira M, Gerow FJ, Hardy SB. Complications of chemical face peeling. Plast Reconstr Surg. 1974;54:397–403.
21. Stegman S, Tromovitch T. Chemical peels, in Cosmetic Dermatologic Surgery. Chicago: Year Book, 1984:27–45.

CHAPTER

16

Facial Peeling: Trichloroacetic Acid

STEVEN S. GREENBAUM
GARY P. LASK

Trichloroacetic acid (TCA) has been in the dermatologist's armamentarium for many years. TCA can be used in high concentrations to destroy localized skin lesions such as actinic keratoses, seborrheic keratoses, and xanthelasma. It has also been used to treat diffuse conditions such as mild inflammatory acne, melasma, and other variegated pigment abnormalities.[1,2]

TCA is commonly employed for chemical peeling of the face. (For an alternative method of facial peeling, see Chapter 15, which concentrates on the use of phenol.) TCA differs from phenol in that it is less toxic, does not require as much stringent monitoring, and often requires less sedation.

Chemical peeling may be classified as superficial, medium, or deep. TCA in strengths of 10 to 20 percent is used for light peels. For medium peels, TCA is used in concentrations of 20 to 40 percent. The effect of these peels is temporary, and they may be repeated every 4 to 6 months to obtain a cumulative affect. TCA 40 to 50 percent is used for deep peels. Medium and deep peels are used primarily to treat actinic damage and pigment abnormalities. Fine wrinkling, mottled pigmentation, leathery texture, gently folded skin, and the localized pigment abnormalities often seen in an aging face can be treated effectively with this modality. Several absorbing agents which enhance the effect of TCA include Jessner's solution (see Table 1), the alpha hydroxy acids, and CO_2 slush or solid.[3]

TCA achieves its effect by destroying the stratum corneum, epidermis, and the upper layer of the dermis. The depth of penetration of the peeling agent into the dermis is the limiting factor for what

TABLE 1
JESSNER'S SOLUTION

salicylic acid 14 g
resorcinol 14 g
lactic acid 14 ml
ethanol QS 100 ml

From G.D. Monheit.[4]

TABLE 2

Type of Peel	TCA Strength, %
Superficial	10–20
Medium	20–40
Deep	>40

Note: TCA in concentrations greater than 40% carries an increased risk of scarring.

can be corrected as well as the variable most related to risk of scarring. It was thought that the effect could be enhanced by occlusive taping but this is being challenged.[5,6] Cosmetic improvement is due to a controlled chemical burn with subsequent healing. This allows new skin with a significantly rejuvenated appearance to form. To select the best chemical for treatment, the physician must evaluate the patient and assess the degree of damage.

For TCA, Table 2 indicates the type of peel required and the concentration needed. TCA in concentrations greater than 40 percent carries a greater risk of scarring, pigmentary change, and infection because these concentrations create deeper wounds. When scarring does occur it is more common on the lower half of the face, especially circumorally and around the jawline. This may be due to the increased facial movement in these areas and the numerous muscle insertions at the modiolus. Since TCA does not have the systemic toxicity of phenol, it can be used in a less sophisticated office setting.

PATIENT SELECTION

Perhaps the most important decision in treating with chemical peeling is selecting the right patient. TCA can be very effective in combating actinic damage where fine wrinkles, mottling, and other sun-induced changes can be dramatically improved. As is the case in all chemical peeling, the best patient for a peel is a middle-aged to elderly blonde, blue-eyed, fair-skinned woman. Because of their slightly thicker skin and general reluctance to camouflage pigmentary change, men are usually not as good candidates.[7]

In the initial consultation, the patient should be informed of the risks as well as the benefits of chemical face peeling. This allows the patient to decide independently whether he or she wishes to go ahead with the procedure.[8,9] Pretreatment with topical tretinoin (retinoic acid, or Retin-A) may also be started, since it is thought by some that this may actually reverse some of the features of photoaging. With TCA the risks include hyperpigmentation, hypopigmentation, variegate pigmentation, scarring, infection, persistent erythema, and a line of demarcation between peeled and unpeeled skin that can be satisfactorily concealed only with makeup.[10] There are different opinions about whether hyperpigmentation or hypopigmentation is more common after TCA peeling. Regardless, all patients are given strict instructions to avoid sun exposure and to use effective sunscreens. A Wood's light can be helpful when used to examine the patient's skin (especially for melasma), since epidermal pigmentation is accentuated under the light, whereas dermal pigmentation becomes less noticeable.[11] Epidermal pigment can be expected to respond considerably after chemical peeling whereas dermal pigmentation may respond only after peeling quite deeply or not at all.

The patient should be thoroughly informed about the actual procedural technique and about what to expect during the recuperative period. The questions most often asked by patients relate to pain. Postoperative discomfort varies depending on the depth of the peel and the areas that are peeled. It is common for patients to have no postoperative pain once the procedure is completed and they leave the office. The deeper the peel, the more edema, the more oozing, and hence more discomfort. For the superficial and medium-depth peels, there is often minimal or no postoperative discomfort. The most uncomfortable area seems to be the eyelids as it is common for them to become red and very edematous. It is not uncommon for the patient's eyes to be swollen shut. Patients should be informed about this so that they will not be alarmed if it occurs. We suggest that patients bring someone with them to the office so that they can be accompanied home, since patients can be preoccupied with what they have been through and groggy if sedation was used.

With the advent of oral acyclovir (Zovirax), it has become possible to peel patients with a history of active herpes simplex infection. In fact, some practitioners routinely administer oral acyclovir 200 mg five times a day to any patient on whom they plan to perform a peel.[12] The risk of significant scarring from a widespread herpetic eruption makes the administration of this medicine quite prudent.

TCA in milder concentrations of 10 to 35 percent is often used for more superficial "freshening" peels and medium-depth peels.[12] As would be expected, recuperation from such a peel is more rapid and less uncomfortable than is the case with a deeper peel. Patients may not have any pain once they leave the physician's office. The desquamation process occurs more rapidly (usually 3 to 7 days) since the wounding is more superficial. In addition, the healing proceeds more quickly and the patient is often able to return to work in a week without drawing undue attention to his or her face. This compares favorably with the two-week period of avoiding unnecessary exposure to the public we recommend to our patients with deeper TCA or phenol peels.[13] Some patients are unable to take two weeks off from work, and they should be aware that this may be desirable for deeper peels. If they are unable to do this, they may be better candidates for a more superficial peel, with the understanding that the results will be more subtle.

TECHNIQUE

Every patient must be seen for a thorough initial consultation prior to a chemical peel. This appointment is used to discuss the patient's desires, the risks and benefits of chemical peeling, and the alternative methods for treating the problem.[14,15,16] Once this discussion has taken place and if the patient's expectations are consistent with the physician's, the patient is asked to sign a detailed consent form. The patient is urged to ask as many questions as needed and is encouraged to schedule a follow-up session to go over any other problems or new questions that arise prior to the peel.

As in every surgical procedure, the degree of anesthesia and analgesia varies significantly with the individual patient. Many patients require almost no sedation and have relatively little difficulty tolerating the peel. Patients with heightened anxiety and a low pain threshold do better with significant sedation. It is best to use the minimum amount of anesthesia possible to perform the procedure and yet keep the patient comfortable. In cases requiring analgesia and anesthesia, sublingual diazepam (Valium) 5 to 10 mg may be given approximately 20 minutes before the actual peel. A combination of intramuscular meperidine hydrochloride (Demerol) 25 to 75 mg and hydroxyzine pamoate (Vistaril) 25 to 50 mg may be given 30 minutes before the procedure but is often unnecessary. This type of anesthesia usually is adequate and is easily administered in an office setting. Once the patient is comfortable, the face is cleaned with chlorhexidine gluconate (Hibiclens) solution. We ask the patient to be NPO (nothing by mouth) for approximately 10 hours before the procedure if we anticipate using heavier sedation.

Although we degrease the face with an organic solvent such as acetone or ether, it is probably more important that whatever cleansing method used is applied uniformly to the entire face. If the cleaning is not meticulous, localized areas of oil deposition may lead to irregular absorption of TCA and hence exacerbate the pigmentary variability that can result. The TCA is placed in a Pyrex dish on a Mayo stand at the head of the surgical table. (We store our TCA in amber glass bottles. Refrigeration may enhance preservation of stability, although this benefit is probably quite negligible.[17]) If a light or freshening peel is to be done, the concentration of TCA is 10 to 20 percent.[18] A medium-depth peel may be enhanced by applying agents such as Jessner's solution or CO_2 slush or solid before the TCA to further remove the epidermis after cleansing and degreasing in order to ensure an even and more thorough penetration of the TCA. See Table 3.

After the acid is applied, mild erythema with a faint tinge of frost appears. The degree of frosting varies directly with the concentration of TCA used. Although there are many methods of applying the chemical to the face, we prefer cotton-tipped applicators and folded 2″ × 2″ gauze squares. It is advantageous to have cotton-tipped applicators with long enough wooden handles so that the operator's hands are able to move freely above the patient's face without actually coming into contact with it. Several cotton guaze squares are placed on the table for wiping away the tears that may form around the patient's eyes. Cool water compresses can be applied to the patient's face to ease any burning sensation if necessary. The

TABLE 3
AGENTS USED IN COMBINATION WITH TCA TO INCREASE PENETRATION AND DEPTH OF PEEL

Jessner's solution applied in 1 or more coats
CO_2 slush or solid
alpha-hydroxy acids

CHAPTER

17

Facial Defects: Flaps and Grafts

RONALD L. MOY

The aesthetic use of flaps to repair facial defects requires the experience and knowledge to anticipate which flap is the best choice for a given defect. The available loose skin used as a donor site and the texture of the skin that is being moved should be considered. Along with the choice of donor skin, surgical placement of the incisions must be carefully planned so that the incisions are minimally evident. Generally, the best site for placement of incisional scars is along cosmetic boundary lines such as the nasolabial fold, the nasomaxillary crease, the hairlines, and the relaxed skin tension lines. The anatomic distortions that can result after the movement of flaps needs to be considered since obliteration of the nasolabial fold or an ectropion can produce unacceptable cosmetic results. Surgeons must take into account differences in skin texture, thickness, and elasticity on the different areas of the face when designing flaps and grafts.[1] This chapter reviews the advantages and some of the disadvantages of the flaps and grafts that are commonly utilized in selected regions of the face.

ADVANCEMENT FLAPS

Advancement flaps (Fig. 1) are best used in areas where tissue must be moved in a single direction, for example, a surgical defect within or above the eyebrow. Vertical movement can cause an upward movement of the eyebrow. An advancement flap where tissue is advanced from the horizontal direction causes little distortion. The preauricular area and upper lip area are also good regions for an advancement flap because the scars can be hidden within the preauricular crease or vermilion border (Figs. 2 through 5). Tissue can be easily moved horizontally on the upper lip without causing an upward distortion of the lip. The forehead region is amenable to reconstruction with a single or double advancement flap. The main disadvantage of a dou-

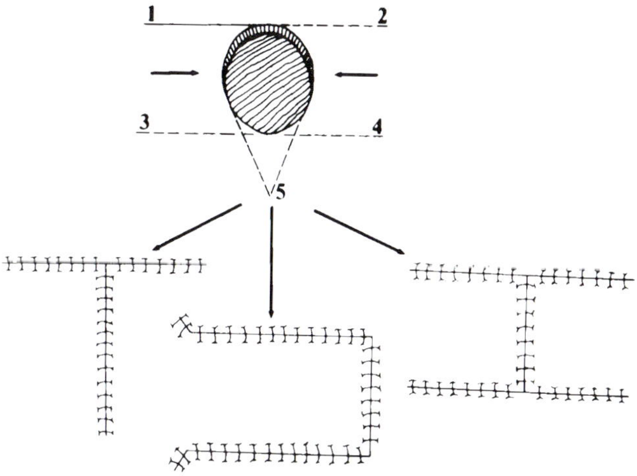

FIGURE 1
Advancement flap. Incising along 1–2 and 3–4 would be a double advancement flap. Incising just from 1 and 3 to the defect would be a single advancement flap. Incising from 1 to 2 and the triangle at 5 would be an A to T advancement flap. (*From Moy,*[14] *with permission.*)

FIGURE 2
Basal cell carcinoma of the upper lip. (*From Moy,*[14] *with permission.*)

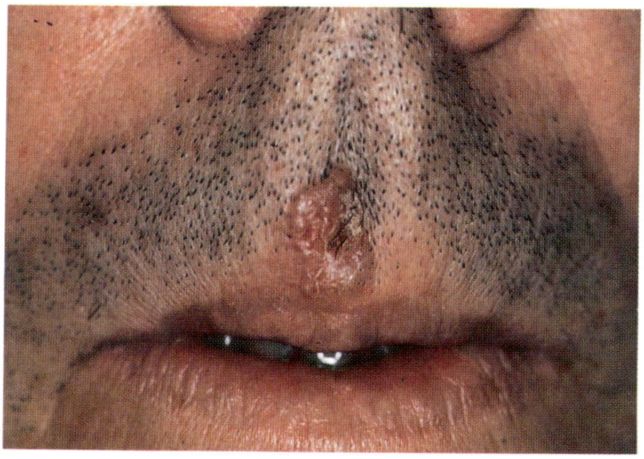

ble advancement flap (H-plasty) is the creation of five incision lines that outline an H (Fig. 1). A single advancement flap can reduce the number of scars and should be attempted before a double advancement flap is created.

A variation of the single advancement flap is the A to T flap or O to T flap, in which only one side of the flap is incised and the final scar outlines a T. This flap reduces the number of scars compared with a single advancement flap. Additionally, the scars in an A to T flap can be easily hidden. A to T flaps are best used in the eyebrow area, the upper lip, and the preauricular area (Figs. 2 through 5). Another form of the advancement flap is the Burow's triangle flap. The incisions for this flap can be placed within a natural fold such as the eyebrow, the nasolabial fold, the hairline, or the lip,

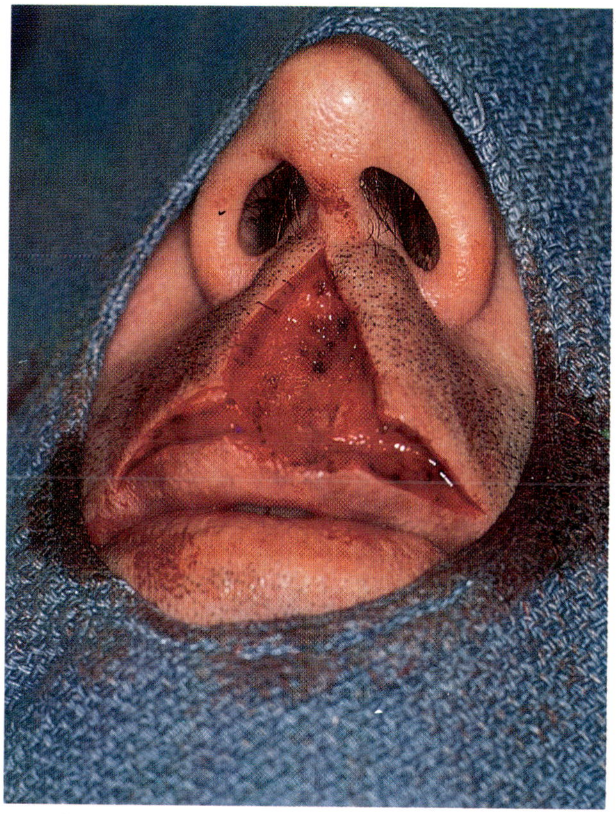

FIGURE 3
Excision of a tumor as a triangular defect and incision along the vermilion border as an A to T advancement flap. (*From Moy,*[14] *with permission.*)

FIGURE 4
A advancement flap sutured carefully with a reapproximation of the vermilion border. (*From Moy,*[14] *with permission.*)

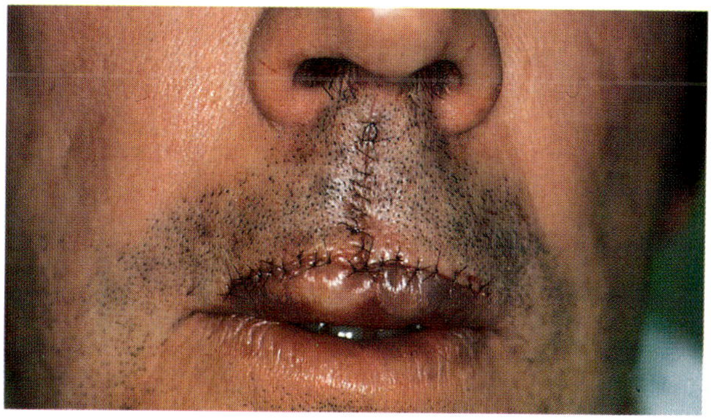

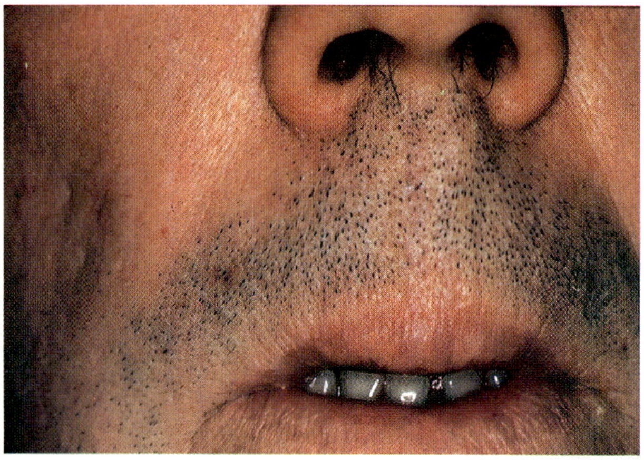

FIGURE 5
Cosmetic result 6 months later. (*From Moy,*[14] *with permission.*)

while the Burow's triangle is placed at some distance from the defect.

With a helical advancement flap, the helix is advanced over the surgical defect on the ear. This flap is useful for repairing helical defects.[2]

ROTATION FLAPS

The rotation flap is a simply designed flap that has limited usefulness on the face. The main disadvantage is that rotation flaps usually require long incisions to mobilize sufficient tissue to fill the surgical defect. This flap is usually best suited for the creation of large flaps on the cheeks but can also be used for the creation of smaller flaps on the nose. Two types of rotation flaps are the O to Z flap and the glabellar turn-down flap.[3]

The O to Z flap is a variant rotation flap that has limited application on the face because it is difficult to mobilize the tissue without creating long incisions. This flap can be used when an elliptical incision would distort anatomic structures since it can be conceptualized as an incomplete elliptical incision.

TRANSPOSITION FLAPS

Transposition flaps are the most frequently used local skin flaps on the face. The most common types include the rhombic flap, the bilobed flap, the nasolabial flap, and the Z-plasty.

The *rhombic flap* is the most versatile type of transposition flap. Ideally, it can be designed so that the tissue is transposed from any direction, although transposition of normal skin should generally be in the direction where the skin is most extensible. Rhombic flaps are best used on the cheeks, temples, and upper dorsal area of the nose, where the skin is loose. They do not work as well on the forehead or scalp, where the skin is tight.[4]

The five most commonly used variations of the rhombic flap are the classical Limberg flap, the Dufourmental rhombic flap, the Webster 30-degree transposition flap, the double rhomboid flap, and the rhombic flap into a round defect.

When one is designing a rhombic flap, the most important consideration is deciding which skin area is available as a donor region. A rhombic flap makes use of this extensible donor skin to fill the defect, while the donor skin should close side to the side. The flap is designed and outlined so that the direction of maximum extensibility is used. Resultant scars, the possible distortion of anatomic structures, and the relaxed skin tension lines should be considered when one is designing the flap.

Once the direction of maximum skin extensibility is determined, the type of rhombic flap can be considered. A round defect can be repaired with a rhombic transposition flap, often without having to trim the corners of the flap. This modified rhombic flap has the advantage that the positioning of the transposed flap is not predetermined, allowing the scar to be placed in the least conspicuous site along the direction of maximum skin extensibility. Tissue does not have to be unnecessarily sacrificed to produce a rhombic flap. The corners of the flap usually fit well into the round defect. The other important aspect of this modified rhombic flap is that the flap can be made smaller than the defect to be reconstructed since the sides of the flap do not have to exactly match the sides of the rhombic defect.[5] Sometimes it is easier to conceptualize the rhombic flap when the surgical defect is a true rhomboid. The Limberg rhomboid flap is the flap that should be mastered first. All the sides of the defect and the rhombic flap are made equal. This flap can be harder to move, and the secondary defect can be harder to close than is the case with the Dufourmental rhombic flap. The Dufourmental flap angles the flap upward instead of just extending the short diagonal of the defect. This upward incision for the first side of the rhombic flap facilitates the transposition of the flap and closure of the secondary defect (Figs. 6 through 12). The Dufourmental flap is useful when closure of the secondary defect is expected to be difficult.

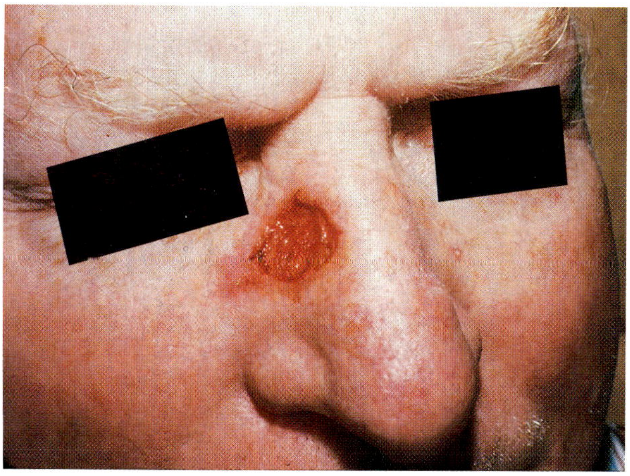

FIGURE 6
A rhombic defect. (*From Moy,[14] with permission.*)

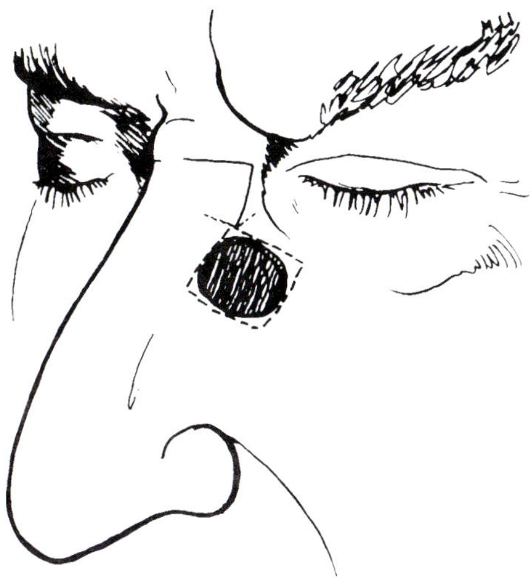

FIGURE 7
Dufourmental rhombic flap designed to facilitate closure of the secondary defect and movement of the flap. (*From Moy,[14] with permission.*)

The Webster 30-degree transposition flap is best used to prevent the dog ears that can result from other rhombic flaps. The base or hinge part of the flap is elongated into a 30-degree angle or incised with a W-plasty to prevent the usual dog ear from occurring.[4]

The bilobed flap is used primarily on the lower third of the nose, when tissue from a loose area such as the upper nose is needed to fill a defect on the lower nose, where the skin is not very extensible. The loose skin on the upper part of the nose is moved into a lobe of the flap on the middle part of the nose while the skin on the middle part is moved into the surgical defect on the lower nose.

Basically the skin is "walked down" from the upper nose to the lower nose. This flap is not very useful on the cheeks, where a single transposition flap such as a rhombic flap can be used. The design of the flap is improved when the dog ear at the base or the hinge part of the flap is excised so that the

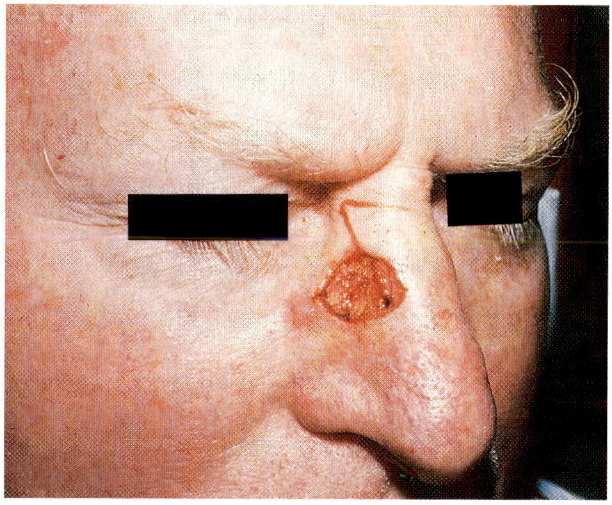

FIGURE 8
Dufourmental rhombic flap. (*From Moy,[14] with permission.*)

FIGURE 9
Flap moved into place. (*From Moy,[14] with permission.*)

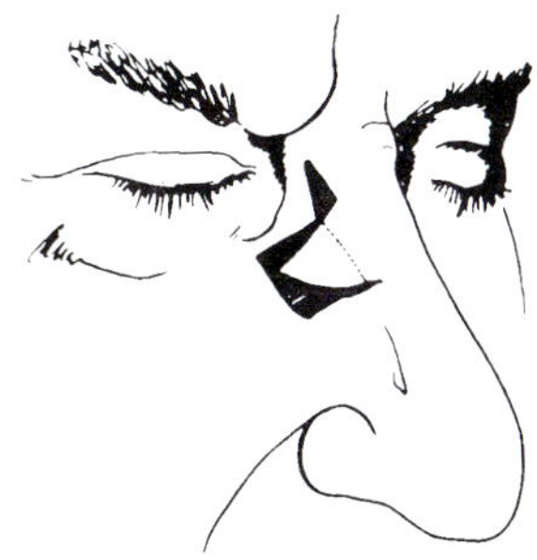

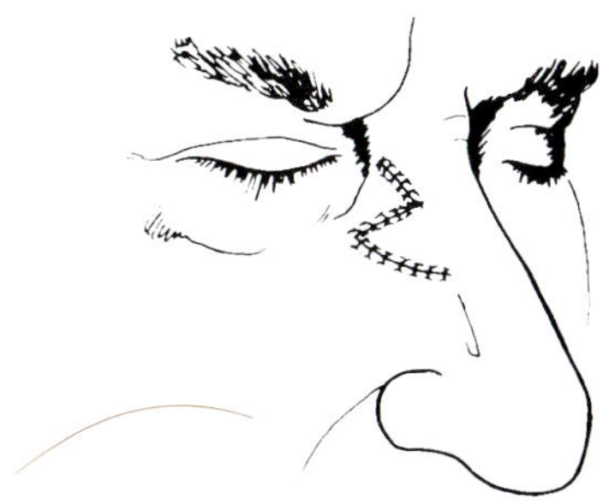

flap moves more easily into place (Fig. 13). The flap also moves more easily when it is designed so that it does not transfer tissue 180 degrees from the donor area. The smaller the area of transposition, the easier the movement of the flap and the less the tension on the flap. The first lobe of the flap can be made smaller than the surgical defect. This flap is very useful for reconstruction of defects on the lower nose (Figs. 13 through 18). Because these flaps are rounded, they have the potential to create a trapdoor deformity or pincushion effect; how-

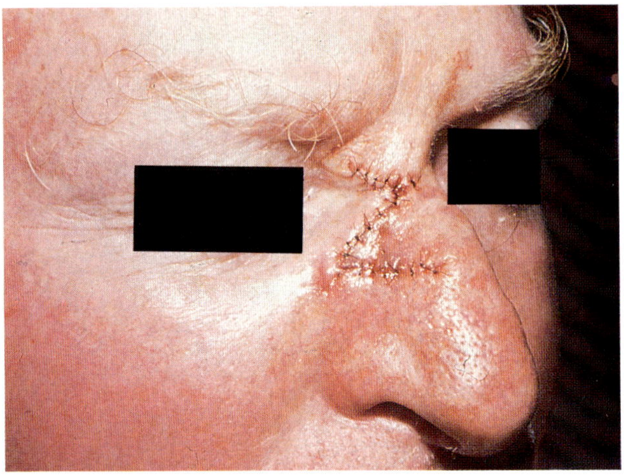

FIGURE 10
Dufourmental rhombic flap sutured into place. (*From Moy,*[14] *with permission.*)

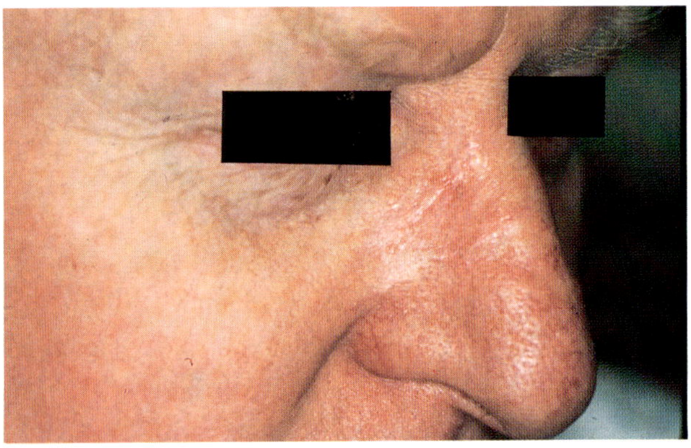

FIGURE 11
Final result, front view. (*From Moy,*[14] *with permission.*)

FIGURE 12
Final result, front view, 4 months later. (*From Moy,*[14] *with permission.*)

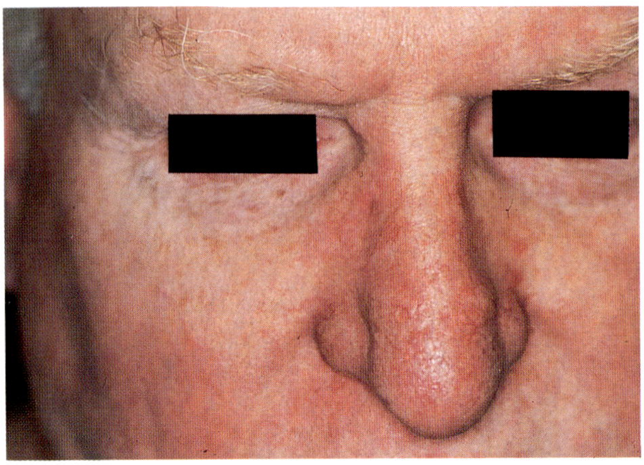

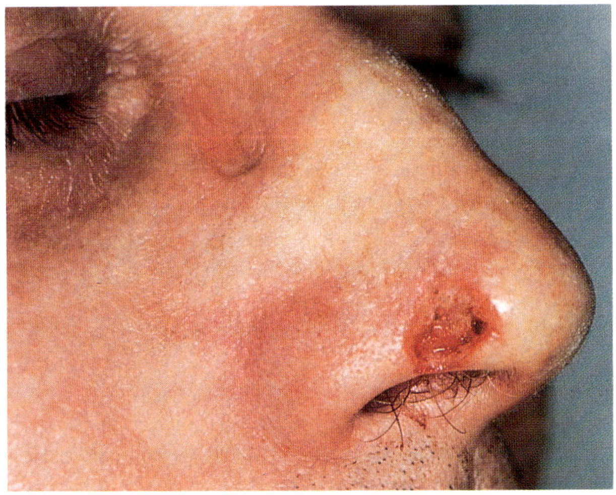

FIGURE 13
A wound after Mohs micrographic surgery. (*From Moy,*[14] *with permission.*)

FIGURE 14
A bilobed transposition flap designed so that the flap does not transfer issue 180 degrees and the dog ear at the base of the flap is excised. (*From Moy,*[14] *with permission.*)

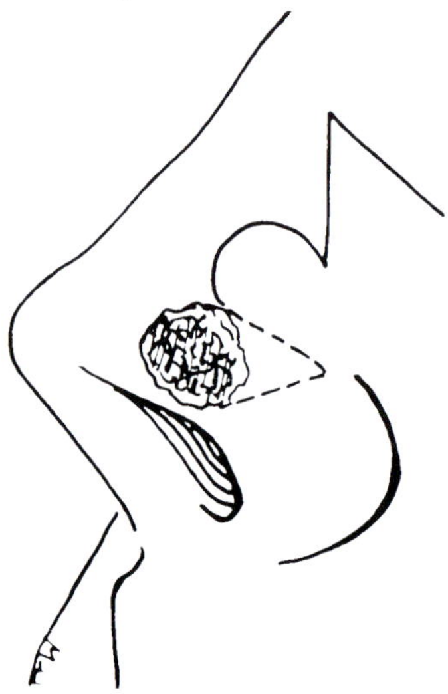

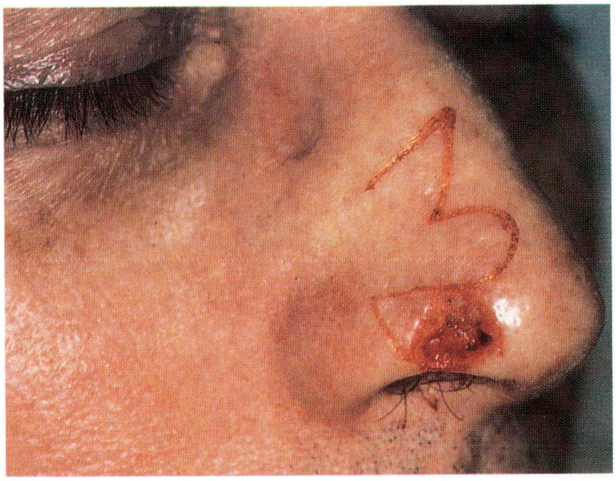

FIGURE 15
A bilobed transposition flap; skin is moved from the upper nose to the lower nose. (*From Moy,*[14] *with permission.*)

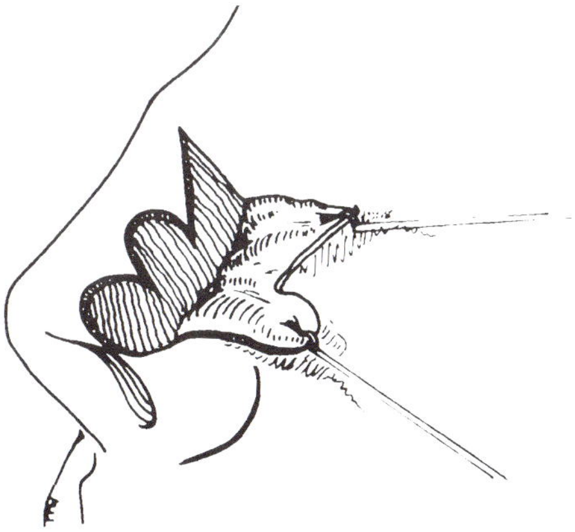

FIGURE 16
A flap moved into place with skin hooks. (*From Moy,*[14] *with permission.*)

ever, this complication can be prevented by means of sufficient undermining.[6]

The Z-plasty is a transposition flap that is useful for lengthening scars and changing the direction of a scar.[1] It is used primarily in attempting scar revision.

Nasolabial Flap

The nasolabial flap is an especially useful transposition flap for large defects on the nasal ala. It can be the best choice for large defects on the sides of the nose. The flap should be minimally transposed and maximally advanced into place by designing it so that it is based high on the nose and not twisted about the pedicle. The nasomaxillary crease needs

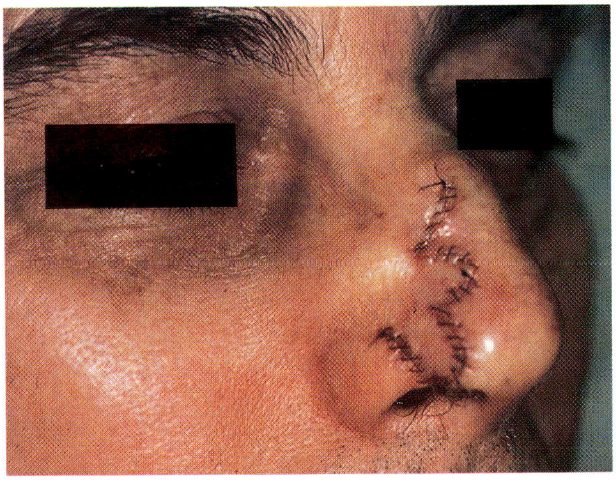

FIGURE 17
A flap sutured. Note the minimal distortion of the alar rim. (*From Moy,*[14] *with permission.*)

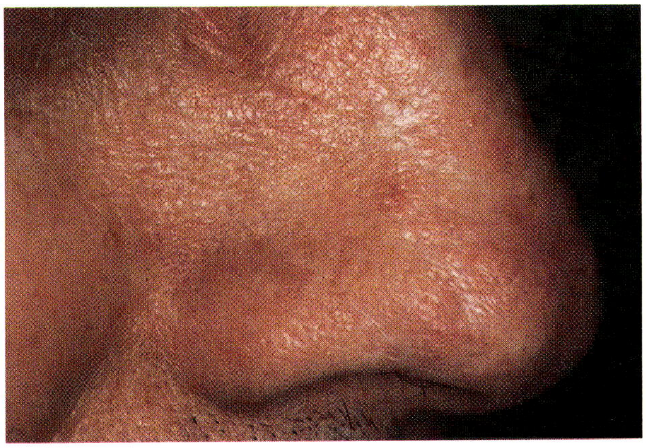

FIGURE 18
Final result 6 months later. (*From Moy,*[14] *with permission.*)

to be re-created as much as possible. The tip of the flap can be turned in on itself to recreate a missing alar rim.[6]

SUBCUTANEOUS ISLAND PEDICLE FLAP

The subcutaneous island pedicle flap is ideally used for reconstructing large defects on the nose. The midforehead and the cheek above the nasolabial fold are areas that allow a fairly long subcutaneous island pedicle to exist so that the donor skin can be moved some distance to the surgical defect.[7] The main problem in these two areas is the bulkiness underneath the island of normal skin, which often has to be repaired at a later date. A subcutaneous pedicle flap without an island can also be used on the forehead above the eyebrow, the nasolabial fold, and the preauricular area.

GRAFTS

Full-thickness skin grafts are easy to perform and often give excellent cosmetic results. The color and texture match may be poor, and their survival is more precarious than that of flaps. They can be the best choice for large defects on the nose and the nasal tip and defects on the helical rim.

The donor site for the skin graft is extremely important in getting the best match of skin color and texture. The most common area used is the postauricular sulcus area. This skin may not be as sun-exposed as skin in other sites, but the skin is thin and the donor site is easily closed primarily. The thin skin on the postauricular area or the upper eyelid improves the survival of the graft. The supraclavicular area and the preauricular area are alternative donor sites. Larger amounts of skin can be harvested from the supraclavicular area. This skin needs to be thinned and defatted to a greater degree than does postauricular skin. The preauricular donor area consists of actinically exposed skin, and so it potentially allows for a better color and texture match. However, this can create a preauricular scar, and the skin may be slightly thicker than postauricular skin. The nasolabial fold can be used as a donor site, but since the cheek skin is thicker, the graft may fail.

Burow's grafts have a number of advantages over other full-thickness grafts that can lead to excellent cosmetic results. Since the donor site is adjacent to the wound, the color and texture match can be better than it is at traditional donor sites. The graft is easily accessed, and the donor site scar can be made inconspicuous with a linear closure. The only disadvantages of Burow's grafts are the limited size of the graft and the slightly higher risk of necrosis due to the skin thickness of some of the donor areas. This graft is superb for reconstructing a loose nasal tip, the upper lip, and the nasal ala. It can also be used to reconstruct the forehead.[8]

Composite skin-cartilage grafts and cartilage grafts can be used for more complicated repairs. A composite graft from the concha can be used to elegantly reconstruct the ear. A conchal cartilage graft can be used to repair large defects of the ear when cartilage is missing. The entire conchal cartilage can be used and sutured into a cartilaginous defect. A two-stage retroauricular advancement flap can then be used to cover the cartilage graft.

RECONSTRUCTION

Nose

Aesthetic reconstruction of the nose requires the replacement of lost nasal skin with skin of similar color and texture. It requires attention to normal nasal anatomy, including the nasal ala, the alar rim, the nasomaxillary crease, the alar groove, and the "nasal subunits."[9] Bilobed transposition flaps and rhombic flaps are the most commonly used flaps for aesthetic restoration of the nose. Nasolabial transposition flaps, rotation flaps, advancement flaps, and grafts are also used for reconstructing defects of the nose.

Bilobed transposition flaps are used primarily for repairing defects on the nasal ala and the lower dorsal area of the nose. This flap allows normal tissue to be moved down from the upper nose, where the skin is looser, to a defect on the lower nose, where the skin is inelastic. This flap can give superior results if it is thinned adequately, the undermining is adequate (to prevent trapdooring), and there is minimal distortion of the alar rim.[6]

Rhombic flaps are used on the upper nose, where the skin is loose. This flap can be designed so that a superior based flap makes use of the looser skin on the upper nose (Fig. 12).

A *nasolabial flap* is required for a large defect of the nasal ala. It has been said that the nasolabial flap is favored by inexperienced surgeons and that the long-term result is usually aesthetically unacceptable.[1] This statement is at least partly true if there is obliteration of the nasomaxillary crease and trapdooring occurs. If the flap is adequately thinned and is based high on the side of the nose so that the transposition is less, the cosmetic results may be acceptable. This flap is especially useful for defects that go through the nasal ala.

Small *rotation flaps* are also excellent for repairing defects on the ala and nasal bridge. They are simply designed and allow the use of nasal skin within the same cosmetic unit.[10]

The axial frontal flap or extended glabellar flap and the heminose flap are different names for the same flap used to reconstruct larger defects on the nose. The skin is incised from the defect up into the glabellar area. The donor site is really the glabellar area, which is closed in a V-Y manner with the donor scar lying in a glabellar frown line. The flap allows for advancement and rotation of nasal skin. The disadvantages are the long scar created and the limited rotation obtained. The limited rotation can result in a significant amount of pulling up on the alar rim.[3]

Large defects on the nose can also be repaired with a *subcutaneous island pedicle flap* from either the glabellar area or the nasolabial area. The flap is incised, leaving a pedicle attached at the base of the defect. The pedicle is designed so that it is centered on the main arteries in the area, the intraorbital or nasolabial arteries. A tunnel is then created between the pedicle flap and the nasal defect. The flap is then moved underneath the island of normal skin into the nasal defect. The main disadvantage is the bulkiness created under the island of normal skin by the subcutaneous pedicle.

Full-thickness grafts are used for larger defects of the nose, where flaps may cause distortion of the alar rim, and for selective lesions on the nasal tip and nasal ala. Grafts can provide an excellent color and texture match in certain patients; however, this is not as predictable as with local flaps. Patients with sebaceous nasal skin do poorly with grafts.

The most commonly used donor sites for nasal reconstruction are the preauricular area and the postauricular area. The preauricular skin can give an excellent color and texture match on the nose because it is sun-exposed skin. The limitation of this donor site is the size of the graft that can be harvested and the creation of a preauricular scar. The postauricular skin can give a good color and texture match in selected patients with thin, smooth nasal skin. The supraclavicular skin is used for large nasal defects when the postauricular skin is not sufficient in quantity. The supraclavicular skin is inferior for use in grafts because it is thicker skin and often ends up wrinkled and shiny. The forehead skin and the nasolabial cheek skin have been suggested to be the best matches for nasal skin; however, they are more risky because they are thicker.

Burow's grafts are full-thickness skin grafts whose donor site is the skin adjacent to the defect. This skin provides a better color, texture, and thickness match than does postauricular or supraclavicular skin. Burow's grafts can be considered when an adjacent donor site can be approximated in a primary fashion. Closing the donor site makes the defect smaller so that the graft can be made smaller than the original defect. Burow's grafts are useful for the nasal ala and nasal tip.

Cheek

The most commonly used flap in cheek reconstruction should be the rhombic transposition flap. Because of the local skin available on the cheek, many large defects can actually be closed in a primary fashion. Bilobed flaps create obvious and unacceptable scars and may result in trapdooring. Rotation flaps create long scars and do not move skin as efficiently as rhombic transposition flaps do. Advancement flaps, subcutaneous pedicle flaps, and nasolabial cheek flaps are usually inferior to rhombic flaps for cheek reconstruction.

Lip

Reconstruction of the lip requires the use of advancement flaps, mucosal advancement flaps, full-thickness grafts, and rarely transposition flaps. The most commonly used flap is the A to T flap with a vermilion border to hide incisional scar lines.

Obliteration of the nasolabial fold, upward pulling of the upper lip, transferring of non-hair-bearing skin to the upper lip in men, and failing to carefully reapproximate the vermilion border are potential problems that should be considered when one is designing flaps for lip reconstruction.

Temple

An inferior based rhombic flap can provide excellent skin coverage in the temple area. Larger defects can be repaired with a double rhombic flap.

Ear

Helical advancement flaps and full-thickness grafts are the reconstructive procedures most commonly used to repair ear defects. *Wedge excisions* are rarely employed when Mohs micrographic surgical techniques are used to remove tumors on the ear because cartilage is usually preserved. Conservation of cartilage avoids the need to use a wedge excision, which can make the ear smaller and cause more anatomic deformity. When a large amount of cartilage is removed, cartilage replacement with a conchal cartilage graft followed by skin replacement with a retroauricular advancement flap can produce excellent results.[11]

The helical advancement flap can be the most versatile and reliable form of repair for helical defects. This flap can be more easily advanced by incising through the postauricular skin, creating a full-thickness flap. This has not proved to result in a higher incidence of flap necrosis. The disadvantages of helical advancement flaps include a slight reduction in auricular circumference and the frequent compromise of antihelical and scaphal anatomic landmarks.[12]

Large surgical defects on the ear with loss of cartilage require that the missing cartilaginous structural support be replaced with a cartilage graft. The entire ipsilateral conchal cartilage can be removed without the creation of a noticeable deformity. Suturing conchal cartilage into the defect can recreate the shape of the normal pinna. There is no resorption of the cartilage years after the procedure if large pieces of cartilage are grafted. A retroauricular mastoid flap can be advanced over the grafted conchal cartilage and sutured into place. This creates a pedicle flap from the mastoid area to the anterior ear that can be severed at a later date. A full-thickness graft can be sutured into the postauricular sulcus or mastoid area 3 or 4 weeks later. It is important to thin this well-vascularized flap to prevent bulkiness and flap edema. The helix can be recreated by using horizontal mattress sutures through the cartilage graft at the site of the helical sulcus. A conchal cartilage graft with a retroauricular mastoid flap is a simple two-stage procedure that can provide acceptable cosmetic results with large defects of the ear.

FLAP REVISION

Every patient undergoing facial reconstruction should probably be advised that all flaps and grafts may require revisional surgery to improve the cosmetic appearance. Many flaps and grafts on the lower third of the nose, where the skin is sebaceous, benefit from dermabrasion within 2 months of the surgery, because the results do not appear to be as beneficial when the dermabrasion is done later.[6] Dermabrasion of full-thickness grafts is usually performed 3 months after surgery.

Trapdooring or pincushioning can occur on all flaps. It has been reported that rounded flaps are prone to trapdooring while rhombic flaps are not. Although there are many theories about trapdooring, wound contraction underneath the flap seems to cause the elevation of the center of the flap and the depression of the edges of the flap, resulting in the pincushioning appearance. If the flap is adequately thinned and the entire region is widely undetermined, the chance of trapdooring is minimized even with bilobed flaps. If trapdooring does occur, intralesional steroids can be of benefit. Lifting up the flap, thinning the flap, and adequately undermining the flap can improve the appearance. Multiple Z-plasties can break up the forces of wound contraction.[6] Much of the trapdooring improves spontaneously in 6 months.

Z-plasties can be used to lengthen a scar or change the direction of an incisional scar. If a flap or graft fails, the forces of wound contraction take place. The result can be improved with the use of convergent triangular flaps or a Z-plasty to restore the normal anatomy.[13,14]

CONCLUSION

Flaps and grafts have progressed to the point where the aesthetic dermatologic surgeon can choose from a number of procedures.[14] The devastation from cancer surgery or the disarray from trauma can be readily mollified with appropriate repair.

REFERENCES

1. Jackson IT. Local Flaps in Head and Neck Reconstruction. St. Louis, Mosby, 1985.
2. Cavanaugh E. Management of lesions of the helical rim using a chondrocutaneous advancement flap. J Dermatol Surg Oncol. 1982; 9:472–477.
3. Marchac D, Toth B. The axial frontonasal flap revisited. Plast Reconstr Surg. 1985; 76:685–693.
4. Bray DA. Clinical applications of the rhomboid flap. Arch Otolaryngol. 1983; 109:37–42.
5. Quaba AA, Sommerlad BC. "A square peg into a round hole": A modified rhomboid flap and its clinical application. Br J Plast Surg. 1987; 40:163–170.
6. Zitelli JA. The bilobed flap for nasal reconstruction. Arch Dermatol. 1989; 125:957–959.

7. Levine PA. Reconstruction of large nasal defects with a subcutaneous pedicle nasolabial flap. Arch Otolaryngol. 1985; 111:628–630.
8. Zitelli JA. Burow's grafts. J Am Acad Dermatol. 1987; 17:271–279.
9. Burget GC. Aesthetic restoration of the nose. Clin Plast Surg. 1985; 12:463–479.
10. Winton GB, Salasche SJ. Use of rotation flaps to repair surgical defects on the ala nasi. J Dermatol Surg Oncol. 1986; 12:154–158.
11. Moy RL, Zitelli JAZ. Reconstructing large defects of the auricle using a conchal cartilage graft and a retroauricular mastoid flap, abstract. J Dermatol Surg Oncol. 1988; 14:108.
12. Brent B. The acquired auricular deformity: A systematic approach to its analysis and reconstruction. Plast Reconst Surg. 1977; 59:475–485.
13. Limberg AA. The Planning of Local Plastic Operations on the Body Surface: Theory and Practice. Lexington, MA: Collamore/Heath, 1983:393.
14. Moy RL. Atlas of Cutaneous Facial Flaps and Grafts: A Differential Diagnosis of Wound Closures. Philadelphia: Lea & Febiger, 1990.

CHAPTER

18

Facelift Surgery

ROBERT W. HUTCHERSON

The facelift is the most commonly performed aesthetic surgical procedure, and commensurate with the acceptable trend to operate on younger patients, it will likely continue to be the mainstay in the cosmetic surgeon's armamentarium. Additionally, the classic facelift is the cornerstone for ancillary procedures such as liposuction, anatomic augmentation, and chemical peeling, all of which are used by surgeons seeking to refine their results and give greater satisfaction to their patients. As the sophistication of the technique(s) used to embellish the results of the classic procedure evolves, so must the judgment of the surgeons, to allow them to effectively apply their skills. Recognizing that sound surgical judgment and experience are implicitly related, the intent of this chapter is to provide readers with knowledge that will assist them in performing the facelift and related procedures.

PATIENT SELECTION, PREOPERATIVE EVALUATION, PREPARATION

The goal of patient satisfaction begins with patient selection. Because of the elective nature of the facelift operation, it is imperative that the surgeon be able to evaluate a prospective surgical candidate and detect why the procedure will or will not be effective. Particularly salient features in a patient's history that could preclude a smooth intraoperative and postoperative course include smoking, diabetes, hypertension, bleeding disorders, abnormal scarring tendencies, history of obesity or rapid weight loss, and other ongoing medical problems. Although chronological age generally is not a limiting factor, patients who are older or have a "positive" history should receive medical clearance prior to the procedure.

Guidelines regarding preoperative laboratory work are not universally accepted; however, routine preoperative testing should include electrocardiogram, complete blood count, PT and PTT, and chest radiograph, depending on the age and history of the patient. Many surgeons also obtain a bleeding time and routine urinalysis.

During the examination potentially compromising anatomic features should be noted by the surgeon. These include overweight status, retrognathia, anterior displacement of the hyoid bone, short or thick neck, abnormalities in the distribution and texture of hair, and facial skeletal asymmetry. A significant finding during the examination could be reason to discourage a patient or to suggest an ancillary procedure, such as chin augmentation. The severity and distribution of facial rhytides, the general laxity of skin, and the presence of platysmal banding, jowling, and submental fat should be noted. One should also evaluate the prominence of the nasolabial and glabellar folds, degree of forehead furrowing, brow ptosis and severity of lateral canthal rhytides.

The best facelift candidates are thin and possess a prominent jawline and cheeks, moderately high forehead, relatively long neck, and good skin elasticity. Other features, such as a flawless complexion and a sense of balance in facial structure and contours, are attributes of a "natural" candidate.

After the patient's history has been taken and the examination completed, the findings should be discussed. This discussion allows the surgeon to assess the expectations of the patient and to review the inherent risks and potential complications of the procedure. The importance of this exchange of information cannot be overstated; the rapport established during this part of the consultation is profoundly important in avoiding postoperative problems. Additional time spent here is not squandered. Most surgeons find it useful to provide the patient with written material that reviews notable features of the procedure, including the expected postoperative course.

Prior to surgery, patients should be advised to avoid aspirin and aspirin-containing products, alcoholic beverages, and prolonged sun exposure. Patients are frequently given oral supplemental vitamin K.

FACELIFT TECHNIQUE

The classic facelift operation involves the mobilization and repositioning of large areas of the cervicofacial skin unit. Anesthesia may be either local standby or general. The procedure is usually performed on an outpatient basis in the surgeon's office. Occasionally, patients are discharged to an extended-care facility for postoperative observation and nursing care.

The main variable in facelift surgical technique is the extent of undermining of the facial and neck skin. Surgical literature is replete with publications espousing aggressive and minimalist approaches. Most procedures are probably performed somewhere in between, with conservative or liberal tendencies being based on the preoperative characteristics of a given patient. For example, a relatively young patient with excellent skin elasticity and minimal jowling and platysmal banding would theoretically require less undermining than an older patient with severe skin excess. An additional consideration in determining the extent of undermining is the surgeon's attitude toward mobilizing the subcutaneous anatomic units in the face and neck [superficial musculoaponeurotic system, (SMAS)/platysma flap]. These procedural modifications usually require less direct undermining of the skin.

Prior to preparing and draping the patient, the patient's hair is parted (not shaved) and held in place with elastic bands, clips, or umbilical tape, anticipating the course of the incision (Fig. 1). After the preparations, the skin is anesthetized according to the surgeon's preference, usually with a dilute solution of lidocaine and epinephrine (1:200,000 or greater). MAC or general anesthesia may be used.

The temporoparietal part of the incision is made first; it should extend slightly forward in a curvilinear direction above the superior helix of the ear. The length of this portion of the incision depends on the amount of anticipated facial skin to be excised, being extended somewhat for larger amounts. The incision may also vary if a temporal component is to be incorporated into the facelift or if the standard incision and subsequent flap rotation could significantly affect the contour of the sideburn. In the latter case, a horizontal extension is made just inferior to the sideburn (Fig. 2).

The incision is then brought downward in the

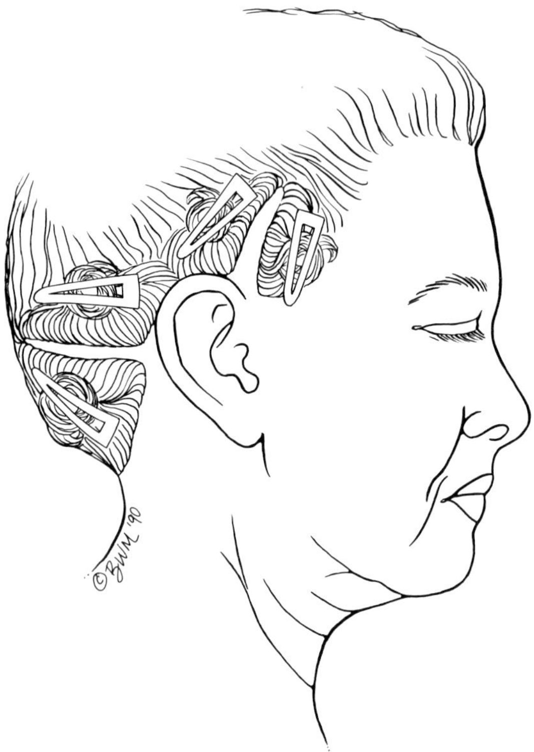

FIGURE 1
The hair is parted along the anticipated incision lines.

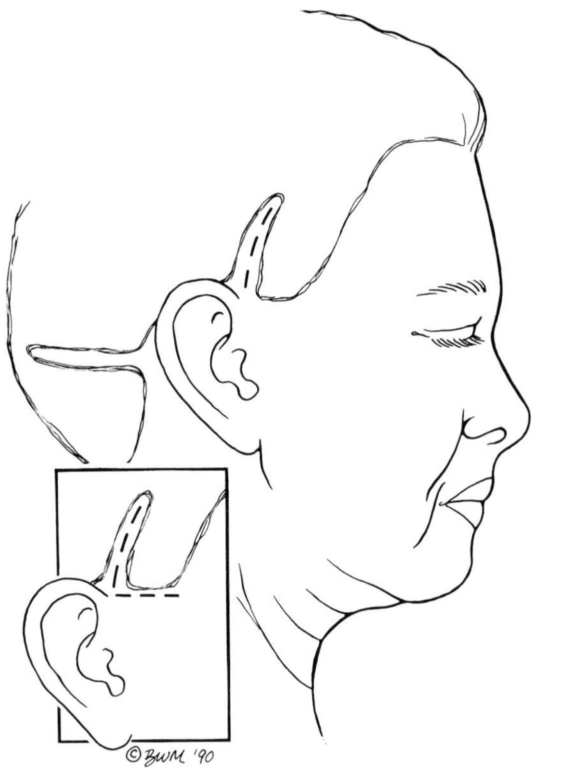

FIGURE 2
The temporoparietal incision is shown curving slightly anteriorly above the helical rim. A horizontal extension of the incision (inset) prevents significant alteration of the sideburn contour.

preauricular crease. Most surgeons prefer to bring the incision to the posterior aspect of the tragus and to return to the preauricular crease as it continues to the earlobe (Fig. 3). This minor variation on the classic depiction of the facelift incision avoids the telltale unbroken line in front of the ear. Opponents of the posttragal incision cite postoperative contour change of the tragus with possible flattening or other anatomic distortion. These concerns can, however, be allayed if care is taken to avoid tension on wound closure in this area.

The earlobe is mobilized and sometimes marked with a suture to allow accurate reapproximation during closure. The postauricular incision is then made in the sulcus, being brought slightly onto the posterior aspect of the concha. At a level that roughly corresponds to the superior aspect of the external auditory canal, the incision is taken posteriorly in the hairline toward the occiput (Fig. 4). The length of this portion of the incision may vary, especially if an extended cervical lift is planned to tighten the posterolateral aspect of the neck, when the nuchal midline may nearly be reached. To perform this extension requires excellent exposure. The surgeon must take great care to avoid trauma to the occipital nerve and an unsightly step-off in the nuchal hairline.

Skin undermining is performed with double-edged scissors, with the dissection being maintained in subcutaneous tissue planes. Temporally, the dissection is lateral to the temporalis facia, which protects the scalp hair follicles. The superficial temporal artery is preserved (Fig. 5).

Anterior to the ear, the dissection becomes more superficial, in a plane lateral to the superficial temporalis fascia (which attaches to the zygomatic arch) and the superficial layer of the cervical fascia (which invests the parotid gland). The transition between the temporal and cheek regions may be facilitated by blunt dissection (Fig. 6). The soft tissue lateral to the zygomatic arch and parotid gland is then elevated. Notably, the plane of dissection is

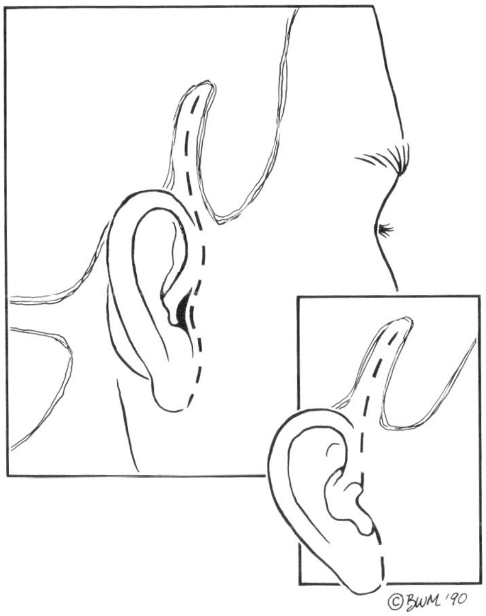

FIGURE 3
The facial incision is depicted in the preauricular crease. Positioning the incision on the posterior aspect of the tragus additionally helps to camouflage the eventual scar.

relatively avascular and easily developed except at the distal parotid region, where vascularity and subcutaneous tissue tensile strength are slightly greater. Mobilization of the superficial musculoaponeurotic system (SMAS) is discussed later.

The neck skin is elevated next, bringing the dissection over the inferior margin of the mandible and lateral to the platysma muscle toward the midline (Fig. 7). In this subcutaneous plane, the marginal branch of the facial nerve is protected, as are larger vascular structures. The posterior part of the neck dissection is performed lateral to the sternocleidomastoid muscle; attention should be taken to avoid trauma to the greater auricular nerve. The length of vertical undermining varies, but may be as great as two thirds of the vertical length of the neck. Fairly aggressive mobilization of skin lateral to the sternocleidomastoid avoids unsightly buckling of the muscle when the skin is repositioned and anchored in the occipital part of the incision.

The wound is meticulously inspected for hemostasis, and the skin flap is then repositioned with

FIGURE 4
The incision is placed in the postauricular sulcus, curving 1–2 mm onto the concha. Tangent to the superior rim of the external auditory canal, the incision is extended horizontally toward the occiput.

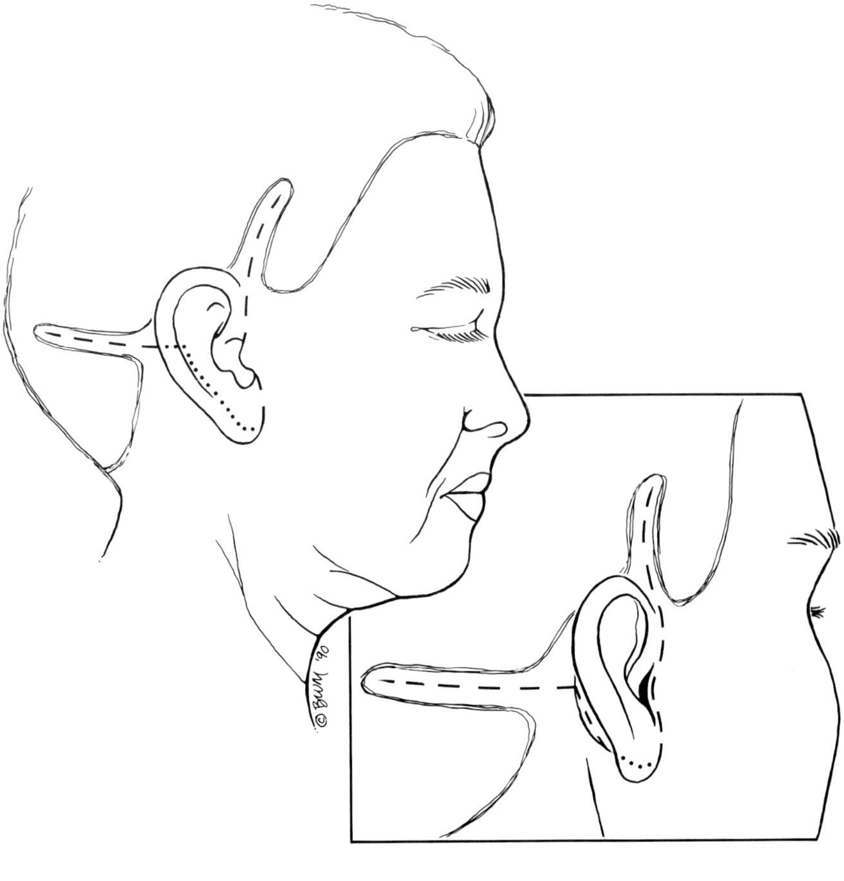

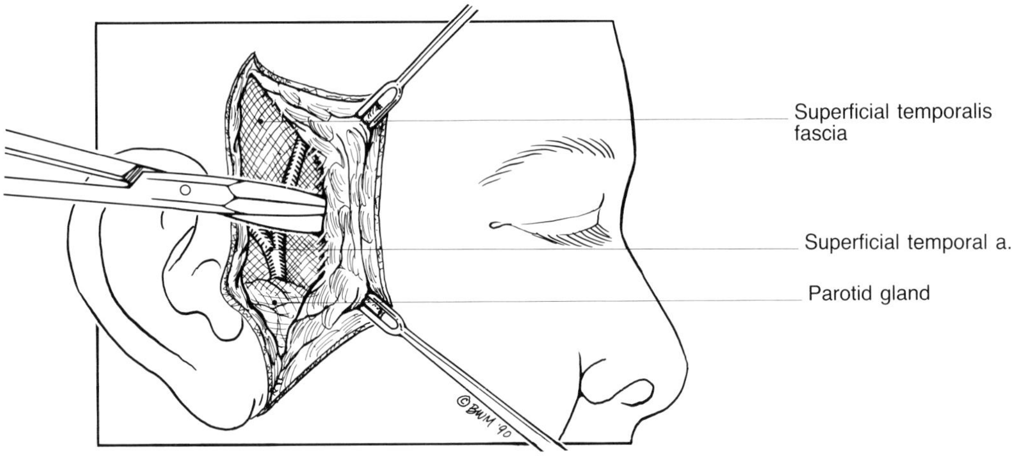

FIGURE 5
The temporoparietal flap is undermined lateral to the temporalis fascia, exposing the superficial temporal artery which is preserved.

FIGURE 6
The facial skin is undermined in a plane lateral to the parotid capsule. The undermining extends over the mandible and may reach the nasolabial fold. The inset outlines the completed flap.

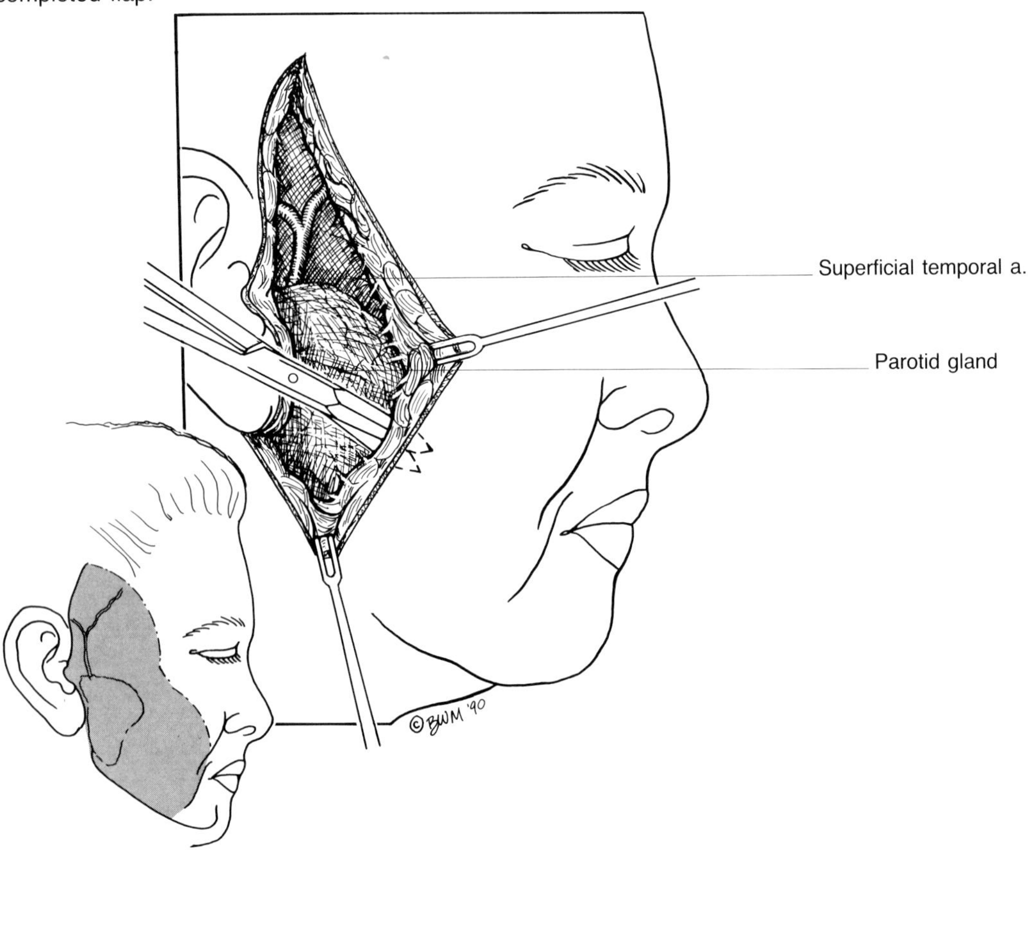

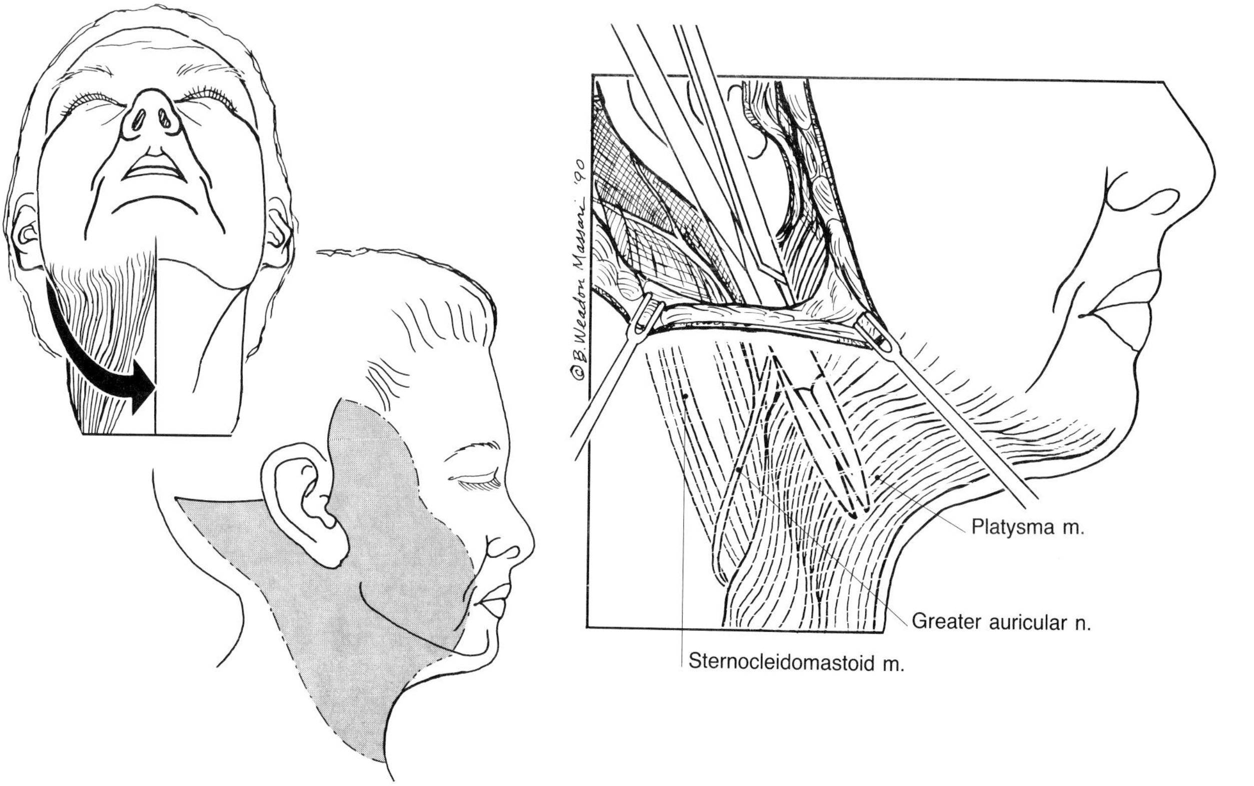

FIGURE 7
The elevation of the neck skin flap is lateral to the platysma muscle. It may extend to the midline and two-thirds down the vertical length of the neck. The shaded area depicts the cervical-facial flaps after completion of extensive undermining. Less aggressive undermining may also be performed.

the patient's head in the midline. The skin reorientation is essentially in a superior and posterior direction. At the areas of greatest tension (temporoparietal and postauricular hairline), the skin is secured with stay sutures or a suitable substitute such as towel clips (Fig. 8). At this point, many surgeons will dissect the contralateral side of the face and neck in a similar fashion. This allows potentially less margin of error in creating skin flap asymmetry during closure. I prefer to close the ipsilateral side after completion of skin flap rotation.

Excision of skin excess is begun in the temporoparietal region (Fig. 9). Here, mild to moderate tension may be placed on the wound margin. The closure can be done sequentially or after completion of the preauricular and postauricular skin excisions. The preauricular and postauricular sulcus wounds should bear no tension after excess skin has been excised. In the postauricular hairline, mild to moderate tension is acceptable and usually necessary. Closure materials in the temporoparietal and postauricular hairline are either staples or moderately heavy nylon sutures (3-0). Surgeons who use nylon say that the sutures give them a better "feel" for tension on the suture line. Undyed absorbable sutures are useful for subcutaneous closure in these areas. Pre- and postauricular closure is with 6-0 and 4-0 nylon, respectively. Although some surgeons do not routinely use drains, drains may be placed in the temporoparietal incision and at the apex of the postauricular sulcus incision (Fig. 10). A pressure dressing is applied at the conclusion of the procedure.

Postoperatively, the patient is started on a suitable antimicrobial and analgesic agent and is seen at frequent intervals. Generally, the pressure dressing is changed on the first postoperative day, and drains are removed. The dressing is replaced and left intact until the third postoperative day. After the dressing has been removed, the wound is

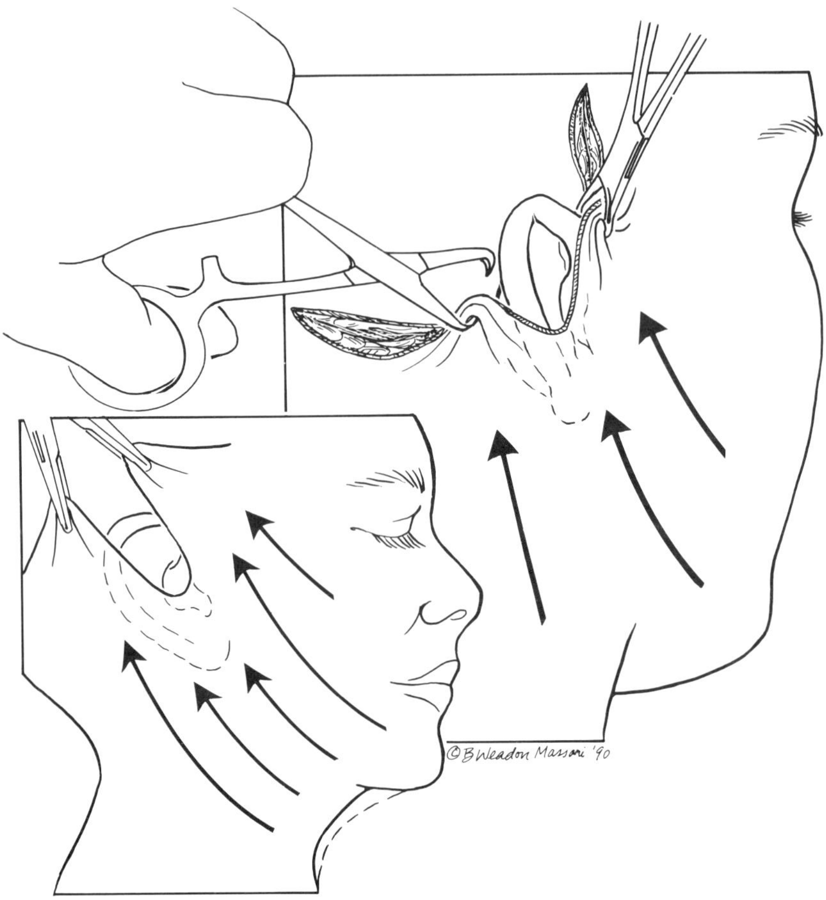

FIGURE 8
Skin flaps are rotated posteriorly and superiorly. Under moderate tension a towel clip anchors the facial flap slightly above the anterior aspect of the helical rim. The cervical flap is anchored at the apex of the postauricular sulcus incision.

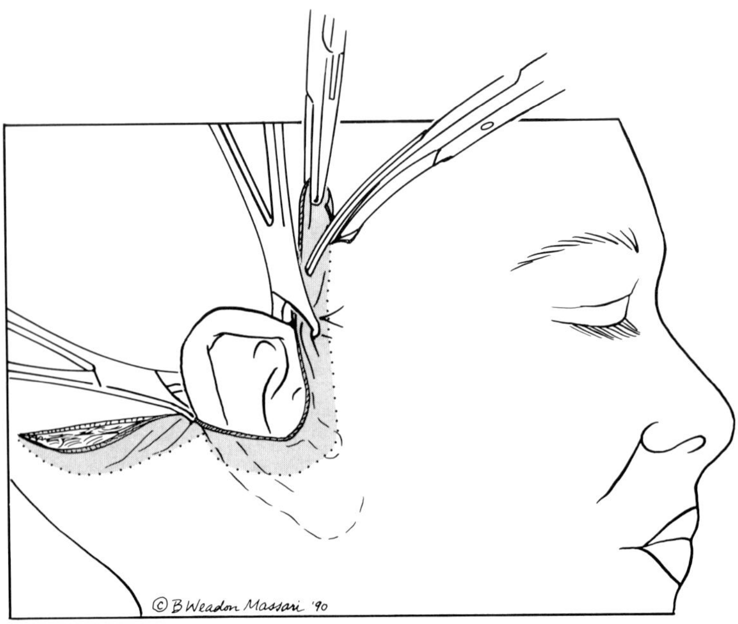

FIGURE 9
Excess skin is trimmed and suturing performed sequentially. Flap excision allows moderate tension on the temporoparietal and occipital areas of the wound. Virtually no tension is placed on the preauricular and postauricular sulcus closure.

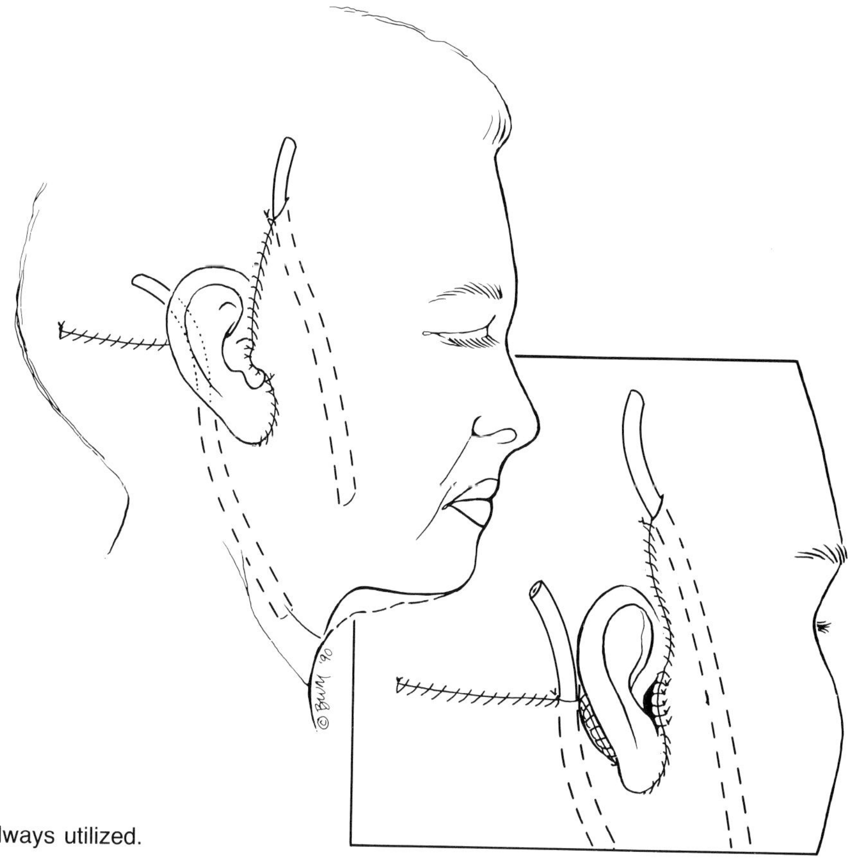

FIGURE 10
Penrose drains are depicted, but not always utilized.

cleaned and treated topically with an antibiotic ointment for several days. Sutures are usually removed on postoperative day 5 (preauricular), day 7 (postauricular, sulcus), and day 10 (temporal and postauricular hairline). Patients are allowed to gently wash their hair after the preauricular sutures are removed. I permit the use of hypoallergenic makeup at that time if the clinical situation is otherwise satisfactory. Activity restrictions are maintained for 3 to 6 weeks depending on the extent of the procedure.

ANCILLARY TECHNIQUES

The enduring desire to improve the aesthetic result has led to modifications of the classic cervical-facial procedure. These modifications are not universally applicable, and not all are enthusiastically welcomed by the surgical community. Depending on the preoperative findings, the following surgical options may be found useful.

Subfascial (SMAS) and Subplatysmal Dissection

In 1974, Skoog described a technique that employed modest undermining of the skin with aggressive mobilization of the subfascial and subplatysmal planes in the face and neck, respectively. Subsequently, cadaveric dissections and clinical trials were used to support the efficacy of this technique. Presently, the number of surgeons using this technique or modifications of it supports the conclusion that it is a useful ancillary cosmetic surgical procedure.

This procedure is based on the concept that the aging process is not confined to the skin, but also affects muscle and related soft tissue (Fig. 11). Hence, extensive undermining of the SMAS in the face and neck, with more limited undermining of the skin, theoretically allows treatment of the entire aging unit. A prominent benefit of this approach is the placement of minimal tension on the cutaneous closure, since most of the suture line

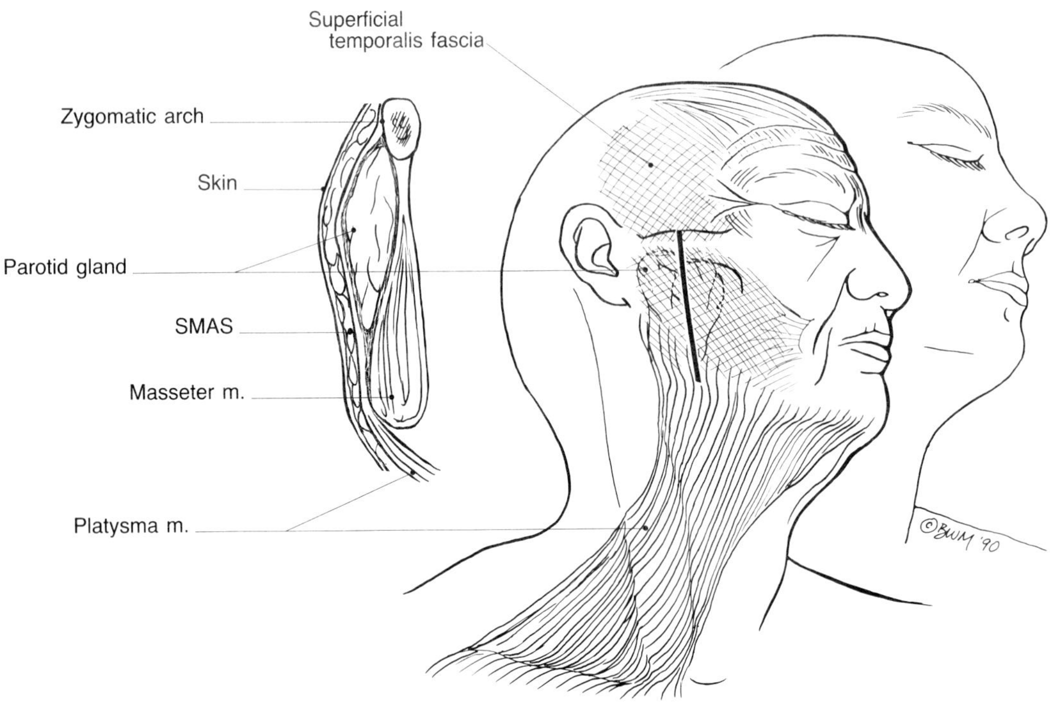

FIGURE 11
The SMAS is shown as viewed laterally and on coronal section. The relationships to other anatomic landmarks are noted.

tension is placed on the musculoaponeurotic closure. This reduces the risk of skin slough and unsightly scarring. In theory, the soundness of this procedure cannot be seriously questioned. At issue, however, is whether the results warrant the potentially greater risk to the facial nerve and other deeper-lying structures. Time has supported the judgment that it does, particularly when preoperative evaluation demonstrates prominent laxity of facial-neck skin, with jowling and platysmal banding. Some feel that the procedure may also flatten the nasolabial fold somewhat.

The technique begins with routine elevation of the cervical-facial skin flaps. Then, with sharp dissection the facial musculoaponeurotic unit is skeletonized, starting at the level of or slightly inferior to the zygomatic arch. In this area, the flap is relatively thin, consisting primarily of the fascial aponeurosis. As the dissection is continued inferiorly, the flap thickens. A clear fascial plane is easily developed over the parotid capsule, and this plane extends down to the inferior margin of the mandible. With a combination of sharp and blunt instrumentation, the dissection can be continued forward, beyond the parotid capsule toward the nasolabial fold. In this area, great care must be taken to avoid trauma to the buccal branch of the facial nerve, which runs transversely in the operating field (Fig. 12). Care must also be taken not to violate the parotid capsule, which could result in a postoperative salivary fistula. The surgeon can gauge the endpoint of the dissection by tugging on the flap and observing the effect on the jowl and perioral-nasolabial regions.

Next, the dissection is carried over the inferior margin of the mandible into the fascial plane beneath the platysma (Fig. 13). This plane is also fairly easily developed, but be alert for the marginal mandibular branch of the facial nerve. Although generally this nerve is not at significant risk until the mandibular notch has been reached, there is enough variation in the course of the nerve that it must be looked for as soon as the posterior part of the platysmal flap has been isolated. The dissection can be carried as far anteriorly as clinically indicated. Hemostasis should be obtained with bipolar electrocautery in areas close to the nerve.

The SMAS and platysmal flaps are then rotated in a posterosuperior direction and anchored with stay sutures, starting with the subfascial muscle

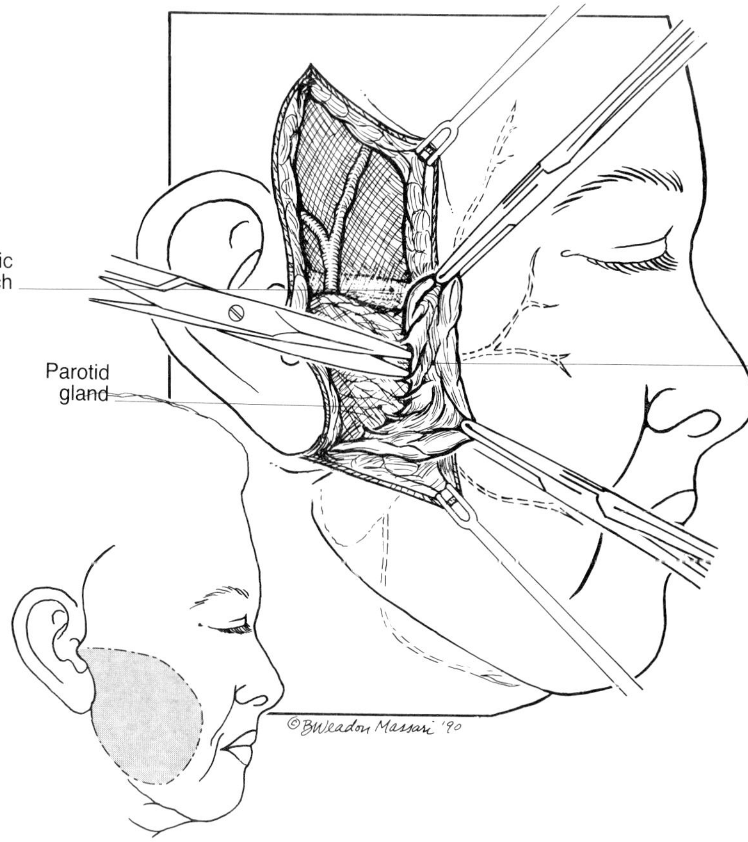

FIGURE 12
The SMAS dissection begins slightly inferior to the zygomatic arch and extends inferiorly and anteriorly in a plane lateral to the parotid capsule. The SMAS may be widely undermined, but branches of the facial nerve must not be traumatized.

FIGURE 13
The platysmal flap is developed anterior to the sternocleidomastoid muscle, usually in continuity with the SMAS dissection as the latter extends over the mandible. Wide undermining can be performed, but the marginal branch of the facial nerve must be carefully avoided.

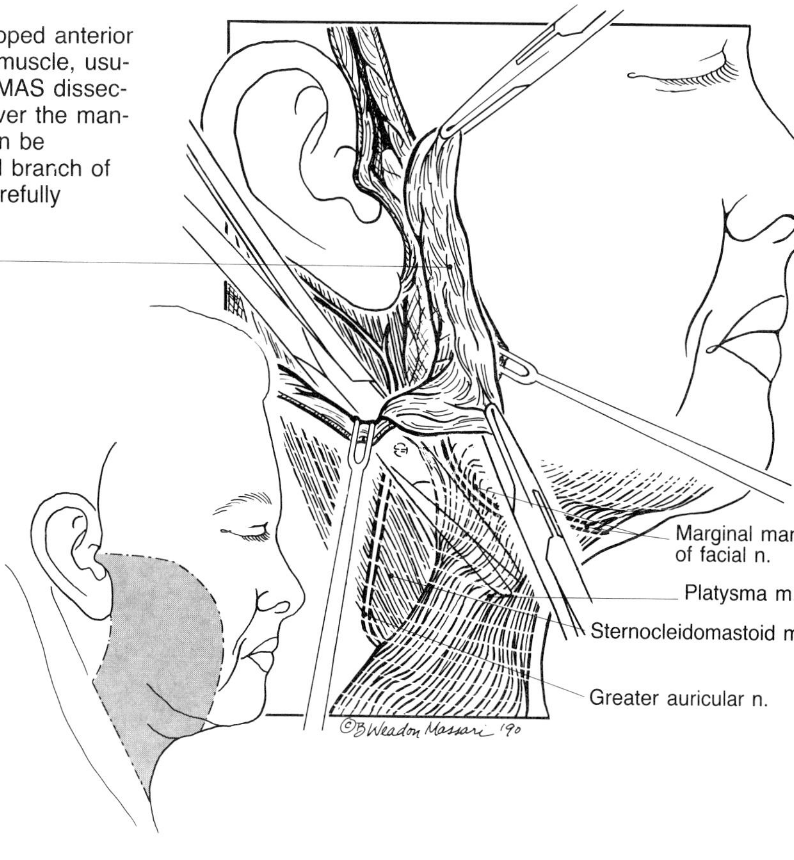

flap in the cheek (Fig. 14). Excess aponeurosis and muscle are trimmed from the flap, and it is then imbricated under moderate tension to the fascia overlying the zygomatic arch. The sutures are buried and can be placed along the arch up to two thirds of the distance between the anterior helical rim and the lateral canthal without jeopardizing the frontozygomatic branch of cranial nerve VII. Either permanent clear nylon or long-lasting disolvable undyed suture may be used.

The platysmal flap is similarly trimmed and imbricated to the tough fascia overlying the sternocleidomastoid muscle (Fig. 15). A variation of the latter is to suture the platysmal flap to the fascia overlying the mastoid tip. The number of sutures used depends on the amount of tissue mobilized. When a lesser dissection of these anatomic units is needed, plication may be used instead of imbrication, but one must guard against creating a visible subcutaneous fold.

Occasionally, a prominent medial band of platysma, present in part because of partial dehiscence of the submental decussation, may be treated by partial excision of the inferomedial portion of the muscle band and midline repair of the decussation (Fig. 16). Additional modifications of platysma surgery are used to refine neck contour, including extensive midline plication, complete inferior transection of the platysma with posterior imbrication (Fig. 17), partial posterior and anterior resection (Fig. 18), and a variety of partial platysmal muscle slings. These techniques are not used by all surgeons, and many surgeons suggest that the results do not warrant the additional potential complications including neck asymmetry and marginal mandibular nerve injury. Weakness of the corner of the mouth can also occur with overzealous resection of the anterosuperior platysma. Dressings and postoperative care after SMAS and platysma surgery are the same as for a classic facelift.

FIGURE 14
The SMAS is repositioned as shown, and excess is excised.

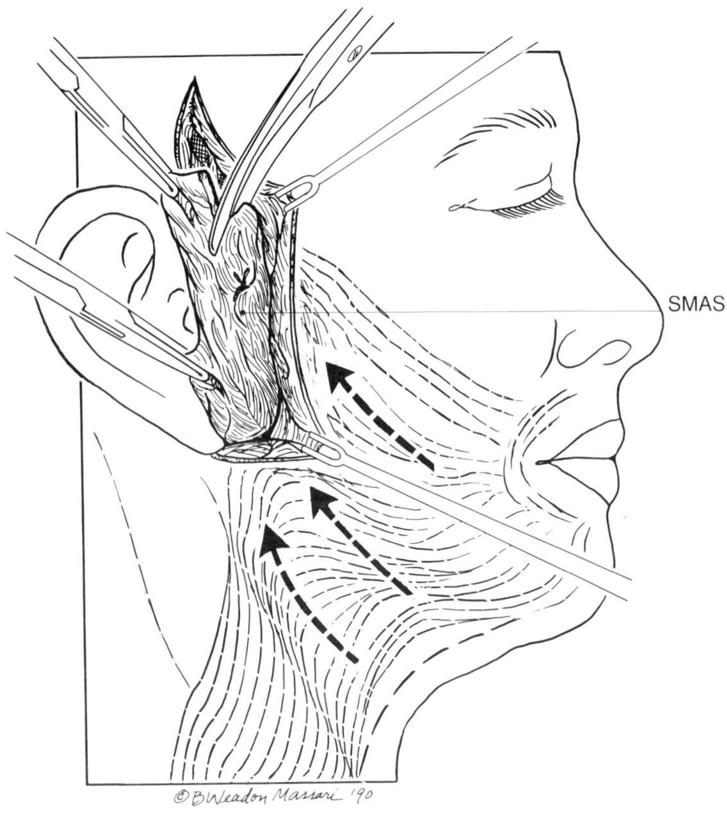

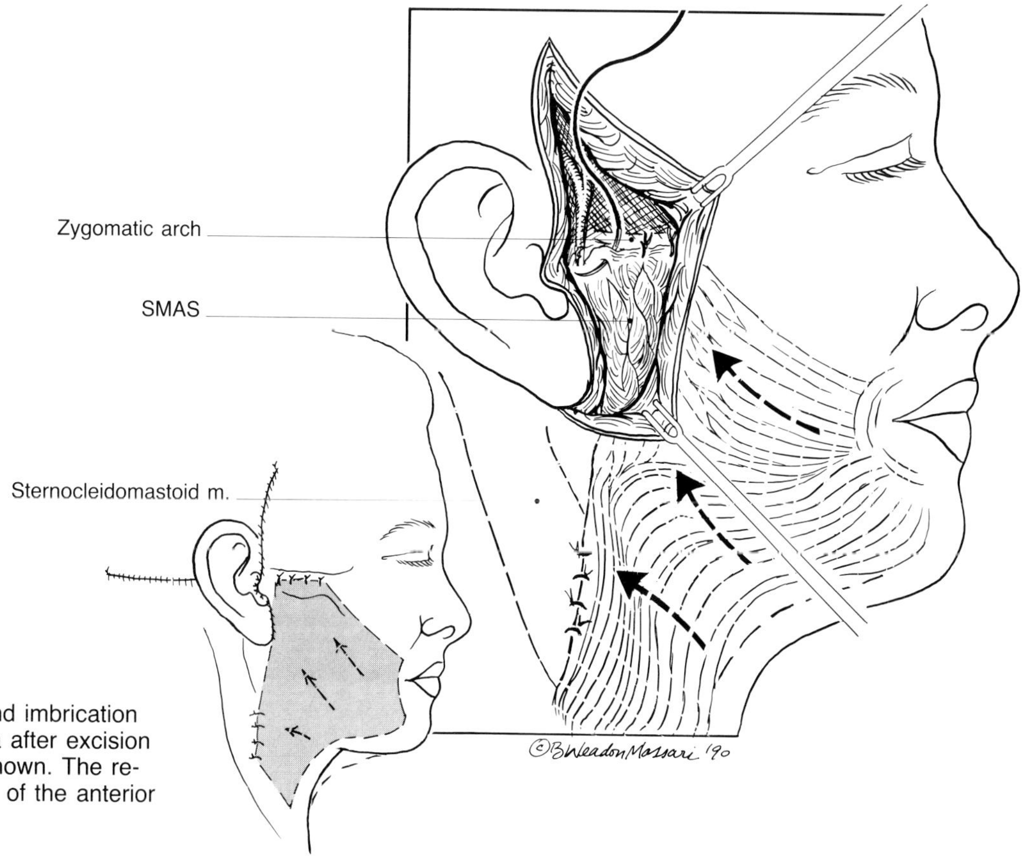

FIGURE 15
The direction of pull and imbrication of SMAS and platysma after excision of excess tissue are shown. The resultant contour change of the anterior neck is shown.

FIGURE 16
The platysma is approximated in the midline after vertical resection of the anterior platysma borders. The procedure is performed when significant medial redundancy of the platysma exists. This anatomic problem is often associated with absence of the platysma decussation.

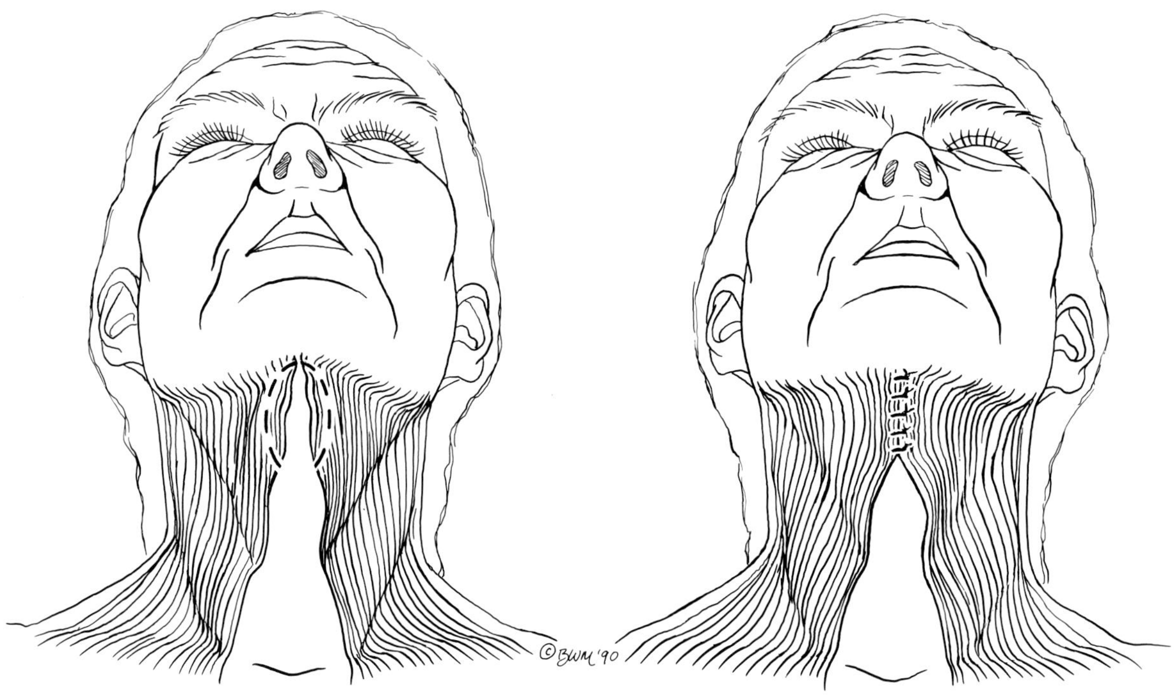

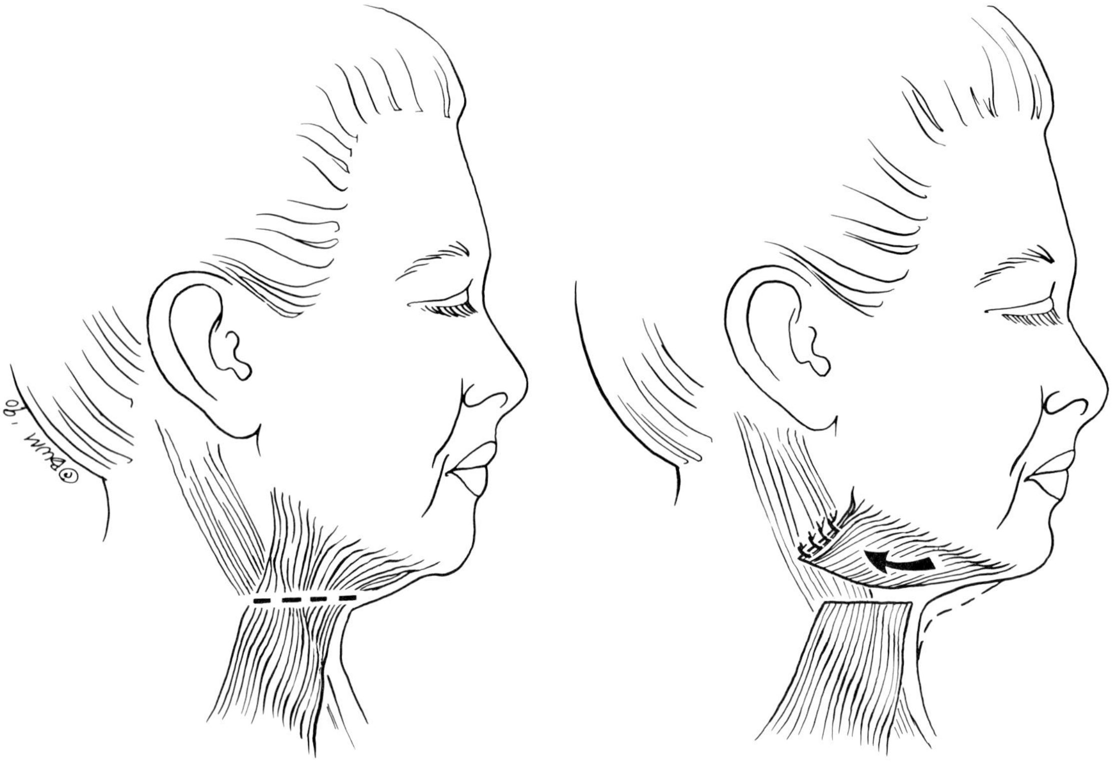

FIGURE 17
The platysma has been completely transected and imbricated posteriorly. This technique is useful in patients with an obtuse cervicomental angle, but may be complicated by puckering of the skin along the line of transection as healing occurs.

FIGURE 18
When significant generalized redundancy of the platysma exists, wedge resection of anterior vertical bands with partial posterior resection and imbrication can be done. The former is useful when midline submental plication still results in residual inferior platysmal bands.

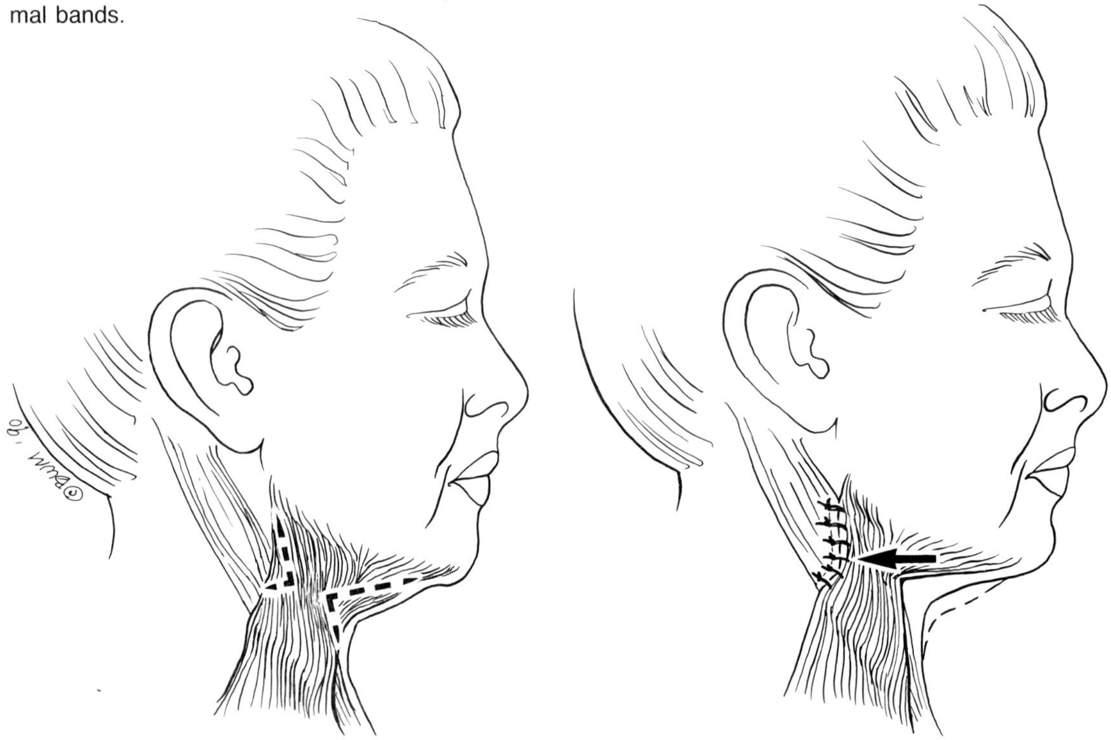

Dissection of the Buccal Fat Pad

The Buccal fat pad is located anterior to the masseter muscle, deep in the soft tissue of the cheek. The pad may give additional unwanted fullness to a cheek and may be excised to subtly improve contour in this region and to lend more relative definition to the malar eminence. Some surgeons advocate its removal through an external approach after the subfascial muscular flap has been elevated over the cheek. The author feels that inherent in this approach are a greater risk of bleeding from a vascular bundle that penetrates the fat pad anterior to the masseter muscle and a greater risk to the buccal branch of the facial nerve (Fig. 19). Another approach to the buccal fat pad is an intraoral one, which is performed at the conclusion of the facelift. A small horizontal incision is made in the buccal mucosa inferior to, but in the region of, the parotid duct. Sharp scissor dissection through the fibers of the buccinator muscle (which should be separated horizontally) produces the thin membranous septum overlying the fat. With gentle external pressure, the fat can be easily delivered through a stab incision in the septum (Fig. 20). The base of the pad can be clamped, and after the excision, a

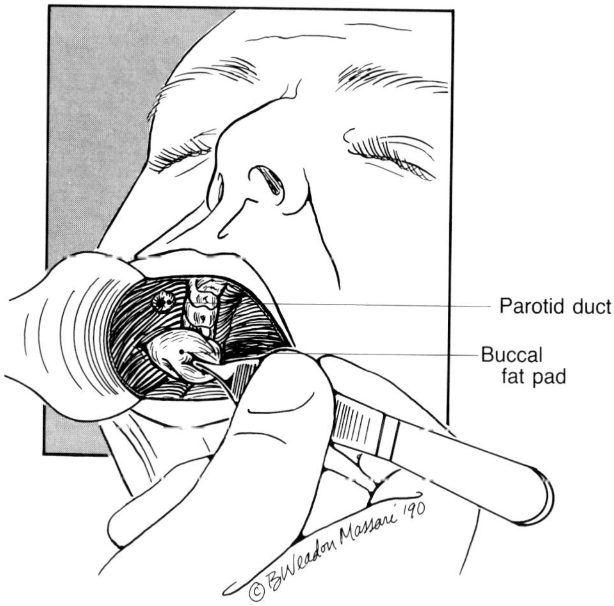

FIGURE 20
The intraoral approach to the buccal fat pad is through a horizontal incision made inferior to the parotid duct in the region of the molar teeth.

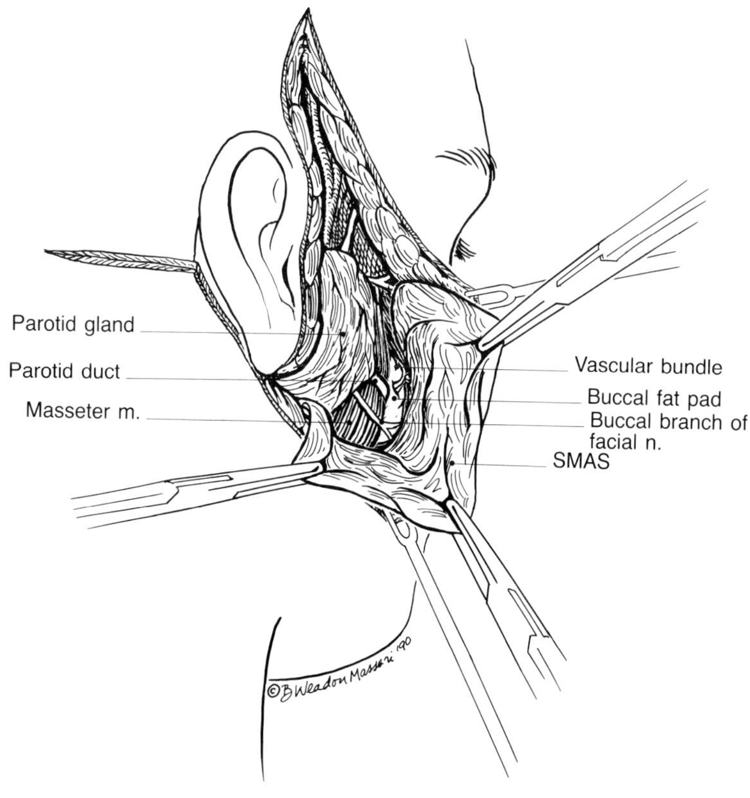

FIGURE 19
The buccal fat pad is found anterior to the masseter muscle and can be reached cautiously through the facelift incision.

free tie or bipolar electrocautery is used on the stump. Bipolar cauterization is particularly important here, to avoid any potential damage to the lip. Dissolvable sutures are used for closure.

Temporal and Coronal (Forehead) Lift

The temporolateral, canthal, and forehead regions require consideration as separate aesthetic units. A cervical-facial operation will not correct significant lateral canthal or forehead rhytides. To address the former, the temporal lift mobilizes the soft tissue lateral to the temporoparietal fascia and allows some flattening of lateral canthal rhytides when the flap is rotated in a posterosuperior direction. Some mild correction of lateral brow ptosis is also possible with this approach. The procedure is frequently performed in conjuction with the facelift by extending the incision superiorly in curvilinear fashion into the temporoparietal scalp (Fig. 21). Undermining must avoid the superficial temporal artery and should remain in the fascial plane to protect the frontal branch of cranial nerve VII. An additional technique advocated to embellish the temporal lift is plication of the lateral portion of the orbicularis oculi muscle. Theoretically, lateral canthal rhytides are more effectively reduced with this artistry. However, it also places the frontal zygomatic branch of cranial nerve VII at greater risk, and this possibility must be weighed against the potential benefit.

The forehead can be treated separately or at the same time as the face and neck. When the forehead is part of a staged procedure, the facelift is usually done first. The coronal incision preferred by most surgeons is placed several centimeters behind the frontal hairline after the hair has been parted. The incision extends in the bitemporal scalp, approximating the superior helix (Fig. 22). Undermining is in the areolar tissue plane lateral to the periosteum. In this plane, the surgeon can carry the dissection to the glabellar region, skeletonizing not

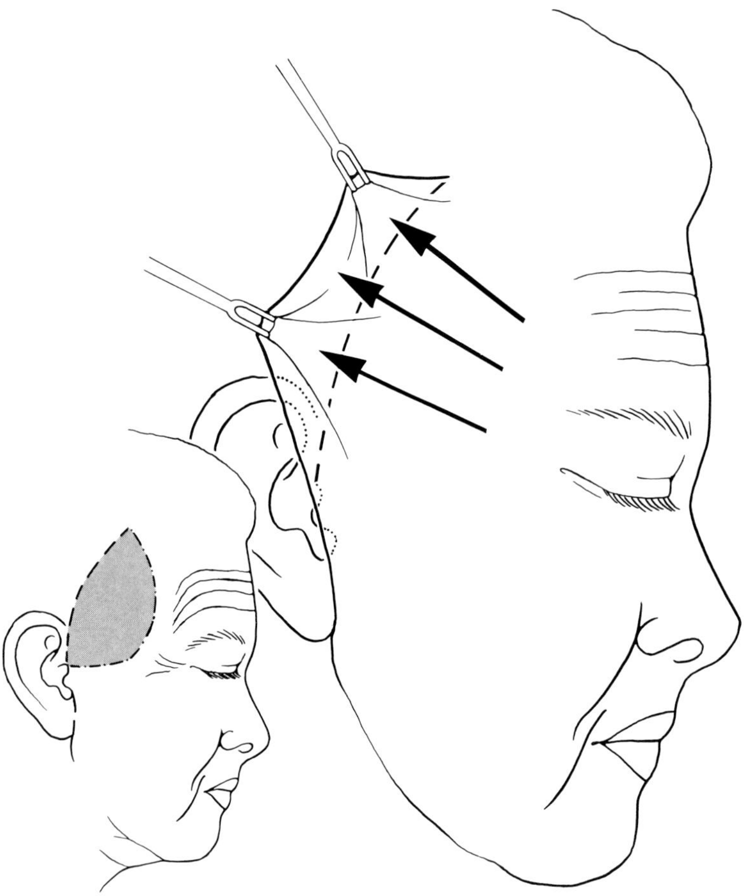

FIGURE 21
The temporal lift incision is depicted as a curvilinear extension of the facelift incision. Wide undermining is lateral to the temporalis fascia and results in a flap which is repositioned by pulling in a posterior and slightly upward direction.

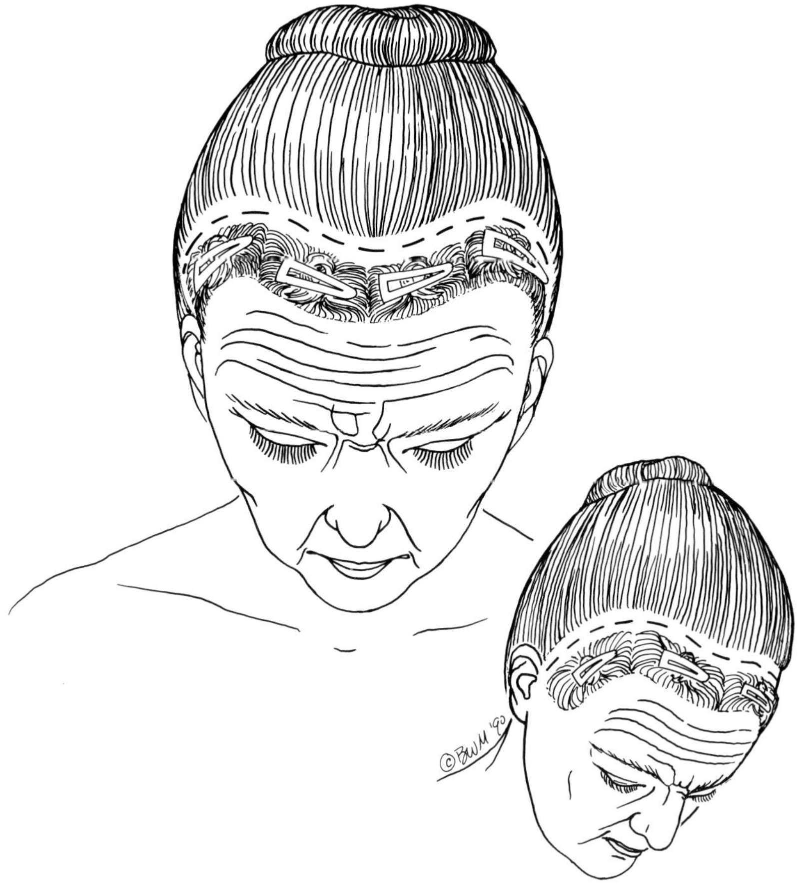

FIGURE 22
The coronal incision is outlined on the scalp through parted hair and is curved slightly forward medially, following the contour of the hairline.

only the frontalis, corrugator, and procerus muscles, but also the supratrochlear neurovascular bundle, which must be preserved (Fig. 23). Suitable retraction is necessary for visualization of these structures: many surgeons use illuminating fiber-optic speculae to improve visualization. Depending on preoperative indications, laxity of the corrugator and procerus muscles can be treated by avulsion or cauterization, which is particularly effective in reducing deep glabellar furrows.

The frontalis muscle has been dealt with by using a variety of techniques including partial excision and checkerboarding of the muscle by either sharp dissection or electrocautery (Fig. 24). The aim of all methods is to diminish the effect of the muscle on horizontal furrows. When the flap is positioned, a ptotic brow is also elevated. Excess scalp is excised after stay sutures are placed at 3- to 4-cm intervals along the flap (Fig. 25). The frontal branch of cranial nerve VII is well protected as long as the surgeon is not fervent in treating the lateral 3 cm of the frontalis muscle, where the nerve usually inserts in the muscle.

A modification of this technique places the incision at the junction of forehead skin and hairline, and it may be extended inferiorly around the sideburn. This preserves the position of the sideburns and avoids excision of hair-bearing scalp. However, if too much tension is placed on the wound, the resultant spreading can be disastrous. A routine pressure dressing is used, and soft drains may be placed if desired.

Patients undergoing a forehead lift might be aware of a mask-like quality to the upper third of the face in the immediate postoperative period. The edema of the flap, which is responsible for this appearance, may also transiently affect function of the frontal branch of cranial nerve VII, especially if the frontalis has been dealt with aggressively. Advising patients of these possibilities preoperatively is imperative.

Liposuction

Liposuction has become an accepted refinement technique. (See also Chapter 30.) It is useful for es-

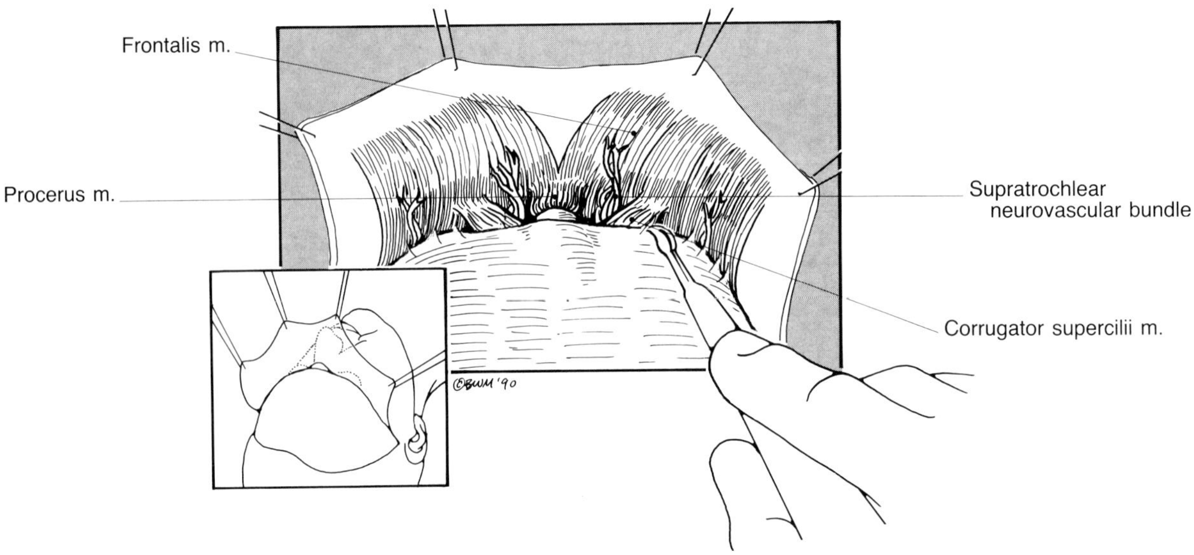

FIGURE 23
The forehead flap is elevated exposing the frontalis, corrugator, and procerus muscles. Aggressive undermining can extend over the supraorbital rim. The supratrochlear neurovascular bundle is preserved.

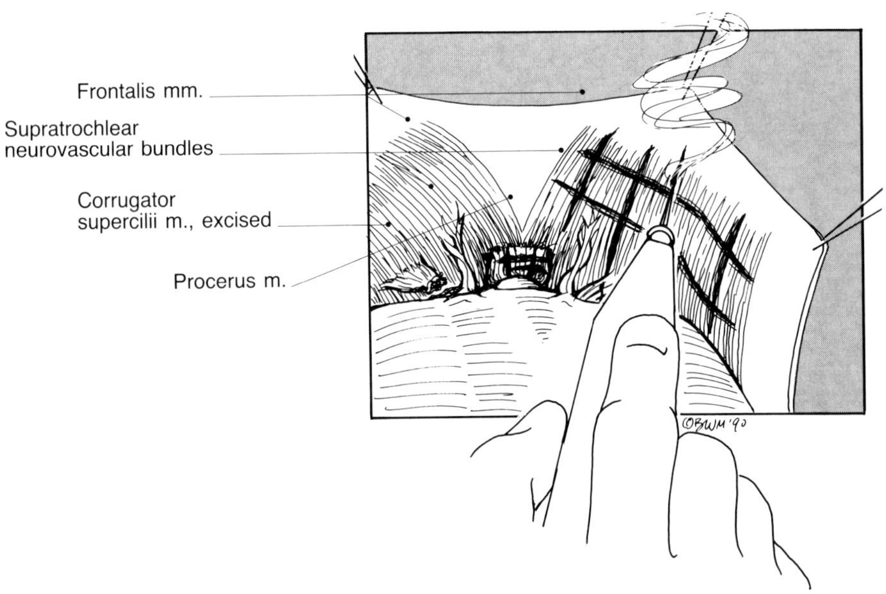

FIGURE 24
Crosshatching the frontalis and procerus muscles with electrocautery is depicted. Partial muscle removal with sharp dissection can also be performed as shown with the corrugator.

tablishing an aesthetic contour in the submental-submaxillary triangles and for removing excess fat superior to the nasolabial crease and lateral to the platysma during the cervical part of the facelift (Fig. 26). The superiority of liposuction over conventional sharp dissection is obvious to any surgeon who has spent significant operating time controlling bleeding from the sharp dissection in the submental area.

A small stab incision is made in the submental skin crease, and a skin flap is minimally developed (Fig. 27). A 3.6-mm shark-nosed, closed-tipped suction cannula is introduced. The fat is then aspirated from the area, which is demarcated prior to injection of local anesthetic. Fat lateral to the platysma is removed similarly, with attention being paid to keep the opening in the cannula tip from traumatizing the dermis.

In the parasymphyseal-jowl region, one must be careful to avoid trauma to the perioral musculature and to the marginal mandibular branch of cranial nerve VII as it inserts in these muscles. As with the jowl, the nasolabial region can be reached by way of the preauricular part of the facelift incision. This area can also be treated via a stab incision in the lateral inferior quadrant of the nasal vestibule (Fig. 28). Here a 2.4-mm cannula is appropriate for removal of more delicate deposits of fat. If submental liposuction is used in conjunction with facelift surgery, elastic support is provided for 3 weeks postoperatively, usually worn nightly. The nasolabial region is treated with cold compresses for 24 hr.

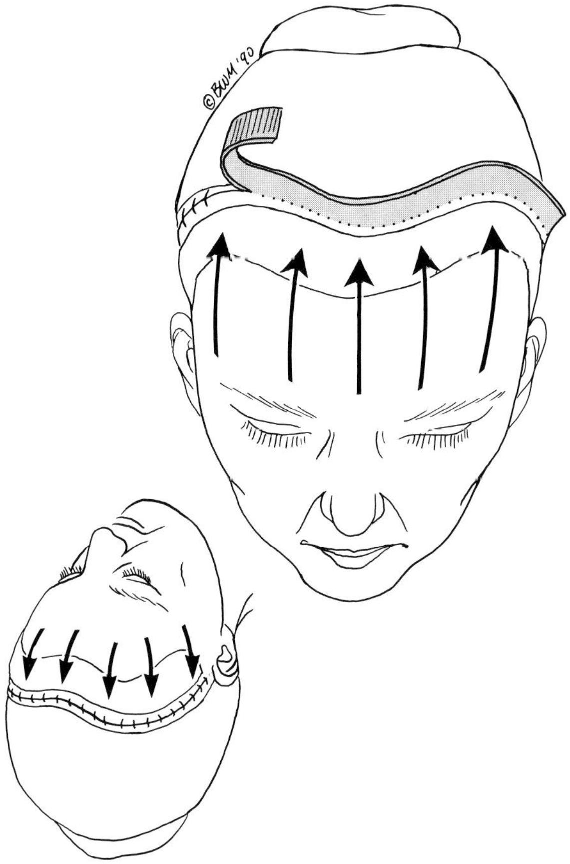

FIGURE 25
The forehead flap is repositioned, flap excess is excised, and the wound is closed with staples under moderate tension.

FIGURE 26
Drawing shows areas of fat deposition frequently treated with liposuction during facelift surgery.

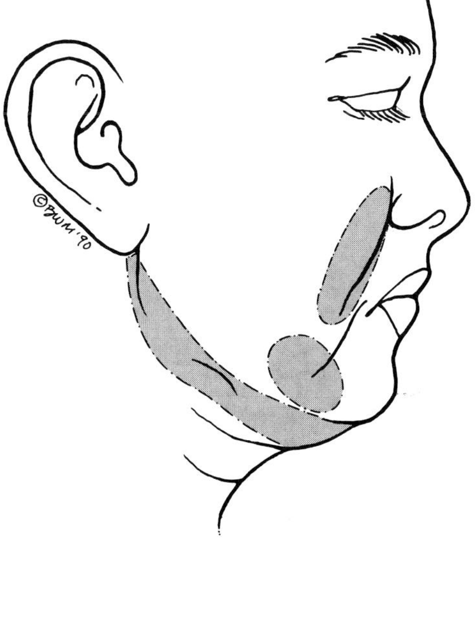

FIGURE 27
The submental skin crease incision is used to remove fat in the anterior and lateral neck, potentially extending as far posteriorly as the angle of the mandible.

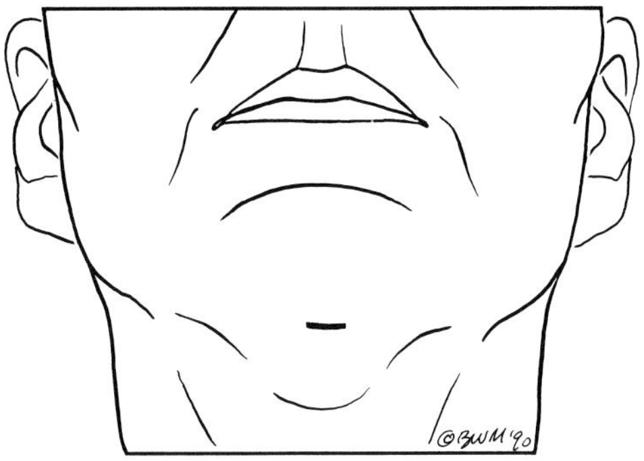

FIGURE 28
The nasal vestibule stab incision is used to reach fat lateral to the nasolabial fold.

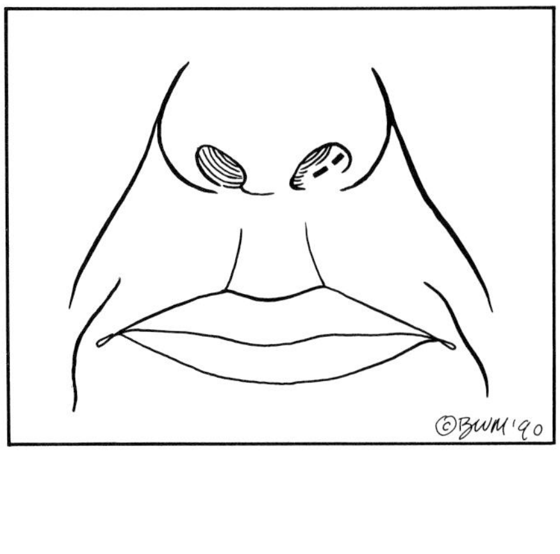

COMPLICATIONS

Complications from facelift surgery are generally minor, with major problems occuring infrequently. Meticulous attention to hemostasis during the procedure and administration of postoperative antibiotics help prevent hematoma formation and infection. Significant bleeding from the skin flap or subcutaneous tissue is heralded by pain and obvious swelling. This situation requires surgical drainage and control of the bleeding vessel(s). It is more likely to occur in patients who are hypertensive or smokers. Usually, if it is treated expeditiously, there are no long-term sequelae; however, if neglected, the circulatory compromise on the skin flap from an expanding hematoma may be calamitous.

Numbness following a facelift is usually short-lived unless the greater auricular nerve has been severed. Female patients must be cautioned about wearing expensive clip-on earrings until numbness of the ear lobe has resolved.

Hair loss and wound spreading in areas of significant wound tension can be causes of great concern to the patient. Their occurrence can be reduced by beveling the scalpel away from the direction of hair follicles and by judicious use of subcutaneous sutures in the temporal and postauricular hairlines to minimize superficial wound tension. When these problems arise, surgical correction can usually be satisfactorily performed at a later date.

The most serious postoperative complications are skin slough and facial paralysis. Partial or full-thickness skin loss can be disastrous and underscores the need for refined surgical judgment in determining excision of skin excess. Red flags in the preoperative consultation include any illness that might affect small vessels and hence wound healing. The slough usually occurs in the postauricular region where wound tension is greatest, although more extensive, preauricular skin loss can occur. Where small areas are involved or partial thickness loss occurs, the wound generally heals satisfactorily by secondary intention. However, larger areas of loss can require grafting. In any case, the occurrence of this complication requires clear communication with the patient, as healing may be prolonged. Residual pigmentation abnormalities, skin texture changes, and unsightly scarring may persist.

Paresis of a branch or branches of the facial nerve may be transient secondary to paraneural infiltration with local anesthetic during the procedure. Short-lived nerve weakness is also occasionally a result of stretching the nerve; however, any facial muscle dysfunction that is present longer than several hours after completion of the procedure must be considered a potential problem. This is particularly true with aggressive subfascial or subplatysmal procedures in which the nerve is in greater jeopardy. Although most incidences of paresis resolve, confirmation of significant nerve injury is made with nerve conduction studies when indicated. Neurorrhaphy can be performed, but success rates vary considerably.

CONCLUSIONS

The classic facelift with many of the attendant modifications has been discussed, and germane diagrammatic drawings of the techniques have been reviewed. These procedures will no doubt continue to be refined in pursuit of the goal of improved surgical results and greater patient satisfaction. Inherent in the effective application of these principles is the mandated expression of sound surgical judgment.

REFERENCES

1. Skoog T. Plastic Surgery. Stockholm: Almgrist and Wicksell International, 1974:300–330.
2. Fournier P, Otteni F. Lipodissection in body sculpturing: The dry procedure. Plast Reconstr Surg. 1983;72:598–609.
3. Illouz YG. Body contouring by lipolysis: A 5-year experience with over 3,000 cases. Plast Reconstr Surg. 1983;72: 591–597.
4. Conway H. The surgical facelift: Rhytidectomy. Plast Reconstr Surg. 1970;45:124–130.
5. Mitz V, Peyronie M. The superficial musculo-aponeurotic system (SMAS) in the parotid and cheek area. Plast Reconstr Surg. 1976;58:80–87.
6. Owsley JQ. Platysma-fascia rhytidectomy. Plast Reconstr Surg. 1977;60:843–859.
7. Parkes ML, Kamer FM, Bassilios, MI. Practical suggestions on facial plastic surgery—How I do it. Treatment of alopecia in temporal region following rhytidectomy procedures. Laryngoscope. 1977;87:1011–1014.

8. Lemmon ML, Hamra ST. Skoog rhytidectomy: A 5-year experience with 577 patients. Plast Reconstr Surg. 1980; 5:283–297.
9. Gonzales-Ulloa M. Facial wrinkles. Plast Reconstr Surg. 1962;29:658–673.
10. Guerrero-Santos J, Espaillat L. Muscular lift in cervical rhytidoplasty. Clinic Plast Surg. 1978;5:29–49.
11. Vistner LM, Souther WG. The anatomical basis for common cosmetic anterior neck deformities. Ann Plast Surg. 1979;2:381–388.
12. Adamson JE, Toksu AE. Progress in rhytidectomy by platysma-SMAS rotation and elevation. Plast Reconstr Surg. 1981;68:23–33.
13. Dingman RO, Grabb WC. Surgical anatomy of the mandibular ramus of the facial nerve based on the dissection of 100 face halves. Plast Reconstr Surg. 1962;29:266–272.
14. Pernkopf E. Atlas of Topographical and Applied Human Anatomy. Baltimore: Urban and Schwarzenberg, 1980;118–126.
15. Mayer DM, Swanker WA. Rhytidoplasty. Plast Reconstr Surg. 1950;6:255–263.
16. Pangman WJ II, Wallace RM. Cosmetic surgery of the face and neck. Plast Reconstr Surg. 1961;27:544–550.
17. Kaye BL. The extended neck lift: The "bottom line." Plast Reconstr Surg. 1980;65:429–435.
18. Connell BF. Contouring the neck in rhytidectomy by lipectomy and a muscle sling. Plast Reconstr Surg. 1978;61:376–383.
19. Rees TD. Aesthetic Plastic Surgery. Philadelphia: Saunders, 1980;600–633.
20. Hamra ST. The tri-plane facelift dissection. Ann Plast Surg. 1984;12:268–274.
21. Baker DC, Conley J. Avoiding facial nerve injuries in rhytidectomy: Anatomical variations and pitfalls. Plast Reconstr Surg. 1979;64:781–795.
22. Kamer, FM. Sequential rhytidectomy and the two stage concept. Otolaryngol Clin N Am, 1980;13:305–320.
23. Huber E. Evolution of Facial Musculature and Facial Expression. Baltimore, MD: Johns Hopkins Press, 1931.
24. Webster RC, et al. Conservative facelift surgery. Arch Otolaryngol. 1976;102:657–662.
25. DeCastro CC. The anatomy of the platysma muscle. Plast Reconstr Surg. 1980;66:680–683.

CHAPTER

19

Blepharoplasty and Related Procedures

ROBERT AXELROD

For at least a thousand years people have undertaken cosmetic and reconstructive eyelid procedures.[1] Intradermal pigmentation techniques for outlining and drawing attention to the eyes predated surgery by several thousand years.[2] This chapter describes recent techniques for improving the appearance and function of the eyelids and adjacent structures.[3–12]

Dermatochalasis, or redundancy of eyelid skin, and bulging of orbital fat are common problems that cause patients to seek surgical treatment. *Blepharoplasty* is the procedure utilized to correct these problems and achieve aesthetic improvement. There are various blepharoplasty techniques, many with different goals, but none is capable of correcting all cosmetic and functional eyelid complaints.

Many factors contribute to unwanted folds or bags around the eyelids that detract from one's appearance. Perhaps the most important factor is heredity; children just seem to grow up and look like their parents. Age, skin quality, health status, and environmental exposure all contribute to eyelid appearance. Anatomic features such as brow ptosis, lid laxity, and blepharoptosis also play a major role in the cosmetic appearance of the eyes.[4,13–15] What may be considered attractive eyelid attributes varies between men and women. These features include brow level and contour and eyelid crease and upper sulcus. In both men and women the goals of blepharoplasty basically involve removal of elements that detract from one's overall appearance. In women the aim is to draw attention to beautiful eyes. This includes the ability to wear makeup better and to use pigments to define and augment the lash line.

PATIENT EVALUATION

As in other areas of medicine, perhaps the most fundamental aspect of the evaluation is listening to the patient's complaints. The patient is best able to demonstrate his or her concern by looking into a simple hand mirror. Patients are frequently unable to detail what they do not like about their eyelids, and so a systemic approach is required. This allows the examiner to evaluate with the patient details of brow and eyelid structure, skin laxity, fat bulging, and skin quality. During the evaluation it may become more apparent to the patient what aspects of the lids and related structures are deficient.

After the cosmetic complaints are elicited, a brief patient history should be undertaken to evaluate whether a disease state such as hyperthyroidism, hypertension, or diabetes mellitus is playing a causative role.

Visual acuity and adequacy of tear function should be assessed. Both Snellen's acuity chart and Schirmer's tear production test packet should be basic items in the blepharoplasty surgeon's office.[9,16]

Eyelid level in relation to the pupil in primary gaze is examined to determine whether blepharoptosis is present. Proper evaluation of lid level with the forehead relaxed provides an assessment of levator integrity.

Lower eyelid tonus should be evaluated carefully. Laxity, when left untreated, is a major cause of postoperative lid retraction and ectropion.[9] When pulled down and released a normal eyelid should snap back to the globe prior to blinking. Poor tonus can be corrected at the time of blepharoplasty with a horizontal shortening procedure.[15,17,18]

GOALS

The most common "complication" of blepharoplasty occurs when the results do not measure up to the patient's expectations. The primary sources of this problem are failure of the surgeon and patient to communicate and a mismatch between what the patient expects and what the surgeon can deliver.

Once the examination is completed, the remainder of the visits before surgery should define the goals of surgery as well as what can and cannot be achieved. Blepharoplasty is *not* surgery for wrinkles. Except for the skin that can actually be removed, eyelid skin containing wrinkles cannot generally be pulled or flattened effectively without compromising lid function and contour.

Lateral canthal lines, or "crow's-feet," likewise cannot be improved with blepharoplasty. In fact, it is a matter of controversy whether any surgical technique for the face can adequately relieve these lines.[19]

Malar folds or festoons cannot be eliminated with blepharoplasty techniques. If the condition is severe enough, direct excision is warranted, but this often results in a noticeable scar.

Excessive skin in the medial canthal region—a multicontoured area consisting of the lid, canthus, brow, and nose—cannot be adequately excised without the trade-off of unwanted scars or lines of traction. Sometimes surgical elevation of the brow can lessen the medial canthal redundancy.

Upper eyelid fullness as a result of brow ptosis is best corrected by brow or forehead elevation.[4] Ignoring a significantly low brow greatly limits the success of blepharoplasty. Likewise, including within the skin excision of the upper eyelid the thicker skin immediately beneath the brow results at best in a noticeable scar and at worst in difficulty closing the eyes during sleep. Suturing thick skin to thin leaves a detracting defect in the surface contour of the lid.

In women a common blepharoplasty goal is the creation or enhancement of the upper eyelid crease. This provides a noticeable platform above the lashes on which to apply makeup. It moves the eyelid fold away from the lashes and contributes to the impression of a more alert individual (Fig. 1). The technique of supratarsal fixation more reliably achieves this attractive result (Fig. 2).[6,7]

In men the eyes are generally not prominent, and usually no attempt is made to create a high lid

FIGURE 1
Blepharoplasty can remove upper lid hooding and expose a broader platform above the lashes.

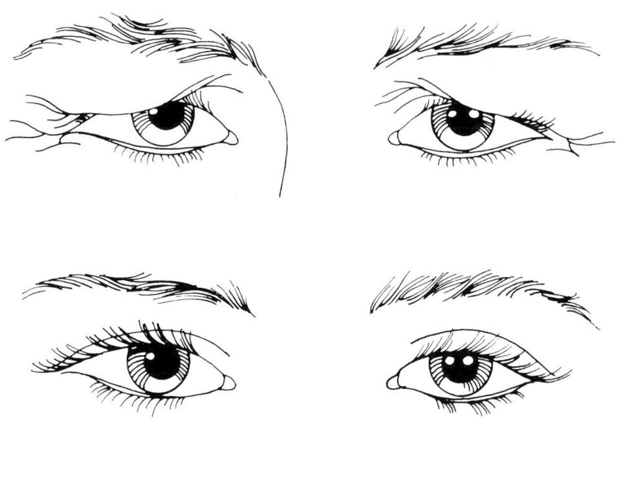

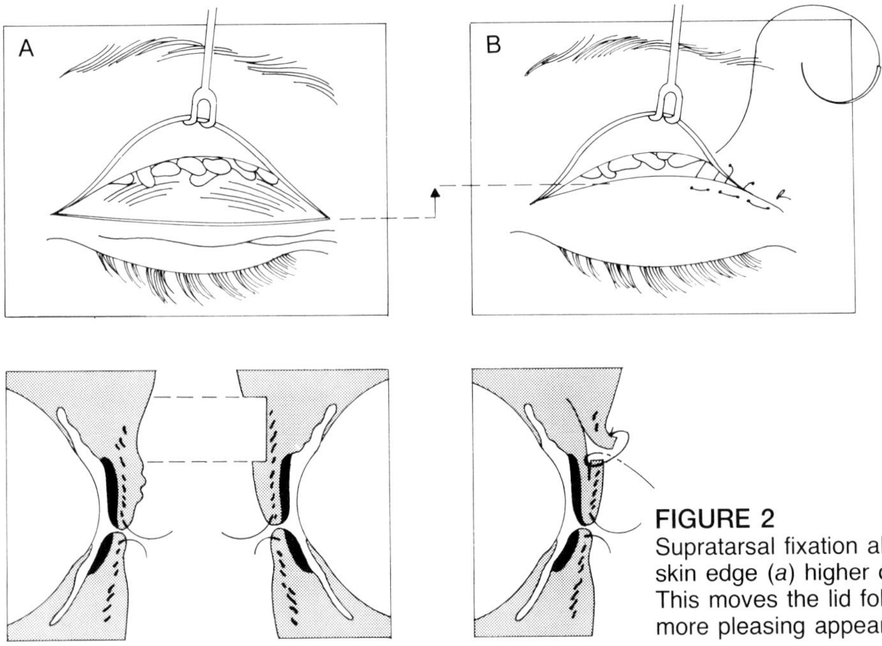

FIGURE 2
Supratarsal fixation allows attachment of the lower cut skin edge (*a*) higher onto the levator aponeurosis (*b*). This moves the lid fold higher on the lid and provides a more pleasing appearance.

TABLE 1
COMPLICATIONS OF BLEPHAROPLASTY

Complication	Causes
Lagophthalmos	Excessive skin excision Deep scar formation with adhesions Suturing of septum
Depressed sulcus	Excess fat excision
Asymmetry of creases	Poor supratarsal excision Asymmetrical fat or muscle excision
Ptosis	Severed levator aponeurosis Supratarsal fixation too high
Pseudoepicanthal folds	Excessive medial upper lid skin removal
Scleral show (lower lid retraction)	Excessive skin excision Deep scar formation Suturing of septum
Ectropion	Excessive skin excision Lax canthal attachments
Infection	Bacterial contamination of skin
Hemorrhage	Usually orbicularis, occasionally vessels in fat

crease. Indeed, a deep upper sulcus and a high crease may be a "feminizing" characteristic. Thus the definition of the crease with supratarsal fixation is generally unwarranted in men.

One of the primary blepharoplasty goals for the lower eyelid in both men and women is the elimination of bags. These unwanted features play a major role in creating a tired, "worn-out" look. They are primarily a result of forward herniation of orbital fat and are familial to a large degree. In younger as well as older patients their removal yields beneficial cosmetic results. When redundant lower lid skin is not present, fat removal can be easily and safely accomplished with the transconjunctival lower lid technique.[8,20]

The goals and limitations of the procedure chosen should be reviewed carefully with the patient prior to surgery. This includes outlining the major risks associated with the procedure (Table 1).[21–24]

EYELID ANATOMY

As shown in Fig. 3, the orbicularis muscle is the sphincter of the eyelids and allows lid closure. Its antagonists are the retractors of the lower lid and the elevators of the upper lid.

The lower lid retractors pull the lid down to permit unobstructed vision in downgaze. They extend to the lower tarsal plate within the fascia arising from the capsule surrounding the inferior oblique muscle (Fig. 4).

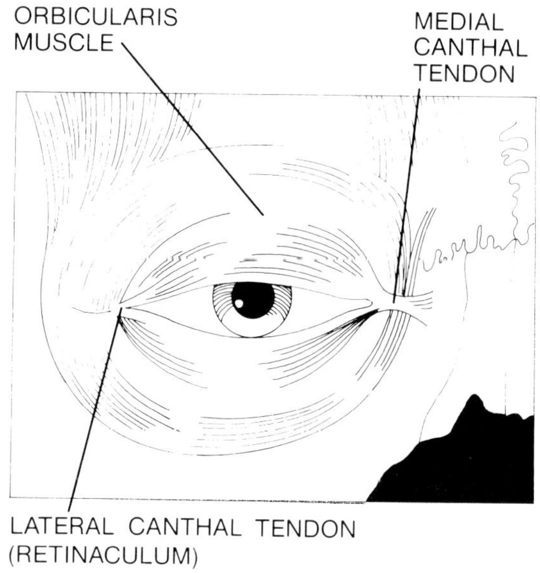

FIGURE 3
The orbicularis muscle is the sphincter of the eyelids, originating and inserting at the medial canthal tendon.

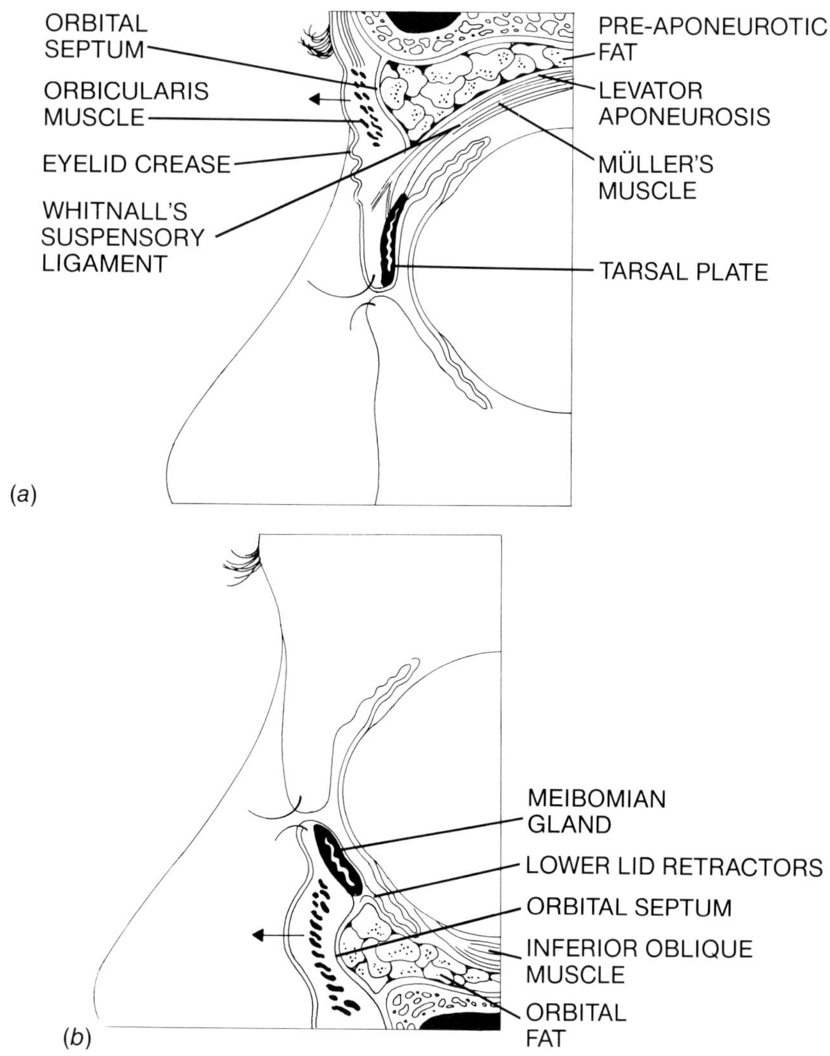

FIGURE 4
Anatomic relationships important for the eyelid surgeon are shown for the upper (*a*) and lower (*b*) eyelids.

The levator muscle is the primary elevator of the upper lid and attaches to the anterior border of the tarsal plate via its broad aponeurosis. The muscle fibers of the levator become connective tissue of aponeurosis at the level of Whitnall's suspensory ligament (Fig. 4). Slips of aponeurosis fibers also attach to the eyelid skin, and the uppermost point of attachment represents the eyelid crease.

The orbital septum is a connective tissue partition that arises from the periosteum of the orbital margin and blends into the levator aponeurosis at a variable distance from the upper eyelid margin.[25] This point of attachment tends to be lower in the eyelids of Asians.[10,11]

Orbital fat is present in the preaponeurotic space and medial to the edge of the aponeurosis in the upper eyelid. These represent the two fat compartments of the upper lid. The lateral compartment, temporal to the edge of the levator, is occupied by the lacrimal gland (Fig. 5).

FIGURE 5
The fat compartments of the upper and lower lids. The lateral compartment of the upper lid is occupied by the lacrimal gland.

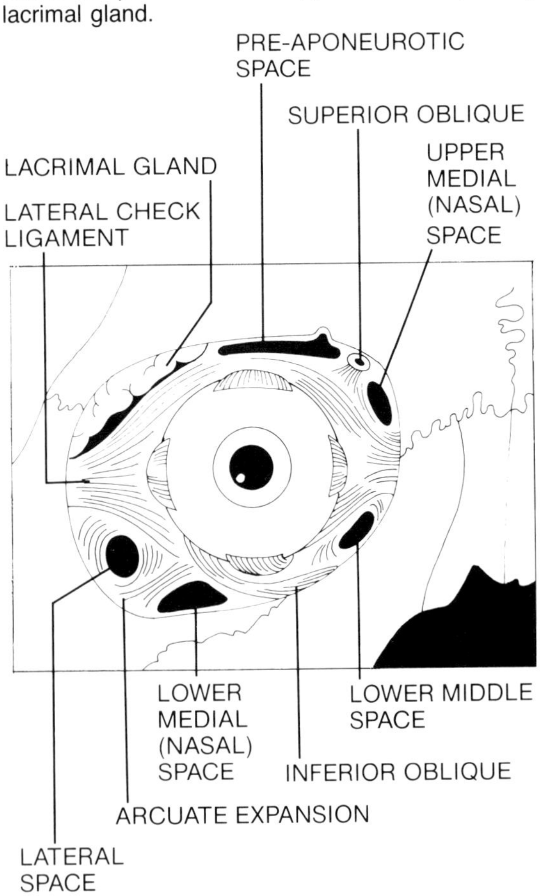

In the lower eyelid the fat is considered to lie within three compartments.[9] The most medial compartment, or nasal fat pad, is separated from the middle fat pad by the inferior oblique muscle. The temporal fat pad is separated from the middle fat pad by a connective tissue band known as the arcuate expansion (of the inferior oblique).

Blood vessels for the most part course on the surface of the fat pads, except in the case of the temporal fat of the lower eyelid, which is penetrated by several vessels. The eyelids in general are nourished by a rich anastomotic vascular supply from both the internal and external carotid systems. This is probably responsible for the low incidence of postoperative infection.

SURGICAL TECHNIQUES FOR BLEPHAROPLASTY

Local Anesthesia

Whether general anesthesia, intravenous sedation, or neither is employed, local anesthetics can assist greatly in minimizing intraoperative problems. When 1% or 2% lidocaine with epinephrine 1:100,000 is used, anesthesia and vasoconstriction persist for up to 1 h. The addition of hyaluronidase 150 IU to 20 to 50 ml of the anesthetic mixture greatly assists in spreading the anesthetic and enhancing the vasoconstrictive effects. Generally 2 to 3 ml of this mixture injected superficially into each eyelid followed by manual pressure on the lids allows sufficient anesthesia for maximal epinephrine effect as well as resolution of the ballooning effect of the injection. Surgery should be delayed at least 15 min from the time of injection. During this interval, the patient can be prepared and draped and the surgeon can scrub.

Skin Marking

Fifteen minutes after the injection, the eyelids are anesthetized, the skin is blanched, and the ballooning dissipates enough to allow skin marking. The design of the upper lid incisions must be symmetrical between the two upper lids with respect to medial and lateral extent, height and contour of the lid crease, and distance from the brow (Fig. 6).

Generally the "lazy S" configuration is applied in order to correct the more common problem of temporal hooding.[9] It should never extend to the horizontal raphe in the lateral canthus and proba-

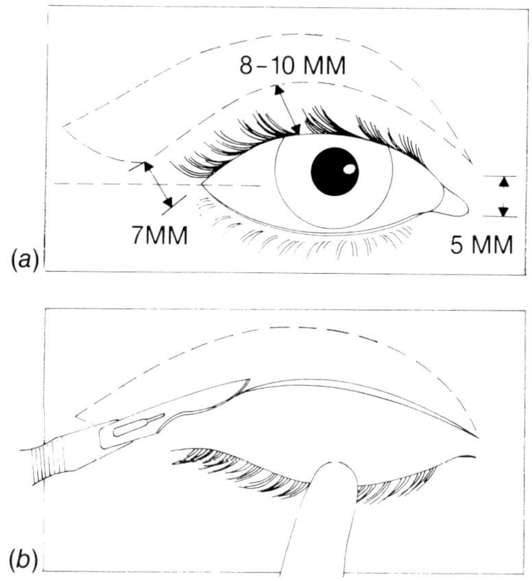

FIGURE 6
(*a*) The "lazy S" markings and approximate relationships to the eyelid margin. A symmetrical design between the two upper lids is essential. Incision with a No. 15 Bard-Parker blade is facilitated by placing the skin on stretch (*b*).

bly should not extend more medially than the level of the upper punctum.

Usually the lower line, representing the eventual lid crease, should be placed 8 to 10 mm above the lashes in the midpupillary line in women and 6 to 8 mm above the lashes in men.

If skin excision is warranted in the lower eyelid, the incision is made immediately below the lashes and extends from just below the punctum virtually horizontally to beyond the lateral canthus.

Upper Lid Blepharoplasty

Once the upper lid excision has been designed with the marking pen, a No. 15 Bard-Parker blade is used to incise along the marks. Stretching the skin with another hand facilitates an accurate cut. As shown in Fig. 4, the lower incision along the lid crease is close to the levator aponeurosis and thus should not penetrate this vital structure.

After incision along the previously marked lines, the skin or skin-muscle ellipse can be undermined and excised. Again, traction on the lid facilitates this excision and keeps the levator on stretch to avoid inadvertent cutting.

The orbital septum can be seen as a thin membrane overlying the preaponeurotic fat once the skin and muscle have been removed. Opening the septum along its entire width is safe and yields excellent exposure so that bulging fat can be removed. An additional advantage of the "open sky" approach is that bleeding vessels can easily be identified and cauterized. Pushing posteriorly on the lid also prolapses the fat forward to aid cauterization. Most bleeding, however, originates in the orbicularis muscle.[22]

Once the lid has been debulked of excess skin, muscle, and fat, closure can be done with the use of a running suture. 6.0 Prolene on a P-1 needle is preferred for its ease of removal.

In women who would benefit from a higher or more sharply defined lid crease, the supratarsal fixation technique can be employed to fixate skin edges to the levator aponeurosis. In this way the crease can be more sharply defined as well as elevated upon levator contraction (Fig. 2).

It is important *not* to close the orbital septum because of the high risk of tethering of the lid and creating an asymmetry of the creases.

Lower Lid Blepharoplasty

Depending on the surgical goals, either a transconjunctival approach or a skin approach can be employed in the lower eyelid.

If herniation of fat is the primary feature, incision into the lower fornix using cutting cautery for hemostasis can be employed. As shown in Fig. 7, an acrylic or glass corneal plate is used to protect the eye and upper lid as well as to ballotte the globe in order to prolapse the fat into the fornix. The lower lid is retracted to aid in visualization. Once the connective tissue partitions enclosing these fat compartments are opened, the billowing fat can be excised. Hemostasis is obtained with electrocautery, and the fat in both lower lids is excised prior to closure of the conjunctivae so that the physician can inspect for symmetry.

Photographs of the patient in the upright position are helpful in the operating room to review areas that require more fat excision, particularly because the recumbent position may hide the bulging. If this occurs, pressure on the globe can reveal the areas where fat will tend to herniate forward.

For redundant skin of the lower lid, a skin-muscle flap generally is created from an infraciliary incision, as shown in Fig. 8. The orbital septum can be opened along its entire width to expose the fat, and the excision can be carried out either directly or after clamping. Opening the septum increases exposure, allowing identification of bleeding sites.

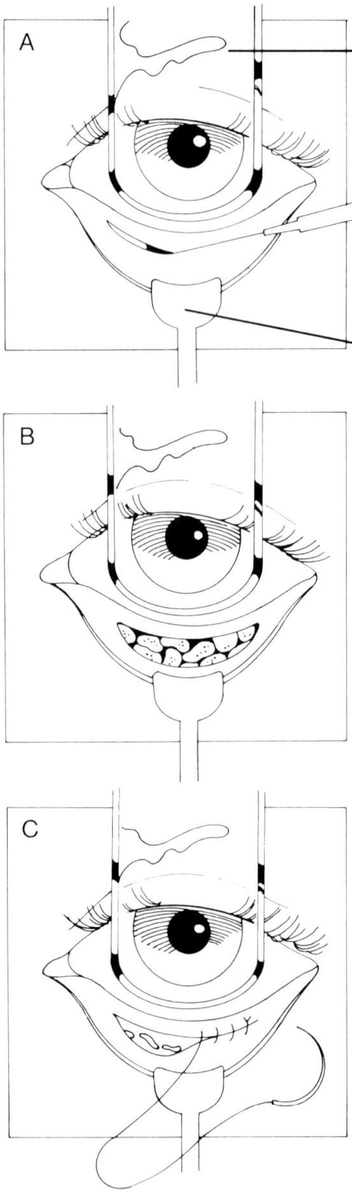

FIGURE 7
(*a*) Transconjunctival fat excision is facilitated by a retractor on the lower lid margin, a protective eyelid plate (Jaeger), and needle point monopolar cautery (cutting mode). (*b*) Connective tissue septae are cut to prolapse the fat into the fornix. (*c*) Fat is excised, and the conjunctivae are closed.

Pressure on the globe can prolapse those sites into view for cauterization.

Once the fat has been excised, the skin-muscle flap is redraped over the lid margin. The margin is positioned at the lower limbus with the patient assuming primary gaze. If the lid margin is pulled down when the patient is instructed to open the mouth, too much skin and muscle probably has been draped over the margin. Generally only a 3- to 4-mm-wide strip can safely be removed without causing lid retraction, even when lid tonus is good.

Pulling the skin-muscle flap superiorly and temporally is associated with a great risk of temporal lid retraction and "rounding" of the lateral canthal angle. This is a most distracting and unacceptable "surgical" look (Fig. 9).

FIGURE 8
The skin approach to lower eyelid blepharoplasty begins with an infraciliary incision (*a*) and may proceed to the construction of either a skin flap (*b*) or a skin-muscle flap (*c*).

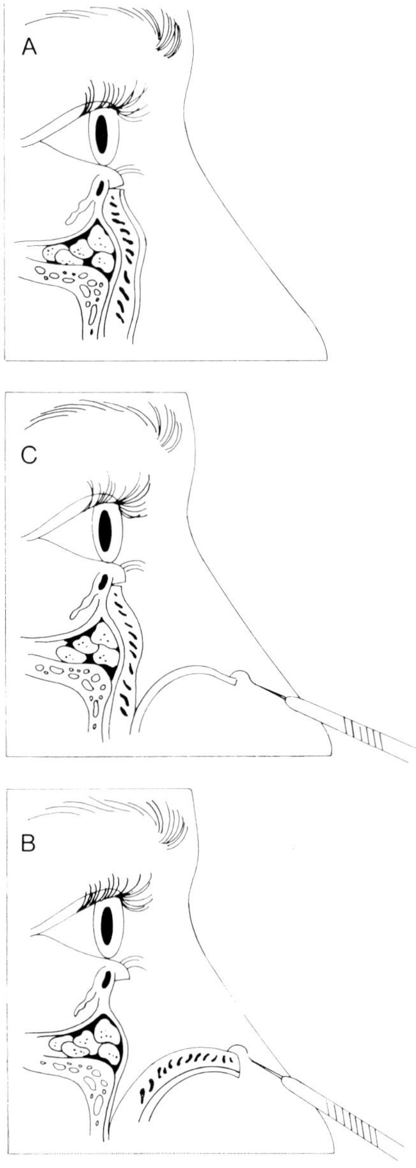

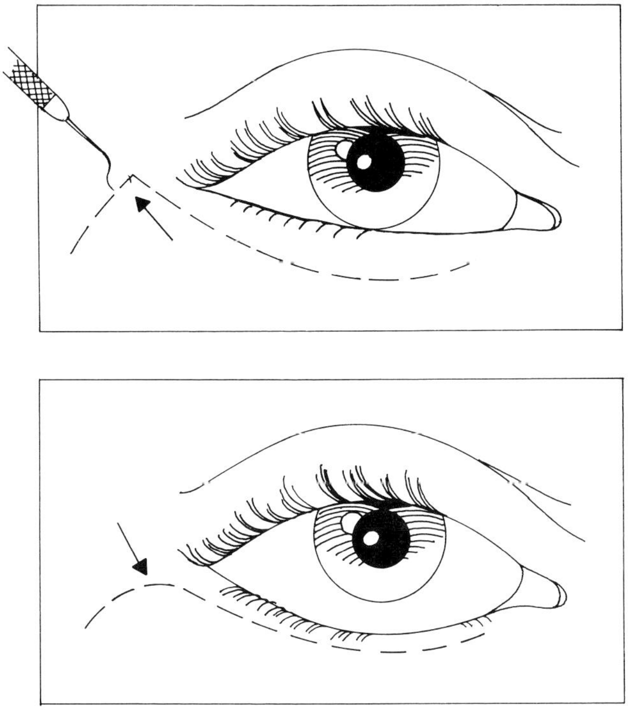

FIGURE 9
Upward and outward pull of the lower lid flap is associated with the risk of subsequent retraction of the lower lid (usually temporal) with rounding of the lateral canthal angle.

After excision of the skin-muscle strip and further cautery of bleeding edges (usually the orbicularis), the skin may be closed with running 6.0 Prolene sutures.

Lateral Canthal Tightening

Recognition of a lax lower eyelid requires correction during lower blepharoplasty, particularly if a skin-muscle flap is to be created (whether or not skin is excised). As shown in Fig. 10, once the flap is dissected and orbital fat has been removed, the horizontal laxity can be corrected. This is done by (1) disinserting the lateral canthal attachment of the lower eyelid, (2) advancing the lid over the orbital rim until the lid is taut, (3) excising the redundancy with a block excision, and (4) resecuring the lid to the rim. Usually only 4 to 5 mm of excision of the lateral canthal portion of the lid is required to effect an adequate tightening.

When the lid is secured to the lateral rim, using 5-0 Dexon sutures on a D-1 needle, the skin-muscle flap can be redraped and excision can be carried out as detailed above. Securing a traction

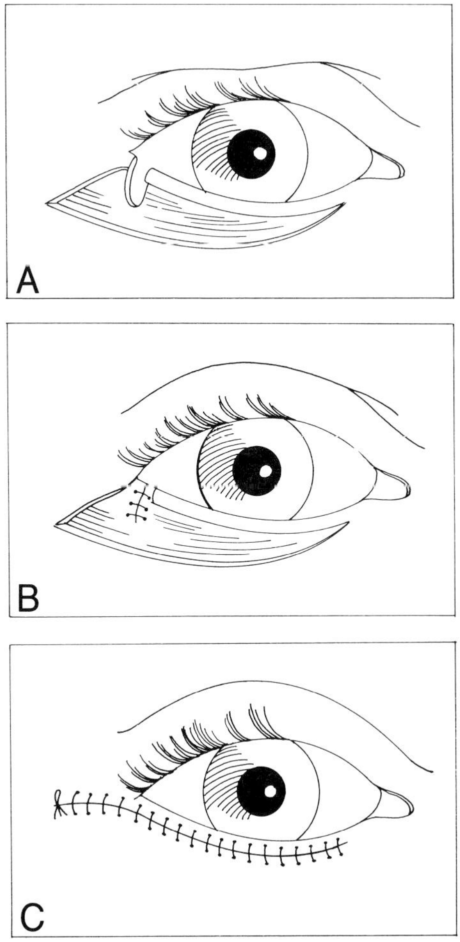

FIGURE 10
(*a*) Block excision after lateral canthotomy under a skin-muscle flap. (*b*) Cut edge of the temporal lid is fixated to the periosteum of the lateral rim to tighten the lid. (*c*) Skin-muscle flap is tailored for closure.

suture of 4.0 silk from the temporal lower lid margin to the temporal brow for 24 to 48 h minimizes the tendency toward vertical retraction of the lid.

PERMANENT EYELINER

General Considerations

There is no doubt that eye makeup in the form of shadow, eyeliner, and mascara can enhance the look of the eyes. Blepharoplasty in women further enhances the look that eye makeup achieves and in no way replaces it.

The use of pigments around the lids is a major component of the average woman's makeup routine that allows her to draw attention to attractive eyes. However, makeup in general, and eye makeup in particular, has the disadvantage of impermanence and can smudge or smear at inopportune times.

In 1984 Angres[12] published a description of his technique of applying an iron oxide pigment between and around the lashes to create a permanent eyeliner. This technique is really designed to simulate a natural look of thicker or darker lashes, not to reflect how one would apply eyeliner makeup heavily for special occasions. Accordingly, the pigment is implanted in lash-bearing regions of the eyelid so as to enhance the look of the lashes (Fig. 11). Heavy implantation of the pigment, particularly in the medial aspect of the lids, is to be avoided.

Consultation with the patient, including an evaluation of her use of makeup, is essential in coming to an agreement on the color and shape of the application. It also serves to educate the patient about the necessity of achieving a look that is natural even when no other makeup is worn.

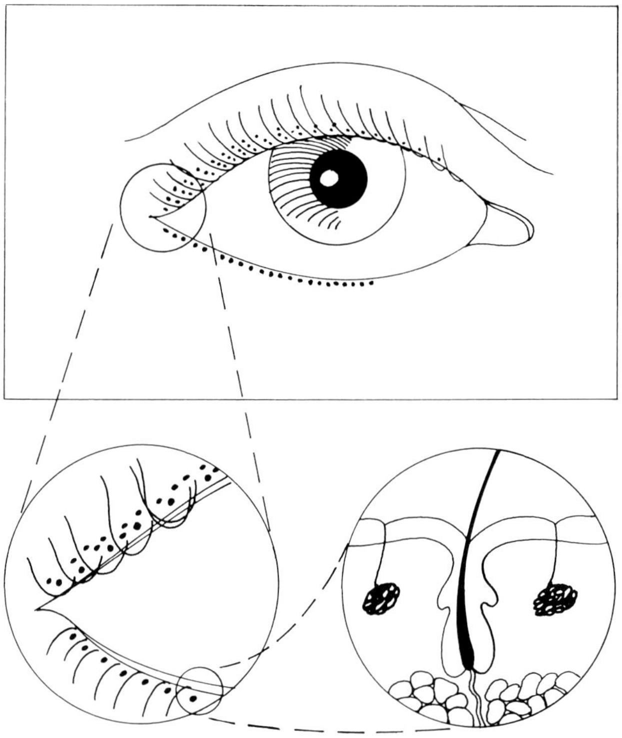

FIGURE 11
Placement of multiple pigment dots within the lash line gives the effect of thicker and darker lashes.

Technique

With the patient recumbent on the operating table, topical tetracaine hydrochloride 0.25% eye drops are applied to minimize corneal discomfort. The eyelid skin adjacent to the lashes is infiltrated with 2% lidocaine with epinephrine 1:100,000 and hyaluronidase. An alternative in the lower eyelid is a regional block from the inferior conjunctival fornix.

The lids are scrubbed with hexachlorophene solution and water, and the patient is placed under the low power (10*x*) of the operating microscope. The use of operating loupes is a satisfactory alternative.

Using either the Angres lid clamp or gentle pressure on the lids from the surgeon's other hand, the handpiece containing the pigment is directed toward the temporal lashes of the upper eyelid. The oscillating needle is engaged, and dots of pigment are created in the skin between the lashes. Once the entire lash line is treated, additional rows of pigment dots can be applied above the lashes, particularly in the temporal one-third to one-half of the upper lid. Intermittently, pigment has to be wiped out of the surgical field with moistened gauze.

In the lower eyelid, a fairly uniform series of pigment dots should be placed between the lashes. Only temporally would one consider a wider series of dots, but care must be taken to avoid too heavy an application of pigment, for it is particularly noticeable in the lower lid.

Intermittently during the procedure the microscope or loupes and the bright overhead lights are removed to assess the heaviness of application of the pigment. The bright lights may bleach the color in the surgeon's perception and thus lead to an application that is too heavy.

At the conclusion of the procedure all loose pigment should be carefully irrigated off the lids and out of the conjunctival sac. The implantation sites are covered with an ophthalmic steroid-antibiotic ointment. The patient is instructed to apply the ointment nightly.

The permanent eyeliner technique can be used concurrently with blepharoplasty. Because of concern about stray pigment getting incorporated into incisions, it is necessary to do the pigment implantation first. At the conclusion of the pigmentation, excess pigment can be washed off the skin and the blepharoplasty can commence. If a skin approach to the lower lid is planned, care must be taken to place the incision immediately below the thin pigment line in the lashes.

The major technical goals of the permanent eyeliner procedure are symmetry of application and avoidance of heavy application of the pigment. The physician must remember that it is easier to apply more pigment later than to be faced with overapplication. If pigment requires removal at a later date, either direct excision (in non-lash-bearing skin) or laser ablation may be warranted.[26]

Postoperative Measures

Ice packs placed over moist compresses for 3 to 5 days after blepharoplasty minimize edema and ecchymosis and provide comfort to the patient.

Occlusive pressure dressings are avoided because of the functional impairment they cause and the risk associated with concealing a vision-threatening complication (see below).

Incision sites are generally covered with an ophthalmic steroid-antibiotic ointment several times daily, and patients are requested to limit activity for 3 to 5 days. The sutures may be removed in 5 days, after which warm compresses may be beneficial in softening contracting incisions and resolving residual ecchymosis.

Complications

Vision-threatening complications are thankfully rare.[23,24,27–29] Nevertheless, blindness after blepharoplasty is well documented and is generally thought to be related to increased pressure on the optic nerve caused by bleeding in a confined space. Symptoms of pain and decreased vision, usually within the first 24 hours, require immediate attention. If the lids are tensely swollen, the globe is palpably firm or proptotic, or vision is reduced, emergency intervention is warranted.

Orbital pressure can generally be reduced by immediately cutting the sutures and opening the wounds or by removing clots and searching for a bleeding site. If this does not result in rapid softening of the eye or lessening of tension on the lids, a lateral cantholysis can be performed as described above (Fig. 10) for the tightening technique.

Acetazolamide (Diamox), osmotic agents, and ophthalmologic consultation are additional measures in dealing with this crisis.

As noted in Table 1, infections, asymmetry, ptosis, and lid retraction can be listed among the postoperative complications of blepharoplasty. Asymmetry can be minimized by careful attention to skin marking; equal excision of skin, muscle, and fat; and symmetrical supratarsal fixation. Generally, the preoperative presence of brow asymmetry makes lid symmetry extremely difficult to achieve with blepharoplasty alone.

Ptosis after blepharoplasty can be due to an inadvertent aponeurosis laceration that was left unrepaired or to the placement of supratarsal fixation sutures too high on the aponeurosis.[9] This can actually tether the levator and pull it down. Often mild degrees of ptosis disappear within 2 to 3 months if treated conservatively with heat and massage.

CONCLUSION

Several techniques can be used in aesthetic blepharoplasty. The choice of surgical procedure depends on the particular cosmetic goals, and this requires the proper informed participation of the patient. In general, the result should be one of improved appearance, lessening of distracting features, and minimal visible signs that plastic surgery has been performed.

REFERENCES

1. Stephenson KL. The history of blepharoplasty to correct blepharochalasis. Aesthetic Plast Surg. 1977;1:177–194.
2. Roenigk HH. Tattooing—history, techniques, complications, removal. Cleve Clin. J. 1971;38:179–186.
3. Rees TD. Aesthetic Plastic Surgery. Philadelphia, Saunders, 1980; 2:479–505.
4. Dingman RO, Peled I, Izenberg P. Forehead and brow lifts and their relationship to blepharoplasty. Ann Plast Surg. 1979;2:32–36.
5. Beard C. Cosmetic blepharoplasty: Anatomic considerations. Trans Am Acad Ophthalmol Otolaryngol. 1969;73: 1141–1149.
6. Sheen JH. Supratarsal fixation in upper blepharoplasty. Plast Reconstr Surg. 1974;54:424–431.
7. Sheen JH. A change in the technique of supratarsal fixation in upper blepharoplasty. Plast Reconstr Surg. 1977;59:831–834.
8. Baylis HI, Long JA, Groth MJ. Transconjunctival lower eyelid blepharoplasty: Technique and complications. Ophthalmology 1989; 96:1027–1032.

9. McCord CW Jr (ed). Oculoplastic Surgery. New York: Raven Press, 1981.
10. Chen WP. Asian blepharoplasty. J Ophth Plast Reconstr Surg. 1987;3:135–140.
11. Doxanis MT. Oriental eyelids: An anatomic study. Arch Ophthalmol. 1984;102:1232–1235.
12. Angres GG. Angres Permalid-liner method: A new surgical procedure. Ann Ophthalmol. 1984;16:145–148.
13. Wilkins RB, Patipa M. The recognition of acquired ptosis in patients considered for upper eyelid blepharoplasty. Plast Reconstr Surg. 1982;70:431–434.
14. Wilkins RB. Evaluation of the blepharoplasty patient. Ophthalmology. 1978;85:703–704.
15. Rees TD. Prevention of ectropion by horizontal shortening of the lower lid during blepharoplasty. Ann Plast Surg. 1983;11:17–23.
16. Rees TD, Jelks GW. Blepharoplasty and the dry eye syndrome. Plast Reconstr Surg. 1981;68:249–252.
17. Tenzel RR, Buffam FV, Miller GR. The use of the "lateral canthal sling" in ectropion repair. Can J Ophthalmol. 1977;12:199–202.
18. Anderson RL, Gordy DD. The tarsal strip procedure. Arch Ophthalmol. 1979;97:2192–2196.
19. Aston SJ. Orbicularis oculi muscle flaps. Clin Plast Surg. 1981;8:679–686.
20. Bourguet J. Notre traitement chirurgical de "poches" sous les yeux sans cicatrice. J Arch Gr Belg Chir. 1928;31:133–136.
21. Wilkins RB, Byrd WA. Complications of blepharoplasty. J Ophth Plast Reconstr Surg. 1985;1:195–198.
22. Sutcliffe T, Baylis HI, Fett D. Bleeding in cosmetic blepharoplasty: An anatomic approach. J Ophth Plast Reconstr Surg. 1985;1:107–113.
23. Smith B, Nesi FA. The complications of cosmetic blepharoplasty. Ophthalmology. 1978;85:726–729.
24. Tenzel RR. Surgical treatment of complications of cosmetic blepharoplasty. Clin Plast Surg. 1978;5:517–523.
25. Putterman AM, Urist MJ. Surgical anatomy of the orbital septum. Ann Ophthalmol. 1974;6:290–294.
26. Tanenbaum M, Karas S, McCord CD. Laser ablation of blepharopigmentation. J Ophth Plast Reconstr Surg. 1988;4:49–56.
27. Heinze JB, Hueston JT. Blindness after blepharoplasty: Mechanism and early reversal. Plast Reconstr Surg. 1978;61:347–354.
28. Stasior OG. Blindness associated with blepharoplasty. Clin Plast Surg. 1981;8:793–796.
29. Lloyd WC, Leone CR. Transient bilateral blindness following blepharoplasty. J Ophth Plast Reconstr Surg. 1985;1:29–34.

CHAPTER

20

Ear Piercing and Repair

MOHAMED AMER
STEVEN GREENBAUM
GARY P. LASK
LAWRENCE CHARLES PARISH

The function of the external ear is to aid hearing. It has also been a focus for cosmetic adornment, from Cleopatra's time to the present. Ear piercing returned to fashion two decades ago and now many people wear several earrings in each earlobe, including men. The ears are relatively large appendages in proportion to the face and attract a significant amount of attention.

PROCEDURE FOR PIERCING EARS

The two most common modalities for piercing ears are manually with a needle as in Fig. 1, or with an ear piercing gun, as in Fig. 2. The materials needed for piercing with a needle include 1% lidocaine (Xylocaine) for local anesthesia, alcohol, a marking pen, a 16- or 18-gauge needle, and earrings made of 14-kt or 18-kt gold or stainless steel.

The patient is placed in an upright position and with the aid of a mirror the patient and physician mark the spots to be pierced. The earrings and the

FIGURE 1
Piercing with a needle (*left to right*): The proposed ostium is marked. The needle is pushed through the lobule from posterior to anterior. After the earring post is placed into the lumen of the needle, the needle and earring are then retracted back through the ostium. The earring is seated firmly in place and the clasp is fastened to the earring.

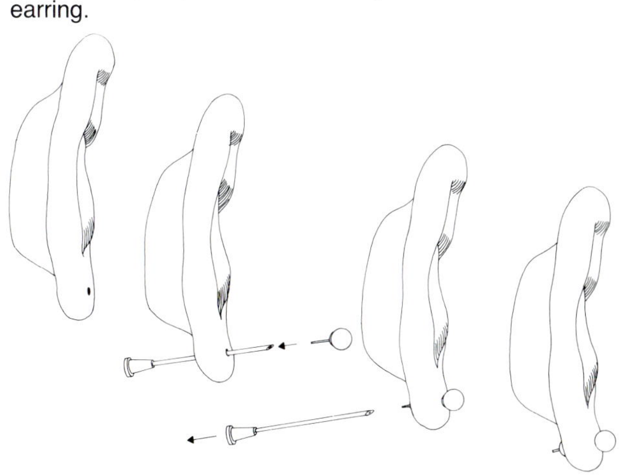

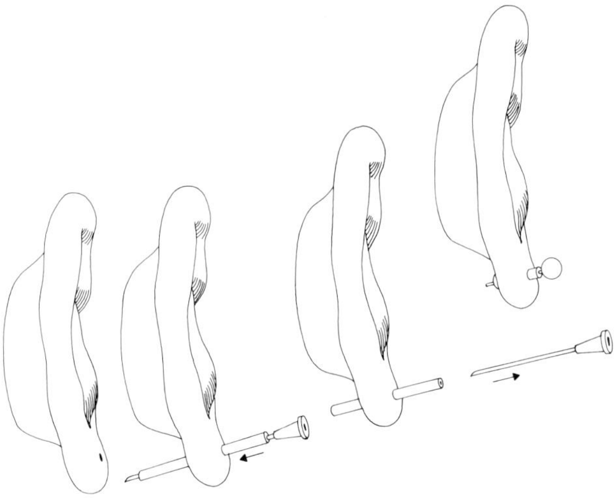

FIGURE 2
Piercing with a gun (*left to right*): Mark the site of the proposed ostium. Introduce an 18-gauge teflon intravenous catheter anteriorly, penetrating the lobule. Withdraw the needle, leaving the teflon catheter in place. Trim the catheter to shorten the length. Insert the earring into the lumen of the catheter and fasten.

lobules are cleaned with alcohol. The sites are infiltrated with 1% lidocaine. With the manual method the lobe is approached from the posterior surface and the needle is pushed anteriorly through the marked point.[1] The post of the earring is then inserted inside the needle and the needle is pulled back through the ear bringing the earring with it. The clasp is then attached to the earring.

Alternatively, piercing can be done with a gun or clamp. The site of the proposed hole is selected. Pressure is slowly and steadily applied to the instrument and the earrings are essentially "shot" through the earlobe. They are left in place for approximately 2 weeks to allow for the formation of the ostium. The patient is instructed to clean the site with alcohol or hydrogen peroxide daily and apply polysporin ointment to the post of the earrings without removing them.

Complications

Keloid formation is one of the most common and most distressing complications of ear piercing. A history of keloid formation is an absolute contraindication to the procedure. The management of keloids is addressed in Chap. 9.

Misplacement of the ostium is another permanent complication. For this reason allowing the patient to participate in choosing the precise spot to be pierced is critical for success.

Allergic reactions to earrings are often caused by nickel, which is found in most gold-plated or gold-filled jewelry, even up to 18 kts. Earrings made of 24-kt gold have so little nickel that allergic reactions are generally not a problem. Areas of allergic reaction can be treated with a topical corticosteroid and the patient is advised to switch to stainless steel or 24-kt gold earrings.

Localized infections caused by *Staphylococcus aureus* or hemolytic streptococci, although rare, do occur. Treatment involves oral or topical antimicrobial agents, for example, cefuroxime axetile (Ceftin) 250 mg twice a day for 7 days.

EARLOBE REPAIR

Once an earlobe has become pierced, it is subject to increased trauma; hence, there is an increased risk of being partially or completely torn. The style of the earring, its weight and configuration, and the ease with which it can be pulled by a child or caught on clothing all may contribute to damaging the lobe.

Many patients are seen in consultation after wearing earrings for several years. Often the opening for the earring has either enlarged to the point of being cosmetically unacceptable or has torn completely through. If the hole has merely enlarged, it is possible to repair the defect completely or still maintain an ostium for the post of the earring.[2–7]

A common method for doing this repair is to first excise the epithelium from approximately 80 percent of the lining of the ostium. The remaining 20 percent is left intact at the superior portion of the hole. Removal of the epidermis can be accomplished using a scalpel or scissors. An alternative method for removing the epidermis is the skin punch, as in Fig. 3. Most partial elongations of the earring hole can be repaired using a 2.0- to 4.0-mm skin punch. It is possible to leave the intact epidermis as described above using this punch method.

Once the epidermis has been removed the opposing skin edges are sutured together with 6.0 suture (nylon, prolene, or rapidly absorbable gut). The ostium may be maintained by inserting a thick piece

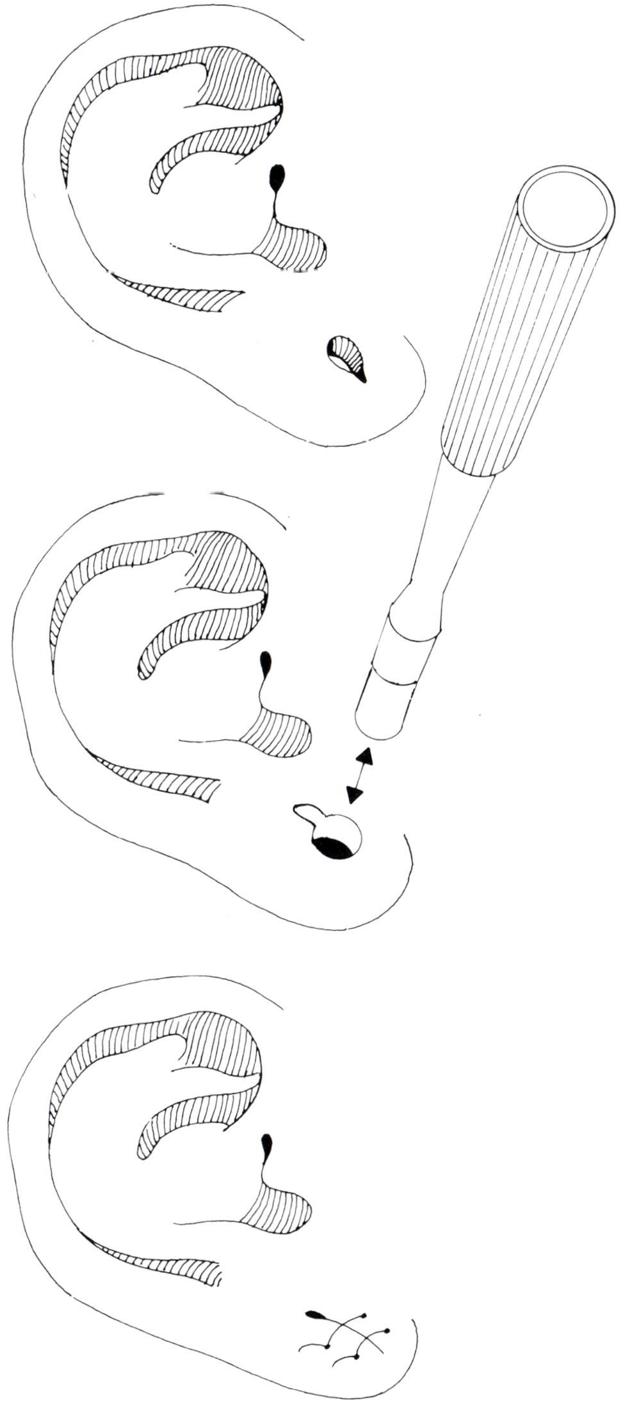

FIGURE 3
On an enlarged ostium, a skin punch is used to remove approximately 80 percent of the epithelial surface. The epithelium at the vertex of the ostium remains intact. The wound is then closed with 6.0 suture.

of nylon suture or even a very light earring or post. The sutures are removed in 5 to 7 days. The patient is asked to wear either no earrings or very light stud earrings for the next 3 months since full wound strength does not occur for 6 months. Only 80 percent of the original strength of the skin will be achieved in this recently sutured area.

If the earlobe has been completely torn there are several methods that may be used to repair the defect.[8] Although the following procedures may be modified to maintain an ostium for insertion of the earring, we often advise repiercing the ear in a slightly different location, either lateral or medial to the incision. The repaired tissue will always be weaker than the surrounding normal skin.

The most common and easiest method for repairing through and through lacerations of the lobule is to anesthesize the earlobe and remove the epidermis from the surfaces of the opposing walls of the earlobe. It is important to make sure that the removal of epidermis extends to the apex of the laceration if complete closure is desired. Leaving the epidermis intact at this vertex will prevent wound approximation, thus allowing maintenance of an ostium at this point. Once this has been completed the skin edges are approximated with 6.0 interrupted sutures. The anterior surface of the lobe is carefully sutured first because this is the side that will be most visible. The posterior surface is then sewn. It is critical to meticulously align the inferior portion of the lobe so that notching is avoided. A Z-plasty at the inferior pole has also been recommended to avoid the dimpling that may occur along the inferior margin of the lobe (see Fig. 4). There should be almost no tension on the sutures. A more acceptable scar may be achieved if there is good eversion of the skin edges since there seems to be a natural tendency for inversion of the edges following this repair.

A second method of repairing the cleft earlobe makes use of the lap-joint principle[9,10] shown in Fig. 5. The epidermis is removed from the inner surfaces of the cleft. Instead of immediately joining the two edges, two complimentary flaps are created. This allows the two sides of the earlobe to interlock. There is only a partial thickness wound created in any axis along the earlobe thus increasing the strength of the wound. The overlap created at the inferior margin of the lobule often prevents the dimpling that may sometimes be found here.

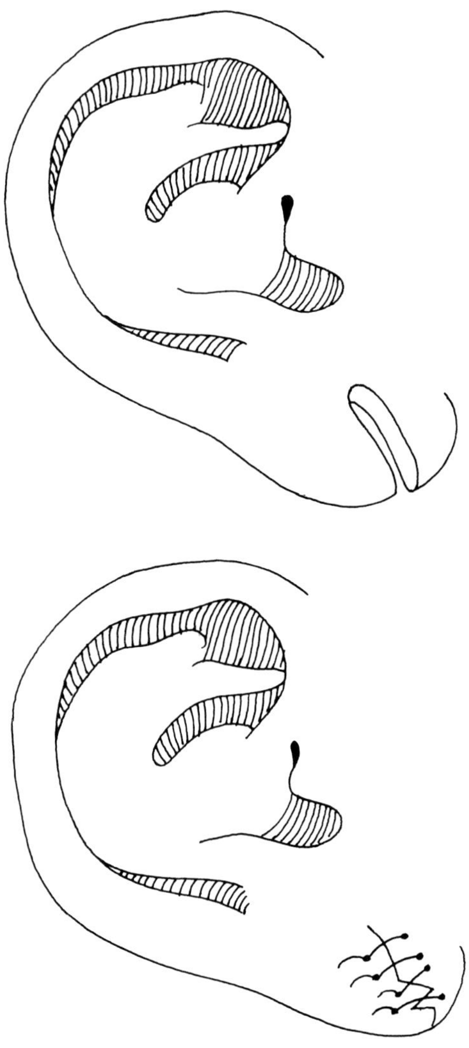

FIGURE 4
Repair of lacerated earlobe using a Z-plasty to avoid dimpling along the inferior margin of the lobule.

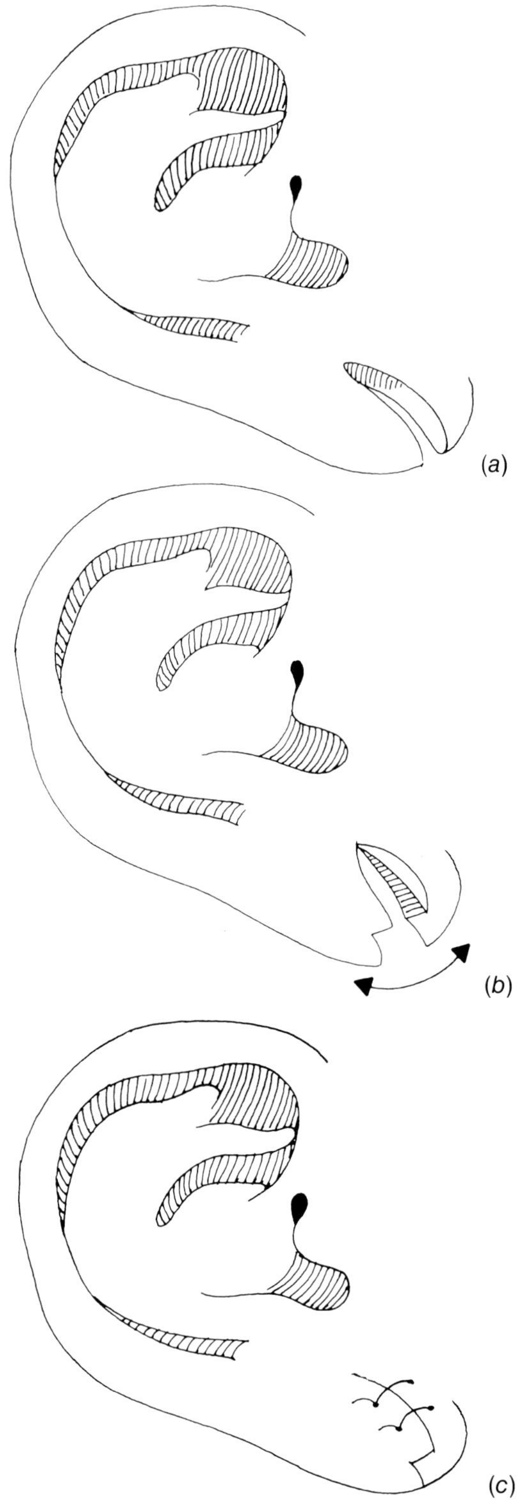

FIGURE 5
(*a*) Lacerated earlobe; (*b*) complementary lap-joint flaps; and (*c*) final result after suturing with 6.0 suture.

REFERENCES

1. Bennett RG. Fundamentals of Cutaneous Surgery. St. Louis: CV Mosby, 1988:611–615.
2. Pardue M. Repair of torn earlobe with preservation of the perforation for an earring. Plast Reconstr Surg. 1973;51:472–473.
3. Buchan NG. The cleft ear lobe: A method of repair with preservation of the earring canal. Br J Plast Surg. 1975; 28:296–298.
4. Hamilton R, LaRossa D. Method for repair of cleft earlobes. Plast Reconstr Surg. 1975;55:99–101.
5. Elsahy NI. Reconstruction of the cleft earlobe with preservation of the perforation for an earring. Plast Reconstr Surg. 1986;77:322–324.
6. Zoltie N. Split earlobes: A method of repair preserving the hole. Plast Reconstr Surg. 1987;80:619–621.
7. Chernosky ME. One-step procedure for earlobe surgical repair and ear post replacement. J Am Acad Dermatol. 1985;12:721–723.
8. Kalimuthu R, Larson BJ, Lewis N. Earlobe repair: A new technique. J Dermatol Surg Oncol. 1982;8:187–190.
9. Argamaso RV. The lap-joint principle in the repair of the cleft earlobe. Br J Plast Surg. 1978;31:337–338.
10. Harahap M. Repair of split earlobes. A review and a new technique. J Dermatol Surg Oncol. 1982;8:187–190.

CHAPTER

21

Leg Ulcers and Lymphedema

TERENCE J. RYAN

The consequences of disease of the leg can most easily be measured by considering the nature of the handicap. The distance one can walk is one measure of such a handicap. It is less easy to measure the amount of discomfort that may be a consequence of corns, calluses, warts, or ulceration; however, the most significant and common problem in dermatology is loss of confidence because of disfigurement which makes one feel "unwelcome." Robert Louis Stevenson gave Long John Silver a wooden leg for the very good reason that he was a pirate, and a villainous one at that. It is a sad reflection on our society that disfigurement is so often associated with evil and that in films and plays the villain is often deformed. There is much evidence that the deformed are shunned, less often touched, and their cry for help less willingly answered.

When members of the public are asked to rate as clean or dirty various bodily traits, scaling exudate and debris between the toes are considered more dirty than many other natural excreta.[1] There is also evidence that for patients, leaving marks of blood on clothing is one of the most distressing consequences of disease.[2] In western society and in places where many eastern religions are practiced, cleanliness is thought to be desirable and market forces have determined that it is essential to have "no odor." Unfortunately, a patient who has a leg ulcer has all these disadvantages.

Loudon[3] drew attention to the early nineteenth-century literature concerning leg ulcers. The following quotation is as relevant today as it was 200 years ago: "Ulcers of the leg form a very extensive and important class of diseases. Inclusion of such cases is generally looked upon as an inferior branch of practice; an unpleasant and inglorious task where much labour must be bestowed and little honour gained" (from the *Edinburgh Medical and Surgical Journal,* 1805).

RECENT ADVANCES IN WOUND DRESSINGS

The aesthetic considerations of the treatment of a leg ulcer require that it be properly managed, with an endpoint of healing being the most desirable feature of all.

A good wound dressing should promote healing, relieve pain, and be aesthetically pleasing. For a wound dressing to succeed, appropriate surgical technique and adequate blood flow must be available to allow the wound to benefit from the dressing. A successful dressing must be well tested on a variety of wounds that have been carefully assessed. Because no two wounds are exactly alike, it is important to have systems of measurement which do not neglect the recording of essential features. In our studies of wound dressings at Oxford[4,5] we have been concerned primarily with leg ulcers, and all legs are first assessed as follows.

1. The physician should first palpate the dorsalis pedis and posterior tibialis arteries.
2. The blood pressure may be taken in the leg using a Doppler stethoscope (Fig. 1). The ratio of the blood pressure in the leg to that in the arm is an indication of the degree of ischemia in arterial disease. A ratio below 0.6 indicates that high elevation and tight stockings or bandages are dangerous to the patient.
3. An assessment of venous incompetence can be made clinically and is best done by demonstration in the clinic. Essentially, blood flow through the veins is measured in the upright and supine positions while reflux is prevented by compression with the hand and some ankle movement is encouraged to induce the muscle pump. In a normal lower limb, foot movement empties both deep and superficial veins through the deep venous system. It is possible to distinguish between superficial and deep vein disease of the valves and postthrombophlebitic obstruction of the deep venous system. A full assessment includes noninvasive blood flow measurement, assessment of the direction of flow, and a venogram.
4. Assessment of the degree of edema should include measurement of the circumference of the leg. The size of the ulcer can be recorded in photographs or by drawing the outline of the ulcer and keeping the drawing as a record (Fig. 2).

(a)
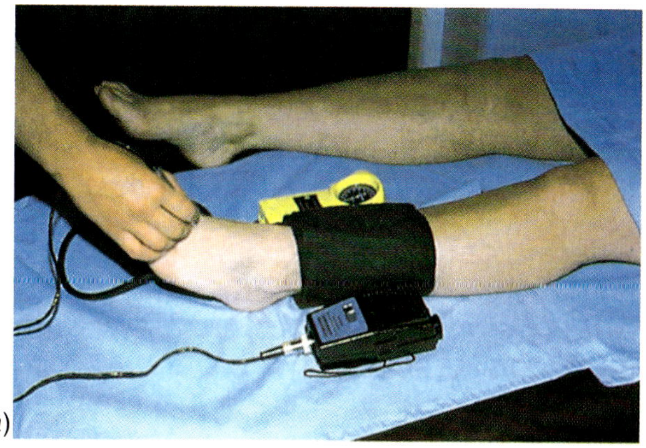

(b)
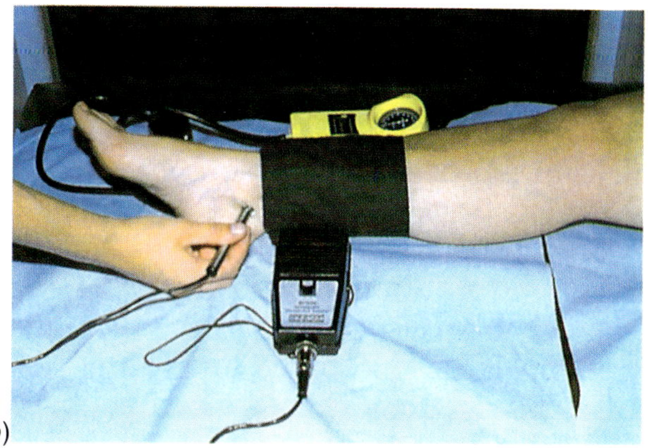

FIGURE 1
(*a*) Detection of arterial dorsalis pedis foot pulse using portable Doppler. (*b*) Detection of posterior tibialis arterial foot pulse using portable Doppler. Attempts should be made to palpate for these pulses digitally. (From GW Cherry and TJ Ryan (eds), Blueprint for the Management of Leg Ulcers. UK: Squibb ConvaTec. With permission.)

FIGURE 2
Tracing of an ulcer to document its size at different time intervals. (From GW Cherry and TJ Ryan (eds), Blueprint for the Management of Leg Ulcers. UK: Squibb ConvaTec. With permission.)

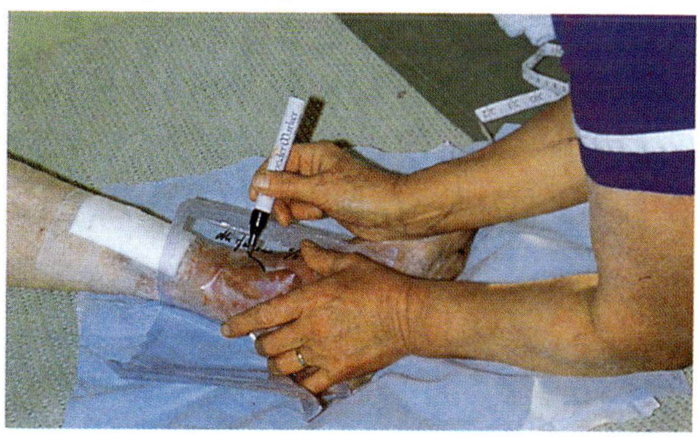

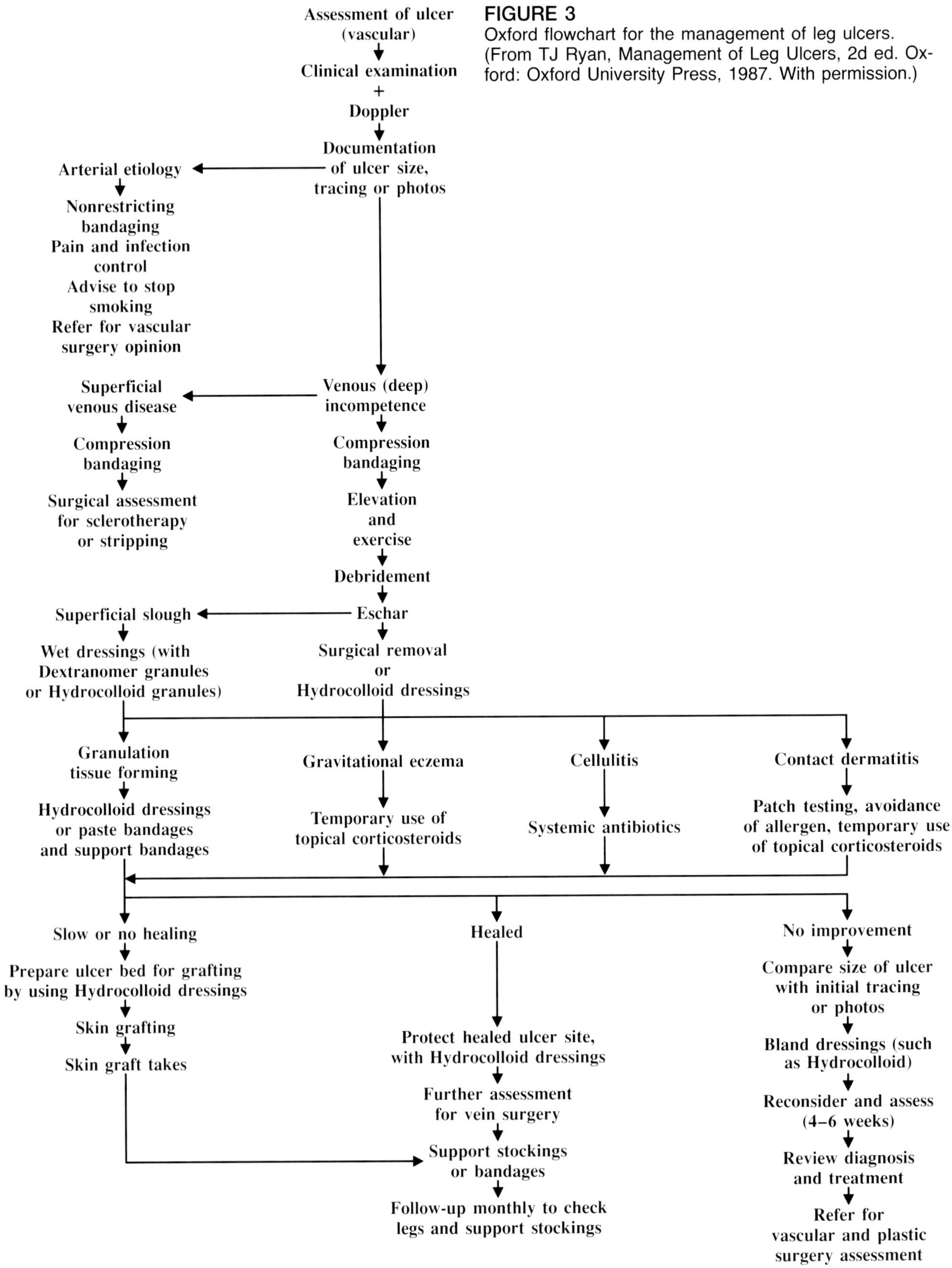

FIGURE 3
Oxford flowchart for the management of leg ulcers. (From TJ Ryan, Management of Leg Ulcers, 2d ed. Oxford: Oxford University Press, 1987. With permission.)

Such examinations are preceded by a full history which takes into account anemia, diabetes mellitus, rheumatoid arthritis, and any other factors which may delay healing.

5. The role of infection and contact dermatitis in regard to a great variety of medicaments must also be assessed. The wound must be measured, and all stages of necrosis and repair must be fully recorded.

When this has been done, it is possible to say whether a new dressing represents a significant advance; only then can one justify aesthetic considerations. The Oxford flowchart for the management of leg ulcers includes the "preaesthetic" management regimen (Fig. 3).

PREPARATION OF THE WOUND

Significant necrotic debris is best removed by means of surgical debridement because dead tissue is often infected. This procedure is painless, allowing the debris to be cut away. Yellow exudate can be removed by applying wet dressings and allowing them to dry so that the exudate is removed when the dressing is removed. Agents such as dextranomer (Debrisan) may be helpful at this state. Varidase can be used to remove necrotic material but may be damaging to surrounding eczematous skin. At this stage antiseptic agents such as hypochlorite, potassium permanganate, and iodides may be helpful. Many of these agents have had a bad press because they can be shown to be cytotoxic or even mutagenic to cells in vitro. In our practice, we do not worry about this until we begin to see healthy granulation tissue, at which point it is desirable to avoid using such agents on the ulcer, although they may still be helpful for the surrounding skin. The good wound dressing comes into its own from the time at which granulation tissue begins to appear. Its value can be measured in terms of pain relief and rate of healing, but it serves a more important purpose in the recognition and recording of an endpoint of total healing. Many leg ulcers fall short of the latter criterion.

EDEMA

Edema always delays healing. It is not always realized that systemic causes of edema such as heart failure have to be distinguished from local venous causes and that lymphatic failure is often a corollary of venous disease. Lymphedema is not very responsive to elevation alone, whereas massage and limb movement are very helpful. Lymphedema is a protein edema leading to fibrosis. It also gives rise to a low-grade inflammation or cellulite which may mimic infection but responds to physiotherapy, including exercise, support, elevation, and massage.

BACTERIAL INFECTION

The techniques for assessing the role of bacteria in preventing or in some cases enhancing healing fall far short of the ideal. The Lancefield type A beta-hemolytic streptococcus is always bad. Several anaerobic bacteria are highly undesirable; they can be picked up using a Wood's light, which detects *Bacteroides melaninogenicus,* which fluoresces a deep red color and is a common accompaniment of anaerobic infection. Bacterial contamination of an ulcer is inevitable, and attempts to make a leg ulcer sterile except immediately before grafting are not recommended because they often lead to resistant organisms or to contact dermatitis. Antiseptic agents may be harmful when there is a very heavy growth of bacteria, but such a growth can be assessed by taking the swab and plating it. The role of infection in tropical ulcers and in immunocompromised patients is of course another matter requiring much greater use of systemic antibiotics.

WOUND DRESSINGS

We have examined many dressings during the past decade. Old favorites for leg ulcers such as zinc oxide paste bandages (the Unna boot) combine support with healing properties. The instructions (Fig. 4) are taken from *The Management of Leg Ulcers.*[6] A carefully applied bandage on a leg that has adequate elevation may be disguised if the color of the covering bandage is approximately matched to the skin and covered with a normal stocking. Any tape used to secure the bandage should be the same color. Some charcoal dressings (e.g., Actisorb) are useful for absorbing excessive exudate and reducing odor, but old-fashioned butter muslin and linen are also useful when applied in generous amounts. From the viewpoint of the dermatologist, the surrounding skin is as important as the ulcer itself.

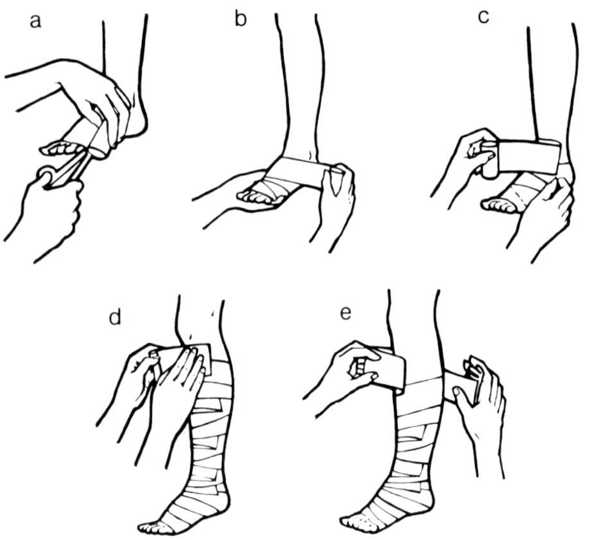

FIGURE 4
Application of medicated paste bandage. (*a*) Take one and a half turns of the bandage around the base of the toes and cut; repeat 2 cm farther up the foot. (*b*) Take the bandage from the base of the toes around the heel and back across the dorsum of the foot. Cut at the level of the base of the toes. Repeat 2 cm farther up to cover the heel properly. (*c*) Take the bandage a final turn around the foot and fold it back at the level of the malleolus. (*d*) Finish by taking the bandage around the leg and folding it back at the sides after each one and a half turns. The bandage should cover the leg up to the tubercle of the tibia and be slightly higher at the back. (*e*) Removal. The bandage should not be cut but unfolded. This avoids skin damage. (From GW Cherry and TJ Ryan (eds), Blueprint for the Management of Leg Ulcers. UK: Squibb ConvaTec. With permission.)

Exudate, pus, and medicaments can do harm, and one always attempts to protect healthy skin so that it will contribute to the healing of the ulcer. Petroleum jelly, silicone water repellents, hydrogen peroxide, and zinc oxide creams may be used.

The Hydrolloid Dressing

The only dressing we have found to constitute a significant advance in the management of ulceration is the hydrocolloid dressing, variously termed Granuflex and Duoderm, which provides a moist environment for wound healing[4,5] (Fig. 5, *a* through *c*). This type of dressing often relieves pain, and it is especially valuable for protecting the surrounding skin since it is closely adhesive but does not macerate.

Its property of promoting granulation tissue has been of great interest.[7] We have noted the richness of the vascular bed of granulation tissue and the surface properties of the granulation tissue which allow epithelium to migrate across it, increasing wound contraction. If the arterial supply to the ulcer bed is sufficient, the capillary bed in granulation tissue is usually very proliferative under the

FIGURE 5
(*a*) Application of a hydrocolloid dressing. (*b*) Typical appearance indicating formation of gel over the ulcer bed. (*c*) Yellow gel is visible on changing the dressing. (From GW Cherry and TJ Ryan (eds), Blueprint for the Management of Leg Ulcers. UK: Squibb ConvaTec. With permission.)

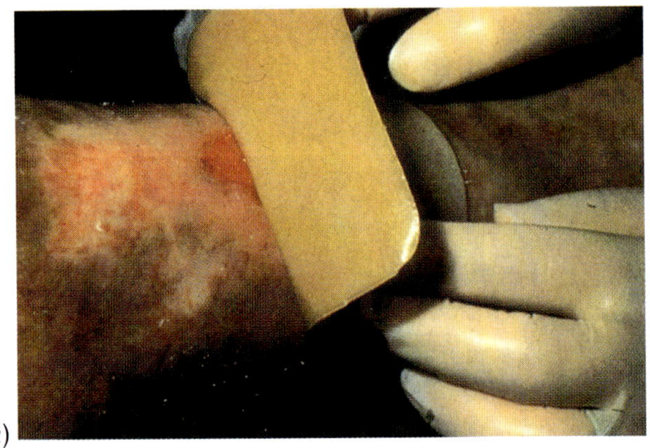
(*a*)

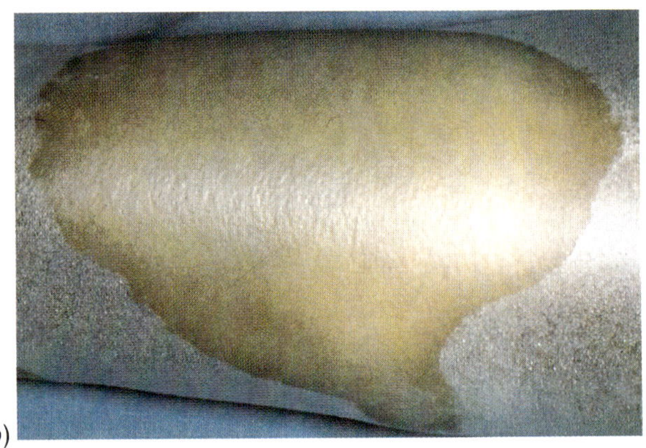
(*b*)

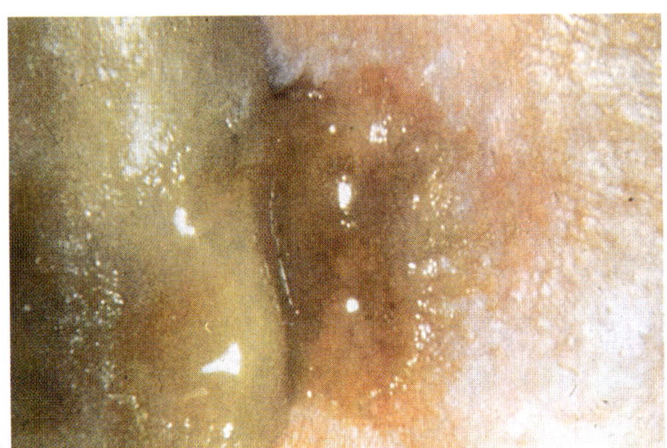
(*c*)

hydrocolloid dressing. We believe the dressing promotes wound contraction, partly through the generation of granulation tissues but perhaps also by eliminating the splinting effect of the dry eschar.

Contraction is a stimulus to wound healing, provided that it does not lead to contracture with associated dense scarring. Fibrinolytic properties may be important; however, there is a stage at which excessive protease activity may prevent the epithelium from sticking to the surface of the granulation tissue. It has become our practice to give the wound a brief respite from the hydrocolloid dressing when the granulation tissue is too rich and the epithelium seems unwilling to migrate.

Do No Harm

This Hippocratic principle requires a realization that some wounds may not heal and that tissues are very easily destroyed by overly vigorous attempts to eliminate bacteria, overtight bandaging, and contact dermatitis. This applies especially to ischemic limbs. Specialists in arterial surgery or radiology and anesthetists concerned with pain relief may preserve an ischemic limb for a year or two and thus maintain the independence of the patient. Aesthetic considerations should rarely be allowed to override safety.

Cost

It is sometimes suggested that modern dressings are too expensive, but this is not so. The burden of an unhealed wound on a family and/or individual and on the community is considerable and costly. A dressing that results in complete healing is better than one that merely accelerates healing for a short initial period. A dressing that can be changed infrequently is less costly than a cheaper dressing that is changed frequently, and a dressing that is aesthetically acceptable increases the compliance of the wearer and the attention of the caregiver.

The Aesthetic Dressing

Some patients need an aesthetic dressing to perform effectively in public, and a larger group of patients have no motivation or preferences but need care. It is a sad reflection on our society that smelly, ugly wounds are a cause of patient neglect. An aesthetic dressing may result in a more willing caregiver.

The aesthetic management of an ulcer consists largely of disguising it with a dressing that not only covers and contains the wound but does not "dirty" the overlying clothing or the environment. The dressing should contain odor so that it is not a burden to the patient, the family, or the community. Coping with an ulcer, however, is closely linked with motivation and patient preference. Some elderly patients lack motivation and seem unaware of the odor, and some prefer to have an ulcer as the only means of attracting attention. This applies to the lonely, old person in the western apartment and to the beggar whose leprous ulcer is a source of income in the east. The well motivated comply with treatment because the rewards of mobility, comfort, and profitable daily living are worthwhile. For those who have no job and are chairbound, putting up with a little discomfort may at least guarantee that a nurse will pay an occasional visit.

The frequency of a change of dressing or of a visit from a nurse may range from a four-hourly wet dressing, which is an enormous handicap for a busy patient, to a once-weekly dressing, which is too infrequent for the lonely. A dressing which permits normal grooming and allows a daily bath is good for the patient's morale. It is also good for hygiene, though in emphasizing this to a patient, one must be careful not to add to the patient's fear of being thought "unclean" or contagious. Real dirtiness is a sign of the uncivilized, the immature, the demented, or the intellectual who believes that dirt is irrelevant. A good dressing is comfortable to apply, maintain, and remove and is malleable and disguiseable. For a busy or poorly motivated patient, the time taken to keep oneself well groomed may be a factor that determines the choice of therapy. When the procedure is time-consuming, it may still be worth prescribing if it is cosmetically acceptable. For patients who are anxious about this and are angry about their disfigurement and the lack of anything that can be done to ameliorate the situation, it is helpful to prescribe even time-consuming measures which add to attractiveness. For example, camouflage of vitiligo or even of a dressing on a leg (Fig. 6, *a* and *b*) can be achieved by prescribing a material such as Covermark or Dermablend. In the United Kingdom, support stockings for men are now marketed in black rather than the more feminine flesh color.

In managing ulcers of the leg, the patient's general well-being and good looks must not be ignored. An elderly patient with dementia who is allowed

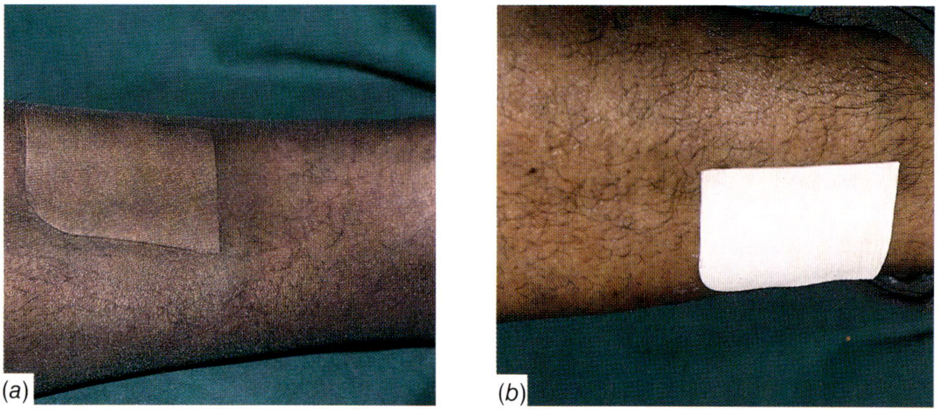

FIGURE 6
(*a*) On a dark-skinned patient, a white dressing has been camouflaged with Covermark and covered with a dark stocking. (*b*) Compare with the untreated dressing.

to go without teeth and with the hair unbrushed can benefit from a little beauty care. Caregivers are easier to obtain for the attractive than for the unattractive; when patients have lost motivation and are unable to declare their preferences, others must be brought in to care for them.

THE SWOLLEN LIMB

Patients with swollen limbs should also be viewed as requiring psychosocial assessment. Although sometimes congenital, a swollen limb can also be a consequence of filariasis, cancer, and radiotherapy of the pelvic organs and can be a late consequence of lymphatic fibrosis around venous leg ulcers. The deformity, the weight, the discomfort, and many of the secondary changes that occur in a swollen limb constitute a disfigurement that severely erodes a patient's confidence and makes the patient less able to perform effectively. The advice given to patients is often inadequate. This is a condition in which self-help based on good advice often brings about complete control.

A recent study of Bendova et al[8] divided those with lymphedema into the ignorant, the perfectionist, and the realist. Unfortunately, ignorance can be due to a lack of good advice, and lymphedema is greatly neglected in most societies; however, some patients remain ignorant because they prefer to ignore a disability or are unwilling to submit to an exacting therapeutic regimen. The perfectionist manages to keep the limb aesthetic, but at the expense of other roles in life, and often indulges in expensive regimens. Such patients obsessively check the condition, clamor for frequent medical opinions, read much literature, and seek foreign medications, alternative medicines, and expensive apparatus. It is the realist who is fully aware of all aspects of the disease, accepts the therapeutic plan and participates in it, supports it by his or her own effort, and is rational rather than emotional about its consequences.[8]

The management of lymphedema includes careful protection of the limb from trauma (Table 1). With exercise, massage, and careful compression bandaging or stockings and with care and much time spent on the limb, even severe lymphedema can sometimes resolve and gross disfigurement can be contained.

It is sometimes argued that surgical forms of therapy are mostly mutilating, and those who advocate conservative therapy argue against surgical interference. Some people simply do not have the time for conservative management; particularly in the developing world, a disfigured but usable limb that results from surgery is sometimes more desirable as a means of retaining employment or supporting a family than is the imposition of a full program of westernized conservative care.

REWARDS FOR REMAINING WELL HEALED

When healing has been effected, there should be rewards for maintaining healing and continuing care; for example, for watching a patient's weight

TABLE 1
MANAGEMENT OF LYMPHEDEMA

Skin toilet
- Emollients: restore and maintain skin suppleness
- Hygiene: reduces risks of infection
- Keratolytics: diminishes hyperkeratosis

Pneumatic compression, preferably sequential multichamber

Massage: generally should be gentle effleurage unless skin fibrosis demands mobilization of tissue and therefore kneading massage (care needed)

Compression hosiery
- High-compression e.g. >30 mmHg
- Graduated compression
- Well fitting and comfortable with no constriction points

Exercises to strengthen muscle pumps

Penicillin (long-term) or another antimicrobial to prevent recurrent erysipelas

Surgery for removal of redundant skin

Elevation, while helpful, does not confer the same degree of benefit as it does in venous edema

Diuretics: largely unhelpful but may produce some benefit, particularly when there is coexisting venous and/or cardiac edema

or preventing pressure sores in a paraplegic.[9] A patient who as a result of healing receives fewer visits from the nurse may give less attention to regimens that maintain good health. A "well ulcer clinic" is a social service that is much appreciated and thus is worthwhile. Unfortunately, a healed leg often needs the support of a bandage or stocking; however, there is no reason why bandages should be aesthetically displeasing. Of course, men have a slight advantage in concealing disfiguring bandages since they can always wear trousers; women can wear pants most of the time. But aesthetically appealing bandages should be prescribed where appropriate. The "confident nude" of the Greek ideal of beauty might not have worn bandages or stockings, but aesthetic drapery such as that which covers the legs of the Venus de Milo constitutes a solution to the problem of disguising disfigurement (Fig. 7).

FIGURE 7
(*a*) Ruben's Bathsheba has plump legs and a pretty face. (*b*) An Unna boot is not aesthetic and her expression seems inappropriate. (*c*) An attractive skirt hides the problem. (Dresden Art Gallery, with permission.)

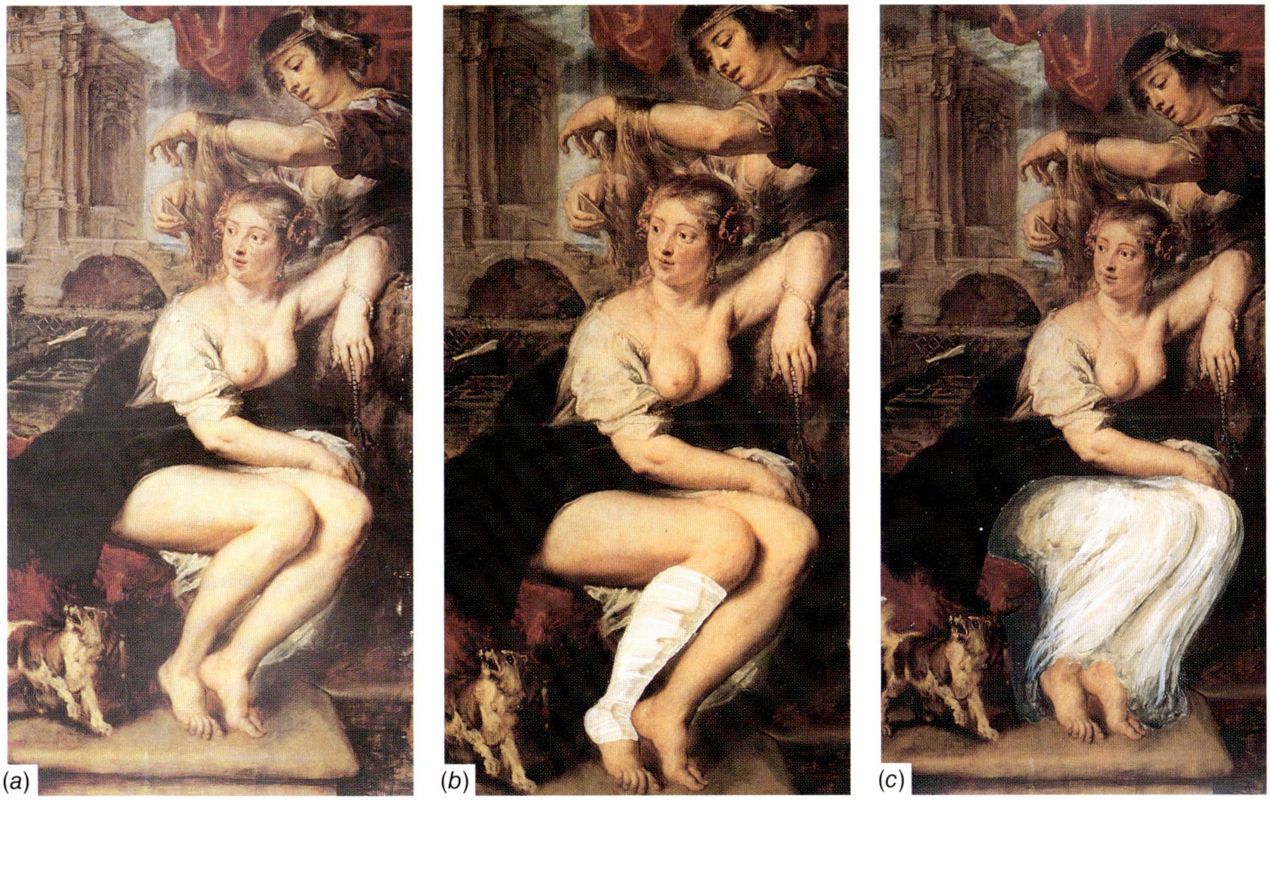

(*a*) (*b*) (*c*)

The look of the legs cannot be considered in isolation in real life any more than it can be in art. A beautiful face can make up for defects in the leg, and success in life, particularly when accompanied by an attractive personality, may allow the owner to ignore the attributes of the leg. In Fig. 7*a* Bathsheba's legs are overly pump and dimpled, but her pretty face and body make up for this. If, as in Fig. 7*b*, the legs are disfigured by ulceration and an overlying bandage, the facial expression seems as inappropriate as the approaches of her attendants; she shows *belle indifference,* and wears a smirk rather than an appropriate smile. After the leg has been disguised with drapery or a skirt (Fig. 7*c*), the expression on her face once more can be enjoyed by onlookers.

REFERENCES

1. Kurtz R: Investigations of the effective meaning of body products. J Exp Res Person. 1968; 3:9.
2. Ginsburg IH, Link B. The experience of stigmatisation in psoriasis, in Farber EM, Nall L, Morhenn V, Jacobs P (eds). Psoriasis: Proceedings of the Fourth International Symposium. New York: Elsevier, Science Publishing, 1987: 549–550.
3. Loudon ISL. Leg ulcers in the eighteenth and early nineteenth centuries. J Roy Col Gen Pract. 1981; 31:263–273.
4. Ryan TJ (ed). An environment for healing—the role of occlusion. International Congress and Symposium Series No. 88. London: Royal Society of Medicine, 1985.
5. Ryan TJ (ed). Beyond Occlusion: Wound Care Proceedings. London: Royal Society of Medicine, 1988.
6. Ryan TJ. The Management of Leg Ulcers, 2d ed. Oxford: Oxford University Press, 1987.
7. Ryan TJ, Cederholm Williams S, Lydon MJ (eds). Fibrinolysis and Angiogenesis in Wound Healing; Highlights of the Second International Forum. New York: Excerpta Medica, 1988.
8. Bendova M, Benda K, Dungleover E. Psychosocial factors in the management of lympoedema of the extremities, in Partsch H (ed) Progress in Lymphology, vol. XI. New York: Elsevier, 1988:545–547.
9. Ryan TJ. Pressure sores: Prevention, management and future research—A medical perspective. Palliative Med. 1989; 3:249–255.

PART

IV

SKIN STRUCTURES

CHAPTER 22

Hair: Medical Aspects

LARRY E. MILLIKAN

As people have become more conscious of their appearance, the association of hair loss with perceived or real aging has increased in importance. A full head of hair often gives the impression of a decade's difference in chronological age. Because of this, the use of therapy to camouflage, stop, or even reverse the progression of androgenic alopecia has become a significant patient concern in the practice of dermatology. Newer techniques offer refinements over older ones and at the same time give a better cosmetic result. While many of the most dramatic advances have been related to surgical therapy, any aesthetic approach to hair care and hair growth must involve a broadly based understanding of the medical aspects of hair and hair growth and in most instances an initial attempt at medical therapy prior to surgical correction.

OVERVIEW

The medical aspects of and patient concern about hair center on the primary complaint of *hair loss.* This situation affects both sexes but traditionally is more of a problem in men. Only recently have there been significant approaches and research findings that suggest the possibility of correcting this problem. During the last two decades surgery has been the primary means of correcting hair loss in men through scalp reductions and hair transplants (see Chap. 23).

An understanding of the physiology and pathophysiology of the interacting factors that result in hair loss is useful in determining the expected response to therapy. Scalp hair grows approximately 0.35 mm a day. Extremes in hair growth include growth of the eyebrows that has been estimated at approximately 0.16 mm a day and growth on the face and axillae between 0.30 and 0.38 mm per day.[1] This rate of growth is important in regard to informing the patient of the timing of expected changes after therapy.[2] External causes of anagen and telogen effluvia are listed in Table 1.

Hormonal Effects

Hormonal effects also may be critical in patients presenting with hair problems. The term *androgenic alopecia* is generally used to describe hereditary hair loss primarily in men but also in women. This relates to a certain extent to levels of androgen in the patient, but sometimes there is no consistent correlation between the various serum levels of the hormones and the extent or rate of hair loss. Hereditary factors seem to be prominent in most families of patients suffering from hair loss.

In general, hormonal effects, especially hereditary effects, have a specific distribution in the bitemporal and vertex thinning that ultimately follows the sequence of the Hamilton scale of androgenetic alopecia in men and in a primarily vertex localization of hair loss in women (see Figs. 1 through 3). Other hormonal effects and certain drugs may have a much more diffuse thinning ef-

TABLE 1
ALOPECIA: MECHANISMS, CAUSES, AND DRUGS

	Basic Pathophysiology Hair growth phases					
	Anagen	%	**Telogen**	%	**Catagen**	%
Scalp	Up to 6 years	85–90	3–4 weeks	10–14	weeks	1
Eyebrow	1–2 weeks		3 months		days to weeks	

Anagen effluvium	*Destruction of growing hairs caused by:* High dose x-ray Cyclophosphamide Thalidomide *Damage to growing hair caused by:* Low dose x-ray Colchicine Cytotoxic drugs Methotrexate Doxorubicin Heavy metals (As, Pb, Bi, Ag) Hypocholesterolemic drugs Bromocriptine
Telogen effluvium	*Shortening of hair cycle caused by:* Androgens* Birth control pills: progestin-dominant Heparinoids Warfarin Vitamin A Oral retinoids Lithium Methysergide Dextran

* Affects only susceptible hairs.
Source: Kligman.[2]

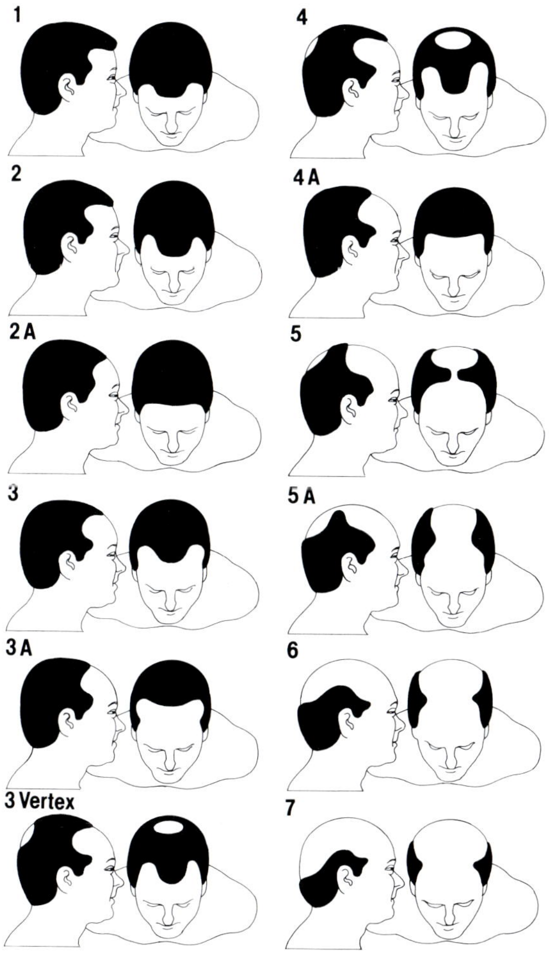

FIGURE 1
Standard patterns of hair loss as defined by the Hamilton scale. (Adapted from Bergfeld[11]; with permission.)

FIGURE 2
Widespread alopecia due to fungal infection, a problem rare in adults but extremely common in children.

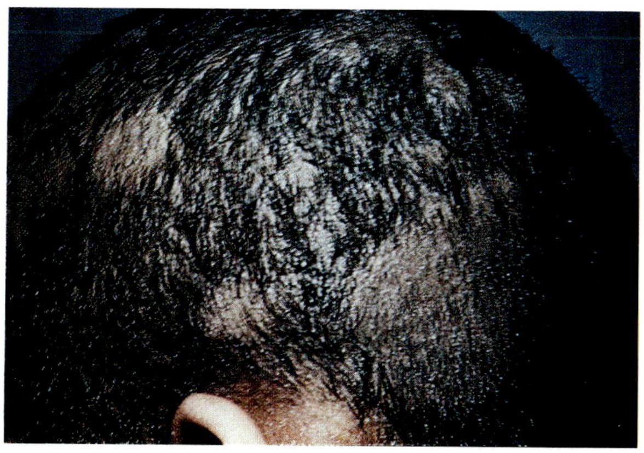

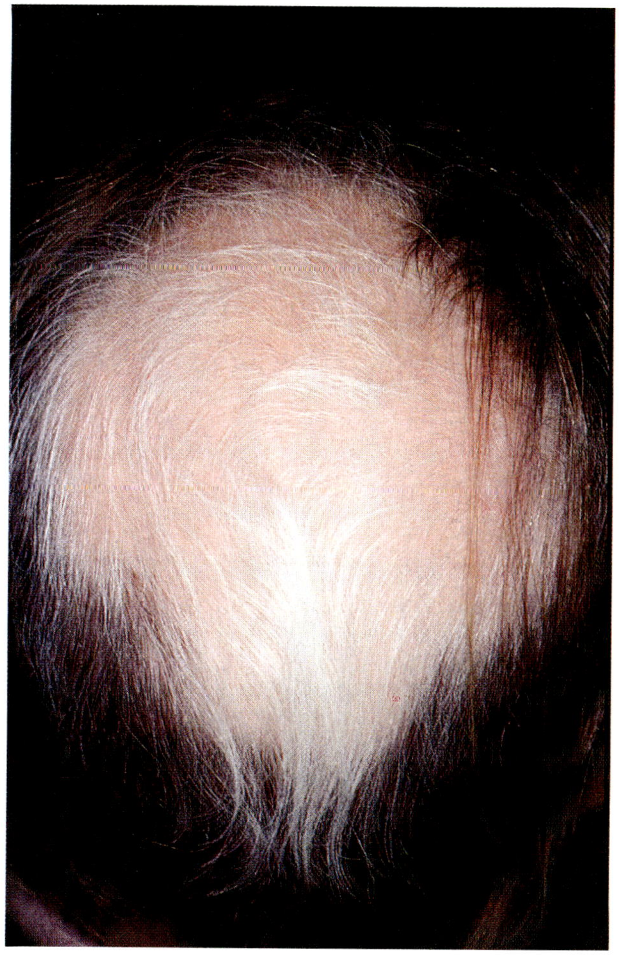

FIGURE 3
Vertex alopecia (alopecia areata) in a pattern where the differential in a female is androgenetic alopecia.

fect. Obvious thinning of the hair on the scalp requires a significant loss, generally 15 to 25 percent of hair, before it is clinically apparent. These hormonal, drug, and physical effects (such as from x-rays) can be widespread or diffuse and often are not associated with significant scalp disease.

The increasing clinical problem of a hormonal effect on the hair cycle is seen in female androgenetic alopecia that worsens secondary to progestin-dominant contraceptives and improves after treatment with antiandrogens.[3] The role of serum levels of hormones may be less important than that of tissue receptors and/or levels of 5α-reductase. This enzyme converts testosterone to dehydrotestosterone, which has much greater (5 to 10 times) potency than does testosterone. The en-

TABLE 2
HORMONES AND ALOPECIA

Androstenediol	← (17B HSA (adrenal source)) →	Dehydroepiandrosterone
(3β-HSD) ↓		(3β-HSD) ↓
Testosterone	← (17BHSD) →	Androstenedione
(5α-Reductase) ↓		(5α-Reductase) ↓
5α-Dehydrotestosterone*	← (17 HBSD) →	Androstenedione
(3α-HSD) ↓		(3α-HSD) ↓
Androstenediols		Androsterone, Epiandrosterone

* 1° androgen
HSD = Hydroxysteroid dehydrogenase

zymatic pathways, which are outlined in Table 2, are important in the evaluation of androgenetic alopecia.

Pharmacologic Effects

Certain drugs and chemicals can cause apparent hair loss through a different mechanism. If the level of insult is strong enough, the metabolism and physiology of the hair may be altered dramatically for a short time only. This results in cessation of the production of hair or hair matrix. When the insult has subsided, the body is able to resume hair production, leaving a constricted shaft of hair called the *Pohl-Pincus mark.* This can also be seen in the fingernails and in a thinning of the nail plate characterized by a groove called a *Beau's line.* This is often seen in patients receiving certain types of chemotherapy. Alopecia occurs later as the hair grows out and breaks off at the site of the Pohl-Pincus constriction, leaving growing hairs proximal to the breakage point.

An understanding of this mechanism allowed Anderson and coworkers[4] to use a unique mechanism to prevent hair loss in patients with doxorubicin alopecia. They found that putting a constricting tourniquet and ice bags on the scalp before chemotherapy infusions allows the hair to recover without hair loss or breakage in many instances.

At very high doses of these drugs, the anagen effluvium is induced with severe damage to the hair papilla, a total cessation of hair growth, and fairly rapid hair fall. The use of certain other drugs which have a milder effect on the hair papilla can stimulate a conversion to telogen and the usual telogen effluvium reaction mentioned above. Thus, the amount of hair in a given area on the scalp may relate to hormonal effects and drugs that affect the normal hair cycle and also may relate to immune or inflammatory reactions that occur in specific sites.

Immunologic Effects

Other instances of hair loss can be associated with apparent immunologic reactions, as in the alopecia areata and inflammatory local tissue reactions seen in inflammatory diseases of the scalp. In alopecia areata, on biopsy, the localized areas show a very intense lymphocytic infiltrate around the hair follicles; this has long suggested the probability of an immunologic reaction. The response in these patients to immunologic active agents such as dinitrochlorobenzene (DNCB), psoralen plus ultraviolet A (PUVA), and rhus antigens tends to support this presumed phenomenon. Unfortunately, most laboratory data have not shown a consistent situation with regard to types of inflammatory cells, infiltrating cells, types of lymphocytes, or host immune status. Other inflammatory reactions (infections and others) are usually associated with the formation of scars in the scalp; it is presumed that these dramatic changes in tissue consistency and perfusion leading to scarring alopecia are the simple and primary causes of this situation. See Fig. 4.

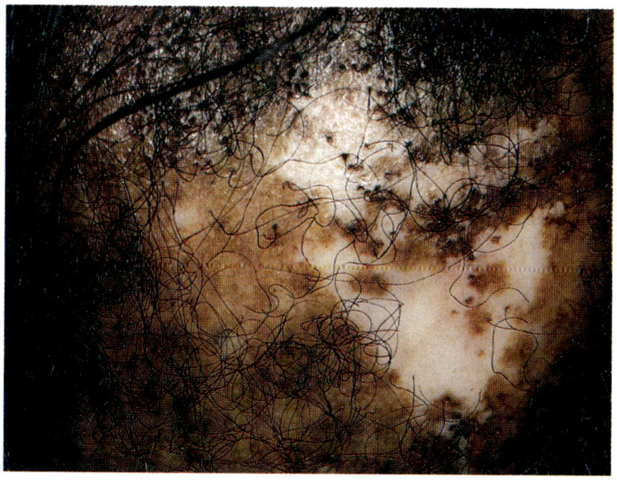

FIGURE 4
Severe inflammatory scarring alopecia. Here the inflammatory reaction was severe, causing not only destruction of hair follicles and production of scars but destruction of pigment cells, leaving areas of hyperpigmentation and areas of total absence of pigment. This type of scarring alopecia is often due to lichen planus or infection and can usually be differentiated on the basis of history.

CLINICAL MANIFESTATIONS

In the overall evaluation of the patient, clinical manifestations are extremely important in making a presumptive diagnosis (Table 3). Any questionable clinical presentation requires thorough evaluation.

EVALUATION OF ALOPECIA

The evaluation of a patient with a medical or preexisting hair problem requires a careful examination. Categorization in regard to localized, pattern, or generalized hair loss as well as separation between the scarring and nonscarring types is the essential first step. The presence or absence of inflammation or concurrent scalp disease is another important aspect of the evaluation on the first visit.

In most instances, evaluation of the current metabolic status of the hair can be accomplished through an organized system of hair plucking known as a *trichogram* (or *trichorhizogram* by Braun-Falco).[5] There is some variation from dermatologist to dermatologist as to the exact procedure used to obtain this sampling. Some feel it is important to sample consistently at least three different regions of the scalp (i.e., parietal, temporal, and occipital). Braun-Falco[5] stated that for this study epilation should be done on the seventh day after the last hair wash. It is very important to note recent manipulation of the hair and/or chemical treatments that may result in some changes in the hair shaft that do not reflect significant underlying problems. This study provides a useful insight into the current status of the hair on the scalp.

An appropriate forceps with rubber over the tips is needed to grasp a proper number of hairs. This is done rapidly to minimize patient discomfort. The hairs are examined under the microscope. From this sampling of hair, one can determine whether the appropriate percentages of anagen, telogen, and catagen hairs are present. This may allow one to make an early diagnosis of telogen or anagen effluvium. Additionally, it is possible with this technique to obtain a good sample of hair for evaluation of potential hair shaft abnormalities. While many hair shaft abnormalities are congenital and present

TABLE 3
EVALUATION OF HAIR LOSS

Hair loss
- Significant?
- Localized: pattern (androgenetic alopecia, trauma) trichotillomania; sectional: bacterial, fungal
- Diffuse (drug, illness)
- Scarring (infection, lichen planus)
- Nonscarring
- Scalp disease? (psoriasis, seborrheic dermatitis)

Hair shaft
- Pull: number of hairs, structural abnormality
- Pluck
  - Trichogram/trichorhizogram
  - Distribution of hair; percentage anagen, telogen
  - Anagen effluvium
  - Telogen effluvium

Responses to therapy against infection: bacterial, fungal
- Seborrheic dermatitis
- Psoriasis

Biopsy
- Immunofluorescence/lichen planus, lupus erythematosus
- Special stains
- Characterization of infiltrate (alopecia areata)

at an early age, a few of these abnormalities are acquired at a later phase in life and relate to dietary problems, chemicals, or hair treatments which may cause hair loss. Such a hair pluck or trichogram also allows the clinician to predict more severe hair loss in the future in the case of a predominance of telogen hairs.

The hair is one of the sites of the most intense metabolic activity in the body; this activity is necessary to form the accessory structures. As a result, the hair is very susceptible to chemotherapeutic agents and to the effects of poor nutrition.[6] As part of the evaluation, signs of inadequate diet, a history of fad diets, bulimia, and anorexia are also very important.

General evaluation of the hands, teeth, and nails can also be helpful, as many metabolic and inflammatory changes that affect the hair may also be manifest in the skin and nails. Abnormalities in the teeth may suggest a more extensive problem, such as certain ectodermal defects with late manifestations. Those inflammatory skin diseases (such as collagen vascular diseases and lichen planus) that result in hair loss may be diagnosed through careful general dermatologic evaluation.

All these phases of the examination can be completed in one to two office visits and then a trial is often in order. First and second visits are usually separated by several weeks to allow the clinician time to see the evolution of the process and the progression of the alopecia, along with the response to therapy. Additionally, by the second visit, evaluation may be at a point where the role of hormones may be seriously considered and can be evaluated with the use of hormone tests (Table 2). This may allow insight into progressing alopecia due to significant changes in endogenous hormones, the presence of a tumor secreting androgens, or another abnormality of hormonal physiology.

Essential to the process of evaluation in the first 6 weeks between the first and second visits is the process of educating the patient about the proper care of the hair and the scalp in order to minimize the effect of such coexisting scalp diseases like severe seborrheic dermatitis and psoriasis. In some instances, the activity of psoriasis in the scalp may cause the hair loss, which then subsides; regrowth occurs upon successful clearing of scalp psoriasis. For this period of time, the response of the scalp to appropriate medication aimed at inflammatory scalp disease (i.e., antibiotics), psoriasis (tar shampoos and steroids), and lichen planus (steroids) is an important supportive finding for the diagnosis.

By the second or the third evaluation visit all the above diagnostic studies have been done and repeated if they are equivocal or questionable; at this point a biopsy is in order. Patients being prepared for scalp biopsy must understand the importance of this procedure in establishing the diagnosis and be reassured of the safety and painlessness of the procedure. In doing a scalp biopsy, it is important to obtain enough tissue to do standard histological studies, studies with special stains, and studies to detect the presence of immunoreactants in the hair and scalp.

Standard immunofluorescence studies can provide supportive evidence for collagen vascular disease characterized by the deposition of immunoreactants at the dermal-epidermal junction. It may also support the diagnosis of some bullous diseases, again with similar findings of different patterns and different types of immunoreactants at the dermal-epidermal junction. Additionally, the presence of colloid bodies and other types of immunoreactants may sustain or support the diagnosis of lichen planus, which is often highly likely on the basis of the histological findings. Some rare instances of unusual infections may also warrant the inclusion of special stains for organisms (acid-fast, Giemsa, Brown Brenn) in this full evaluation.

Table 3 shows an orderly stepwise process that allows one to make a diagnosis of scalp hair loss directly or by exclusion. In virtually all cases the diagnosis of androgenetic alopecia is done by exclusion, based on a lack of other causal diseases and usually a positive family history. Most important, the pattern often is the essential step in the diagnosis.

MANAGEMENT

Medical therapy for localized alopecia is primarily aimed at the cause. Alopecia areata is often very responsive to immunogens such as dinitrochlorobenzene (DNCB), squaric acid, and rhus antigen; irritants such as anthralin; and (often temporarily) topical or intralesional steroids.

Additionally, we have found that cimetidine is

sometimes effective, often as an adjunct to dinitrochlorobenzene or other immunotherapy but occasionally as the sole therapeutic agent. Simple topical immunotherapy using rhus antigen is another valuable approach. The use of psoralens and ultraviolet A or ultraviolet B also is generally successful. See Fig. 5. A sequential approach to therapy as outlined in Table 4 has been successful in our trials.

Topical, systemic, or intralesional steroids may be useful primarily in collagen vascular disease or lichen planus, but these agents are purposely left as a last means of therapy; while usually successful, they result in temporary regrowth with ultimate loss of the hair. Inflammatory or infective conditions of the scalp respond to the appropriate antibiotic. Lichen planus and collagen vascular diseases of the scalp often respond to the use of topical, intralesional, or systemic steroids; however, the ultimate resolution of the process usually requires remission of the disease, which often is difficult to achieve.

In the practice of aesthetic dermatology, most patients present with the problem of androgenic alopecia. As mentioned above, in some instances cyproterone has been useful in the treatment of women. Unfortunately, any agent directly aimed at

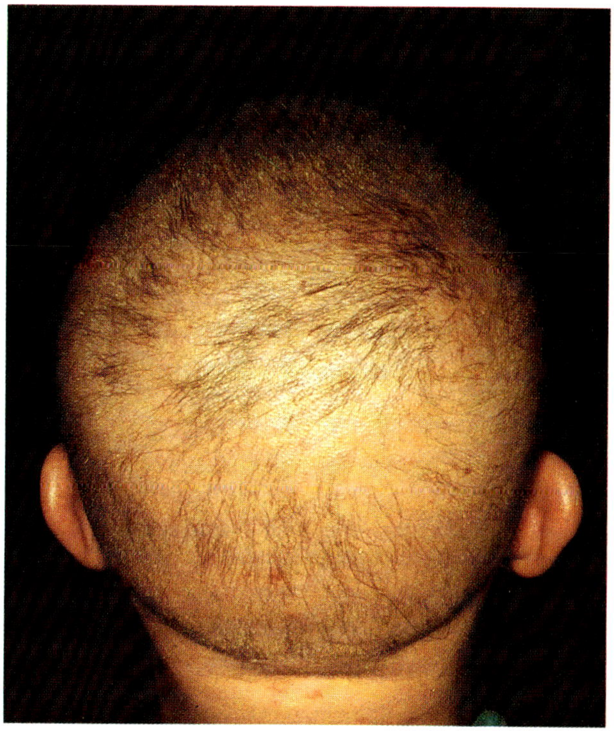

FIGURE 5
Widespread regrowth after ultraviolet therapy in a patient with alopecia universalis.

TABLE 4
THERAPY FOR ALOPECIA AREATA

Irritant
- Hair loss
- Anthralin: apply q d or q 2 d to achieve low-grade erythema
- Phototherapy with ultraviolet B
  - Treatment 2–3 × 1 week; achieve minimum effective dose with each treatment to enhance response
  - Topical: tars; psoralens: use with caution; topical sensitivity persists
  - Systemic: psoralens; used only with widespread hair loss > 48 h for alopecia totalis or universalis
  - UVA: use with topical or systemic psoralens; treat 2 × 1 week

Immunotreatment
- Rhus antigens, squaric acid, dinitrochlorobenzene, and diphencypromine are used primarily to achieve an ongoing low-grade contact dermatitis; applied q 10–14 d; disadvantages: chronic pruritus, irritation

Systemic immunotherapy: cimetidine

Steroid therapy
- This is the last resort with the exception of limited alopecia areata; a topical class I steroid
- Intralesional: used infrequently; scalp atrophy common; rebound hair fall after effect of *depot* steroids has worn off
- Systemic: very rare indications in my practice; used only as adjunct to phototherapy or immunotherapy, primarily in alopecia totalis or universalis

androgenic effects in the body can have an effect on many other organs. This drastically limits the usefulness of cyproterone in the treatment of androgenetic alopecia in men since impotence and gynecomastia are common side effects of this medication.

Newer drugs have been evaluated after the serendipitous finding of hirsutism as a side effect. Minoxidil is perhaps the most famous of these drugs to date. When used for serious forms of hypertension, it has had a major side effect of widespread hirsutism in female patients that has been so dramatic as to deter patients from optimal use of the drug, resulting in severe compliance problems. This side effect was manipulated to obtain a therapeutic effect. Topical use of minoxidil seems to be effective in altering or regressing androgenetic alopecia in certain patients.[7,8] In our experience, it has not been universally effective, but a small number of patients have had a very acceptable response. See Figs. 6 and 7. The vast majority of patients using a 2% minoxidil solution do not obtain the desired reversal of the progression of androgenetic alopecia. Studies that have been under way for long periods of time have involved patients with long-standing alopecia. Studies of minoxidil used in the early stages of hair fall in patients with a strong positive family history of androgenetic alopecia are under way and have indicated that this drug may be far more effective as a preventive rather than as an agent that can reverse established widespread hair loss (i.e., Hamilton classes 4, 5, and 5A). Minoxidil is available in many countries and has been used with some success. In our studies, patients interested in the use of minoxidil often developed a great deal of enthusiasm for the drug, and in some instances we found that their perception of the benefit was far greater than our objective assessment. Minoxidil may have potential utility because it is effective in a small number of patients, and it may represent the first step in a subsequent series of drugs that will allow us to prevent androgenetic alopecia in the future.

Minoxidil is marketed as a 2% solution with three applicators (Rogaine). The drug seems quite safe and may provide a very useful modality for a

FIGURE 6
A patient with Hamilton class 3A male pattern baldness at the initiation of a minoxidil study. Typical pattern for androgenetic alopecia.

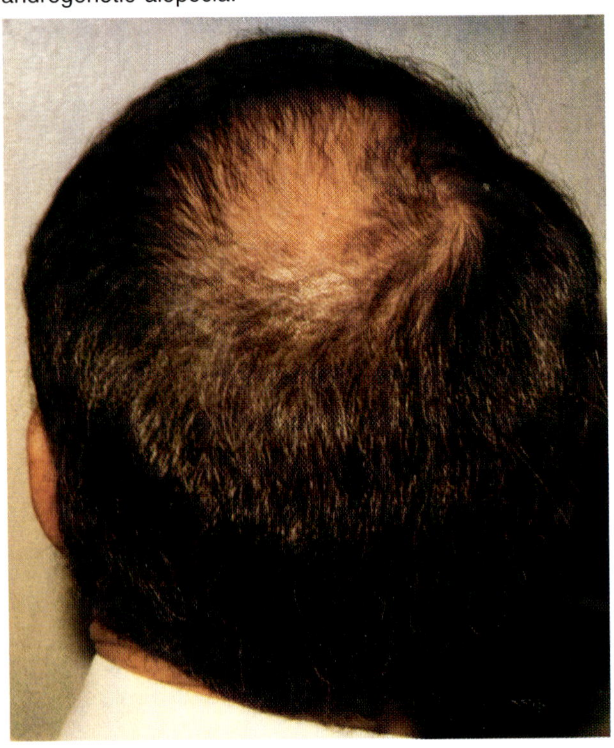

FIGURE 7
Same patient as in Fig. 5 shown 12 months later on minoxidil, with a significant decrease in vertex balding.

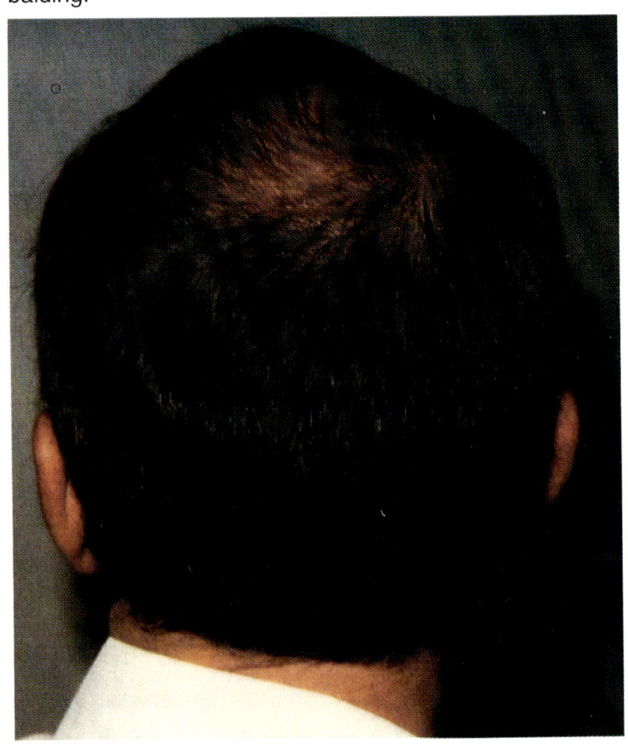

trial of therapy, because nothing else offers any benefit for most patients with androgenetic alopecia.

The safety of minoxidil suggests that minimal laboratory tests are needed. However, our experience with a large number of patients included finding eight asymptomatic healthy young adults with potential cardiac problems, and it is still our policy to screen patients by means of a careful medical history, blood pressure, and vital signs. If there are potential hereditary cardiac conditions, we feel it is important to also include electrocardiograms and even echocardiograms as indicated. We believe that it is necessary to establish a normal baseline in case there are medical problems later in the course of therapy, for this is a drug that will be used by the patient for several years.

The application of minoxidil with one of the three applicators in the marketed package is done twice daily. It is extremely important to emphasize to the patient that application as directed is necessary to achieve the desired effect. It is also important to underscore the necessity of continuous use of the drug. After desirable regrowth has occurred—which may take as long as 7 to 18 months—it is possible to decrease the frequency of application. Based on the Tulane clinical experience, it seems possible to decrease the frequency of application to once daily. Studies of application at less frequent intervals have not established continued efficacy.

When initiating minoxidil therapy, one must emphasize the chronic continuous nature of the therapy. This is not a short-term correction of the problem, and the patient's commitment and compliance are essential. The clinical diagnosis of androgenetic alopecia may include a number of disparate conditions that cannot be clinically separated at the present time, and it is entirely possible that variable responses to minoxidil may be a function of differing etiologies.

The exact mechanism by which minoxidil works remains unclear. The simplistic analysis of its vasodilating effect does not seem sufficient to explain the clinical response; however, the use of another vasodilating drug—diazoxide—which also may stimulate hair growth, lends some support to a vasoactive mechanism for minoxidil. Other effects of minoxidil on cells and tissue in culture have suggested the possibility of other modes of action. Spironolactone was once used widely, but I employ it very rarely in my practice now.[9]

Other drugs that have been studied, include viprostol, which is a prostaglandin analog. This drug has been withdrawn from studies because of inconsistent and/or minimal effectiveness. Cyclosporin and diazoxide may ultimately be evaluated for potential use in treating hair loss. The public's response to minoxidil has been sufficient to encourage further searches for drugs useful in the treatment of androgenic alopecia.[10] Recently, minoxidil therapy has also been reported to be associated with telogen effluvium,[11] another cause for concern even though very rare. Until consistently effective medications are available, surgical approaches will remain the most effective means of dealing with the condition.

REFERENCES

1. Millikan LE. Hair loss in women, in Pechtran B, Shapiro S (eds). Signs and Symptoms in Gynecology. Philadelphia: Lippincott, 1983:419–432.
2. Kligman AM. Pathologic dynamics of human hair loss: Telogen effluvium. Arch Dermatol. 1961;83:175–198.
3. Dawber RPR, Sonnx T, Ralfs T. Oral anti-androgen treatment of common baldness in women. Br J Dermatol. 1982; 20(suppl 22):20.
4. Anderson JE, Hund JM, Smith IE. Prevention of doxorubicin induced alopecia by scalp cooling in patients with advanced breast cancer. Br Med J. 1981;282:423–425.
5. Braun-Falco O, Heilgemin GP. The trichogram, structural and functional basis, performance and interpretation. Semin Dermatol. 1985;4:40–52.
6. Stroud J. Drug-induced alopecia. Semin Dermatol. 1985;4:29–34.
7. Storer JS, Brzuskiewicz J, Floyd H, et al. Topical minoxidil for male pattern baldness. Am J Med Sci. 1986;291:328–333.
8. Olsen SA, Delong ER, et al. Safe response study of topical minoxidil in male pattern baldness. J Am Acad Dermatol. 1986;15:30–37.
9. Coruol P, Michaud A, Menard J, et al. Anti-androgenic effect of spironolactones: Mechanism of action. Endocrinology. 1975;97:52–58.
10. Bergfeld WF. Etiology and diagnosis of androgenic alopecia. Clin Dermatol. 1988;6(4):102–107.
11. Bardelli A, Rebora A. Telogen effluvium and minoxidil. J Am Acad Dermatol. 1989;21:572–573.

CHAPTER 23

Hair: Surgical Aspects

WALTER P. UNGER

Surgical treatment for androgenic alopecia can be conveniently divided into three alternatives: punch hair transplantation, alopecia reduction, and flap surgery. Detailed descriptions for each of these can be found in appropriate texts.[1,2] This chapter describes the basic concepts and techniques employed and their respective pros and cons. Although the procedures are most commonly performed on men, women can also benefit.

PUNCH HAIR TRANSPLANTATION

The basic technique of *punch hair transplantation* is simple. A 4-mm to 5-mm trephine is used to remove skin from a donor area that is judged to be permanently hair bearing. A hole made with a slightly smaller punch is then cut out of the bald or balding recipient site, and the prepared graft is placed in it. After an initial period of effluvium (2 to 3 months) the hair begins to grow again and will survive in its new site as long as it would have in the original location. This simple procedure has almost as many variations as there are practitioners. Outlined below is the technique I currently use.

Principles

Any bald area can be virtually solidly filled during four punch transplant sessions (Fig. 1). During each operation, regardless of the general graft distribution plan, grafts within a treated area are placed approximately one graft apart from each other. Ultimately, some bald areas will be filled solidly, while others will be treated during one, two, or three sessions, depending on the location and the hair density required for a site. Even with experience, it is difficult to anticipate which areas will need two, three, or four sessions. Approaching the problem by dispersing grafts in such a way that ultimately one could do any given area solidly in four sessions allows for whatever degree of filling is later deemed necessary.

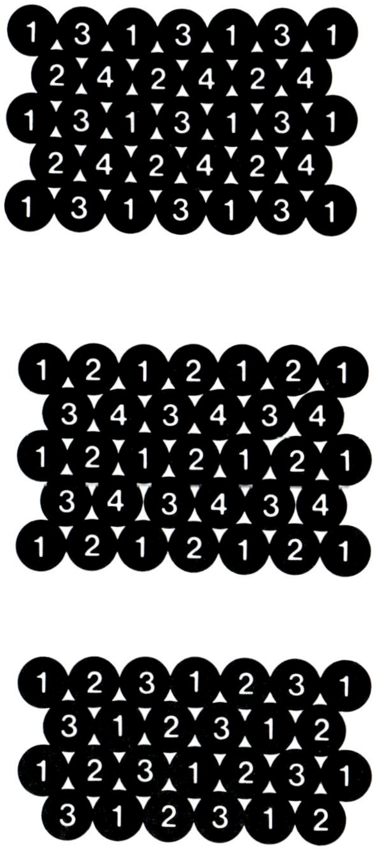

FIGURE 1
Any area of alopecia can be solidly filled in one of three different ways. The method shown at the top is the usual four-stage approach. Areas that are still hair-bearing are treated as shown in the middle. The approach shown at the bottom is the three-stage filling described by Orentreich and Orentreich.[3]

Orentreich and Orentreich[3] described a three-session method of filling a bald site solidly (Fig. 1). I do not have sufficient experience using this technique for large bald sites, as 130 to 150 grafts are necessary in each of three sessions to deal with the anterior one-third to one-half of the average bald area, and sessions of this size are larger than I feel comfortable carrying out. The standard graft size is 4 mm. In a study reported in 1977,[4] 4.5-mm and 4.0-mm grafts were taken from adjacent and clinically similar donor sites. It was found that with regard to hairs per surface area and hair yield per donor area, 4.0-mm grafts were more efficient. In the first sessions, all grafts are obtained with a 4-mm punch. In subsequent sessions, approximately 30 4.5-mm grafts are taken, with the balance being 4-mm grafts. The purpose of the 30 larger grafts will be discussed below. Occasionally, a 5-mm graft or a graft smaller than 4 mm is employed. Larger grafts may be divided as an alternative method of getting 1-mm to 2-mm grafts.

The basic pattern employed is a four- or five-row U-shaped recipient area (Fig. 2). The anterior two rows are punched out with a 3-mm or, more often, a 3.25-mm punch, whichever produces the best donor plug–recipient site fit. The posterior two or three rows are prepared with a 3.5-mm punch, with the exception of the first four recipient sites on the part side of the same rows, which are cut with a 3-mm or 3.25-mm punch to produce greater hair density in the "part" corner.

Usually 90 to 110 grafts are transplanted per session. This number can be increased by extending the U-shaped pattern posteriorly on one side to produce more of a J shape. Sessions of 130 to 150 grafts thus can be done safely without embarrassing the blood supply of the grafts; however, as indicated earlier, I prefer to avoid such large sessions. Studies have shown that four- and five-row patterns of this

FIGURE 2
A typical four-row pattern in the recipient area. Recipient sites are prepared with a 3-mm or 3.25-mm punch in the anterior two rows and for the first four grafts of the most lateral aspects of each row on the part side. All other sites are prepared with a 3.5-mm punch

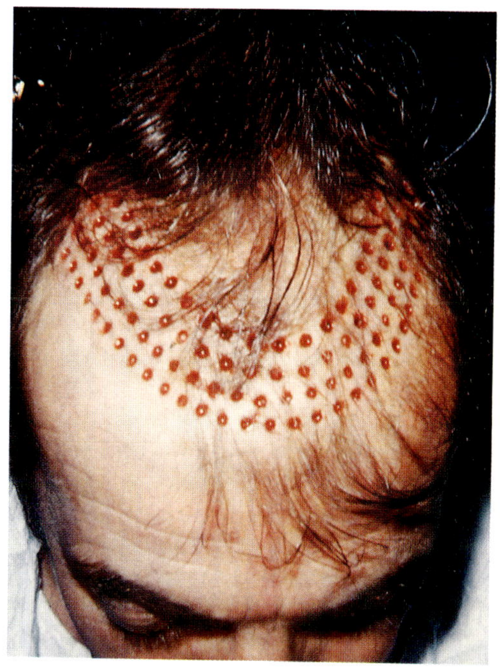

type produce excellent hair yields.[5] Occasionally, if one is anticipating doing a U-shaped alopecia reduction later, an island of grafts may also be inserted in the center of the peninsula between the arms of the U. Alternatively, if the physician is planning an elliptical or Y-shaped alopecia reduction, a minireduction, as described below, may be done concomitantly with the punch transplanting session.

The same U-shaped pattern is repeated in the second session and then is varied, as described below. The second session is done 6 weeks after the first, while 3- and 4-month intervals are left between the second and third and the third and fourth sessions if one is dealing with the same area. These periods may be lengthened, but it is best not to shorten them. When one is transplanting into areas of early male pattern baldness, the sessions are 6 months or more apart, allowing each transplant to grow in and thicken the recipient sites before subsequent sessions are carried out. A detailed description of the advantages and disadvantages of "early" punch transplantation has been published.[6,7]

My office personnel now employ gloves, masks, and glasses when operating, as the incidence of hepatitis continues to be significant and to ward off the potential threat of acquired immunodeficiency syndrome (AIDS). If one uses a hand punch in the recipient area, rubber gloves tend to "catch" as the punch is turned. We have found that Arbrook utility gloves (Surgikos) catch very little. The use of a power punch in the recipient area avoids this problem entirely, but power instruments at this site have other disadvantages, including "catching" of adjacent hair, less accurate spacing, and tedious frequent changes of punch sizes to completely excise the spaces of different sizes left between previously transplanted grafts.

Patients in our office are operated on in a prone position for the donor area and in a supine position with the head of the bed raised to a 45-degree angle for the recipient area, except if the vertex is the recipient site. In this latter case, the patient is usually placed in a sitting position. A "prone pillow" (Fig. 3) is useful when working on the donor area. The patient places the face into an aperture that allows the patient to breathe freely while facing directly into the bed.

The rest of the equipment typically employed for punch transplanting is listed in Table 1.

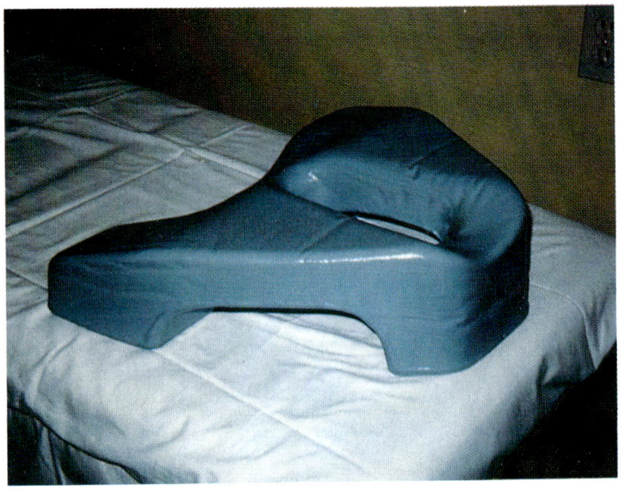

FIGURE 3
To maintain a neutral position, the head is placed in a "Pron-Pillo" when one is harvesting from the midocciput.

TABLE 1
CONTENTS OF INSTRUMENT TRAY

7 Syringes, 10 cc each
1 Syringe: 2% lidocaine, 1:100,000 with 30-gauge needle
2 Syringes: 1% lidocaine, 1:100,000, one with 30-gauge needle, other with 25-gauge needle
2 Syringes: adrenaline, 1:200,000 prepared solution with 25-gauge needle
2 Adson forceps
1 Iris scissors
1 Needle driver
1 Straight Metzenbaum scissors
1 Power punch, 4.5 mm
1 Power punch, 4.0 mm
1 Hand punch, 3.5 mm
1 Hand punch, 3.25 mm
1 Hand punch, 3.0 mm
2 Packages Supramid sutures 2-0, cable-type suture
2 Rolls Kerlix bandage
Baciguent Ointment
1 Vigilon primary wound dressing, 4 × 4 cm
Gauze, 4 × 4 cm
24 Pieces Nu Gauze, 4 × 8 cm

(From WP Unger, RE Nordström[1]; with permission.)

Planning

While most people begin punch transplanting only when they have an area of completely developed alopecia, increasingly large numbers of individuals are being seen before they are totally bald. Such patients can and should be operated on as long as one is certain that the end result will be denser hair. In my experience, "early" transplanting, i.e., transplanting before the area is totally bald, does not accelerate the rate at which the patient is losing hair and may even retard it. Starting early has the advantages of avoiding the embarrassment of total alopecia and allowing the patient to camouflage the recipient area postoperatively much more easily and sometimes completely by the following day. It also enables the individual to proceed with transplanting at a more leisurely rate, keeping pace with the rate of hair loss.

The disadvantages of starting early include an initial thinning of hair in the recipient area (for approximately 3 months) and the difficulty of accurately forecasting the eventual extent of the fully developed area of alopecia. A family history, careful examination, and experience can help minimize the latter problem. It cannot be overemphasized that punch transplanting in patients who are not yet bald should be carried out only by physicians who have considerable experience and expertise. When it is done properly, however, the effects are very gratifying to both patient and doctor (Fig. 4).

FIGURE 4
(*a*) Before the first session. (*b*) After five sessions, top view (471 grafts). (*c*) After five sessions, side view. (*d*) After five sessions. Completed hairline with micrografts.

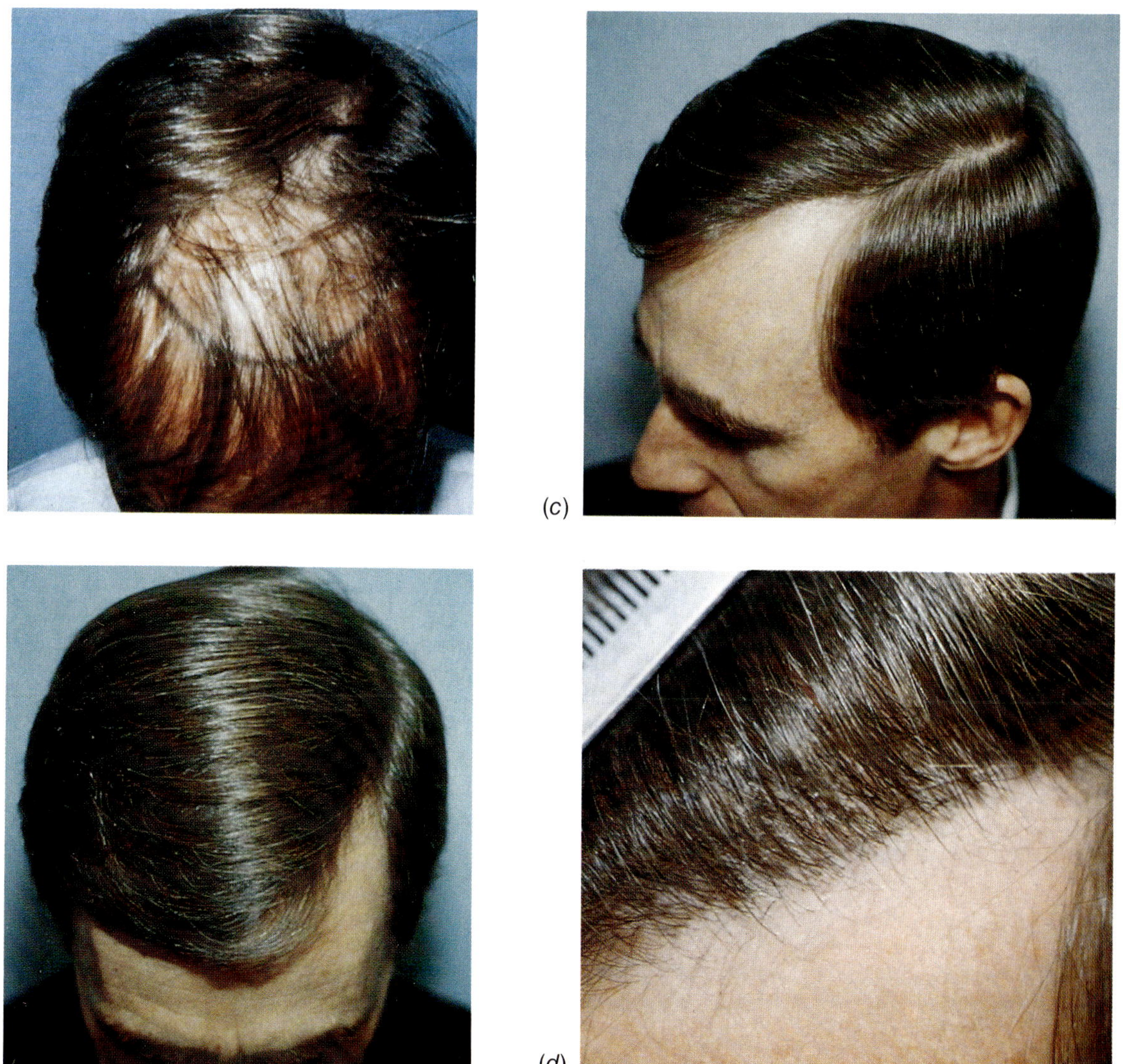

(*a*) (*c*) (*b*) (*d*)

All these comments on early transplanting apply equally to women. In addition, of course, be certain that the woman has good prospects for maintaining a male pattern of androgenetic alopecia, that is, maintaining a relatively dense donor rim while thinning centrally. Some variations in approach are recommended.[8] The most important changes are the treatment of only the left or the right side of the recipient site in each session and the use of smaller sessions; for example, 50 to 60 grafts per session. Both variations allow for easier postsurgical camouflage.

In general, the lighter the color and the finer the texture of the hair, the better. White or salt and pepper hair is ideal, with the second best color being blond (Fig. 5). In addition very coarse and tightly curled hair produces an appearance of greater than actual density, and one can adequately transplant any recipient site with fewer grafts than would be required in a straight-haired white pa-

FIGURE 5
(*a*) Before transplanting. This patient had fine-textured salt and pepper hair, ideal for punch transplanting. (*b*) After transplanting; 335 plugs have been transplanted in four sessions. (*c*) Hair combed up to expose transplanted hairline after four sessions. (*d*) Close-up of hairline after transplanting. The texture and color of the hair resulted in a less abrupt hairline than is usually produced by punch transplanting, even though no micrografts were used.

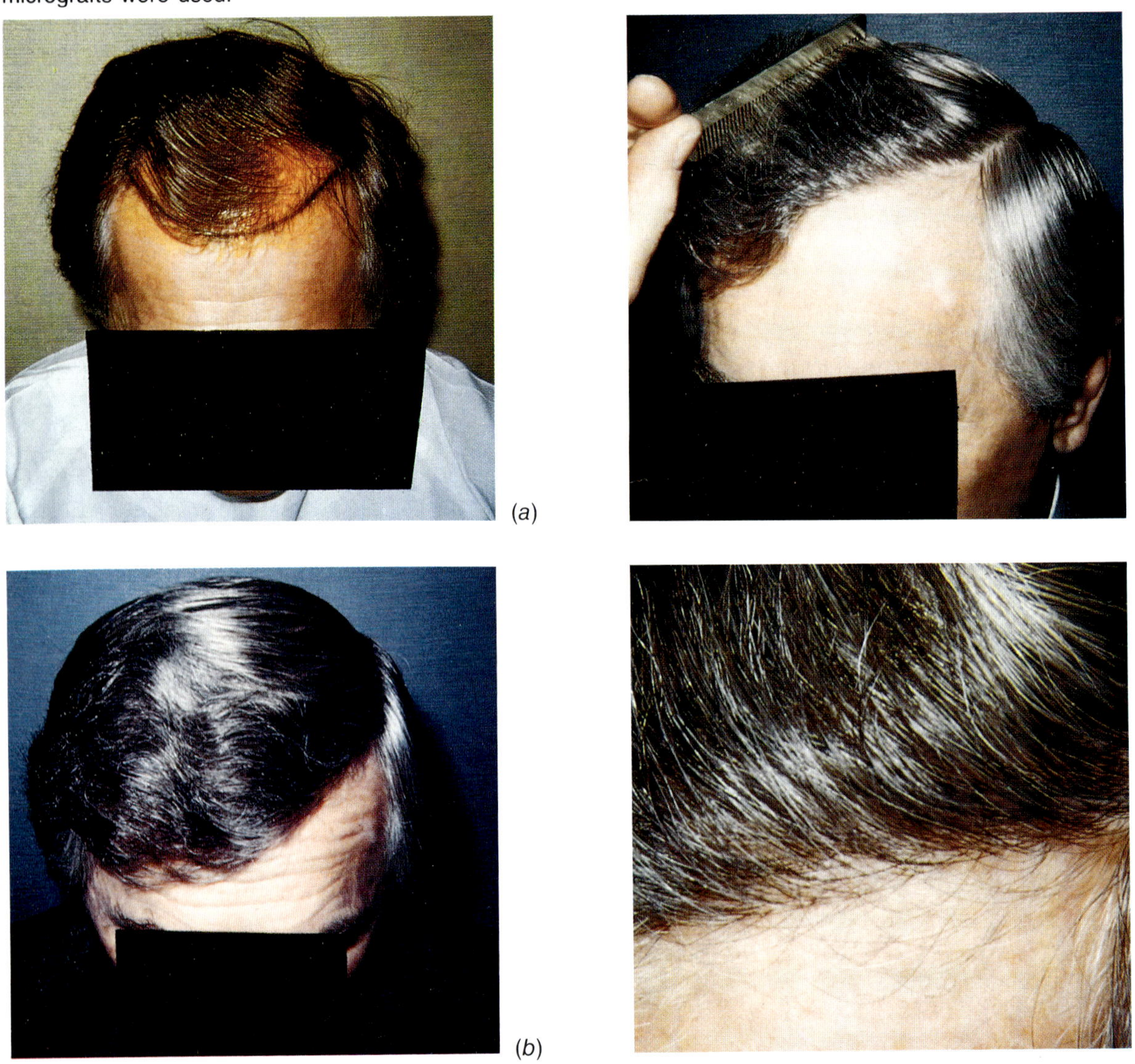

(*a*) (*c*) (*b*) (*d*)

tient. The subject of transplanting in black patients is covered in detail elsewhere.[9] Orientals tend to require significantly fewer grafts than does the average white patient because the diameter of their hair shafts tends to be larger and therefore provides more coverage. The most difficult patients to treat are those with dark, coarse hair and light colored skin. The contrast between the color of the hair and that of the skin accentuates the sparsity in areas that are not densely transplanted. Also, the hairline is more abrupt. Micrografting (see below) is useful in minimizing this problem.

Choosing the hairline pattern begins with an estimate of where one expects the anteriormost and superiormost points of the permanent temporal hair to be. These points are marked, and a third point is chosen anteriorly in the midline, through which a line can be drawn, joining the two temporal points and producing a natural-looking ovoid or slightly bell-shaped hairline. If the third (midline) point is placed too far posteriorly, the hairline will be too flat; if it is placed too far anteriorly, the hairline will be too "peaked." Ideally, the hairline should be as high and conservative as the patient can accept. It will look more natural as the patient ages and will conserve grafts for use more posteriorly, thus increasing the physician's chances of being able to transplant the entire fully developed bald area. The reader is referred to a complete discussion of this subject.[10]

The objectives of physicians and patients vary. One can aim to produce enough hair so that with hairstyling the results are acceptable. If the goal is this modest, it allows for larger areas of alopecia to be covered less densely. The disadvantage is that considerable hairstyling may be necessary to avoid a "cornfield" appearance, and swimming or active sports may become embarrassing. Others prefer to transplant areas more densely so that a minimum of hairstyling is required. More grafts are required to do an area of the same size more densely; therefore, one may be unable to cover a large bald area completely because not enough donor grafts are available. Both objectives are reasonable as long as the patient is aware of the consequences of the route that is chosen. I prefer smaller areas transplanted more densely, but the physician's role is to advise how many donor grafts are available and what variations of use are possible. The advent of alopecia reductions has greatly simplified this aspect of planning, because most patients who combine alopecia reductions with punch transplanting can cover all or most of their bald areas with reasonably dense hair. An idea of the numbers of grafts I use to cover given areas can be gleaned from Figs. 4 and 5.

Whenever alopecia reductions are contemplated during the course of treatment, allowance must be made for the effect they will have on the chosen hairline and part line. Ideally, grafts should not be put into areas that could be excised instead. Alopecia reductions are discussed in greater detail below.

Patients should not wear hairpieces for a week after a transplant session and then as little as possible for an additional week. While most practitioners allow patients to wear a hairpiece the day after transplanting, the warmth and moisture beneath it are conducive to infection. Hats should be worn as little as possible postoperatively for the same reason. If they have holes allowing for circulation of air, they can be worn for short intervals. Individuals who work in occupations or have hobbies that expose them to dirt or debris are advised to avoid these circumstances for 1 week postoperatively.

Preoperative Instructions and Anesthesia

Patients are advised to let their hair grow long enough before surgery to allow for adequate camouflage of the donor site postoperatively. In addition, some patients prefer to change their hairstyles, for example, by growing one portion of the hair longer so that they can comb it over the recipient area and camouflage that area as well. They are asked to start erythromycin 250 mg four times a day beginning the night prior to or 2 h before surgery. Antibiotics are discontinued 5 days postoperatively. Aspirin-containing drugs and vitamin E are avoided for 3 weeks before surgery. No alcohol should be consumed for 1 week preoperatively.

We use diazepam 15 mg orally 30 min before surgery for its sedative effect and to minimize lidocaine toxicity. Atropine sulfate 1/150 4 mg intramuscularly preoperatively is used in the very few patients who are prone to syncope. Side effects include dry mouth and eyes (contact lenses should be removed), aggravation of glaucoma, some prostatic disorders, and cardiac effects. This drug is useful in approximately 1 of 500 patients.

Lidocaine with epinephrine 1:100,000 to 1:200,000 is the anesthetic of choice. It acts rapidly in 3 to 5 min and, when used with epinephrine 1:100,000, lasts approximately 2.5 h. A 1% solution is used to produce a field block in the donor area, while a 2% solution is usually used as a field block for the recipient site. The use of a 30-gauge needle and preoperative diazepam minimize the psychological and physical trauma of the anesthetic technique. In addition, I generally inject four or five spots along the proposed line of the field block and wait for those areas to be totally anesthetized before finishing the field block by injecting through the already anesthetized sites. In this manner the patient only feels four to six injections in the donor area and three or four in the recipient site. Superior to the field block in the donor and recipient areas, I use a 1:200,000 solution of epinephrine in saline for its vasoconstrictive effect. A few people, usually of Celtic heritage, tend to require stronger anesthetics, such as 3% or 4% lidocaine or carbon dioxide lidocaine, as supplements to the original injections.[11]

The hazards of an inadvertent intravenous injection of lidocaine can be reduced by keeping one finger anterior to each site of injection so that one can feel the solution traveling interstitially. If lidocaine with epinephrine is accidentally injected intravenously, the patient becomes pale, begins having waves of uncontrollable shaking, feels faint or nauseous, and may have trouble breathing. Such a reaction can be aborted promptly by administering 10 to 20 mg of diazepam intravenously, providing oxygen, placing the patient in a prone position, and raising the patient's legs to a 45-degree angle. Management of other acute complications during local anesthesia is explained elsewhere.[11]

The Donor Site

Donor grafts should be removed from areas that have reasonable prospects of maintaining hair growth for the life of the patient. The scalp should be examined carefully with the hair wet to aid in delineating areas of thinning. An appropriate family history should be taken. If a patient is young, it is wise to leave an extra 2.5 to 5.0 cm beyond areas of thinning as a margin of safety before the most superior line of donor grafts is harvested.

Curved scissors are used to clip the hair to a length of approximately 2 mm in 4- to 5-mm wide lines separated by rows of uncut hairs 2- to 3-mm wide. The clipped rows provide the donor grafts, while those which are uncut are used to camouflage the donor site after the procedure. The area is rubbed with alcohol swabs, and povidone-iodine or chlorhexidine gluconate is applied and left in place to provide continuing antibacterial activity. Anesthesia is carried out as described above. Additional injections of saline are used at various stages of harvesting to keep the tissues taut. In the average patient, between 20 and 40 ml of saline is injected.

The grafts are cut, angling the punch in the same direction as the hair at that site. Two or three rows are harvested, and then an area of intact hair is skipped and another two rows are harvested. After the grafts are removed, the sites are sutured using 2-0 Supramid Extra CL-20 half-circle reverse cutting needles. Routine suturing of donor sites has been almost universally accepted among transplant surgeons. The exact pattern of donor site harvesting that I employ has been described in detail.[12] Six basic donor areas are employed: the temporal, superior occipital, and inferior occipital areas bilaterally. Grafts used in the hairline are specifically taken from similar though contralateral areas of the donor area to produce a uniform density and quality of hair in the hairline.[12] Other operators prefer a two-line donor site which they extend from one temporal area as far posteriorly and around to the contralateral side as is necessary to yield the desired number of grafts. As many sessions consist of 80 to 100 grafts, such two-line patterns may have to extend virtually the entire length of the circumference of the donor site. Both methods have advantages and disadvantages.[13] Figure 6 is a schematic drawing of the general pattern of harvesting I use.

Punches should be razor sharp at all times. In addition, the skin should ideally be kept taut with injections of saline. This allows for a more accurate angling of the punch, as the tissue "gives" less when pressure is applied. Consequently, there is less of a chance of inadvertently cutting or fraying bent hair follicles at the periphery of the grafts. Most 4-mm grafts yield between 8 and 20 intact hair follicles, though some may yield as many as 30.

The total harvesting of a donor area and its subsequent excision and suturing have been recommended as producing superior donor site scars.[14] Unfortunately, this results in an "alopecia reduction in reverse" and therefore should not be used often. If one excises substantial portions of the donor rim, the ultimate result will be a narrowing of that rim and a stretching of any present or future bald area in the vertex, central scalp, or both.

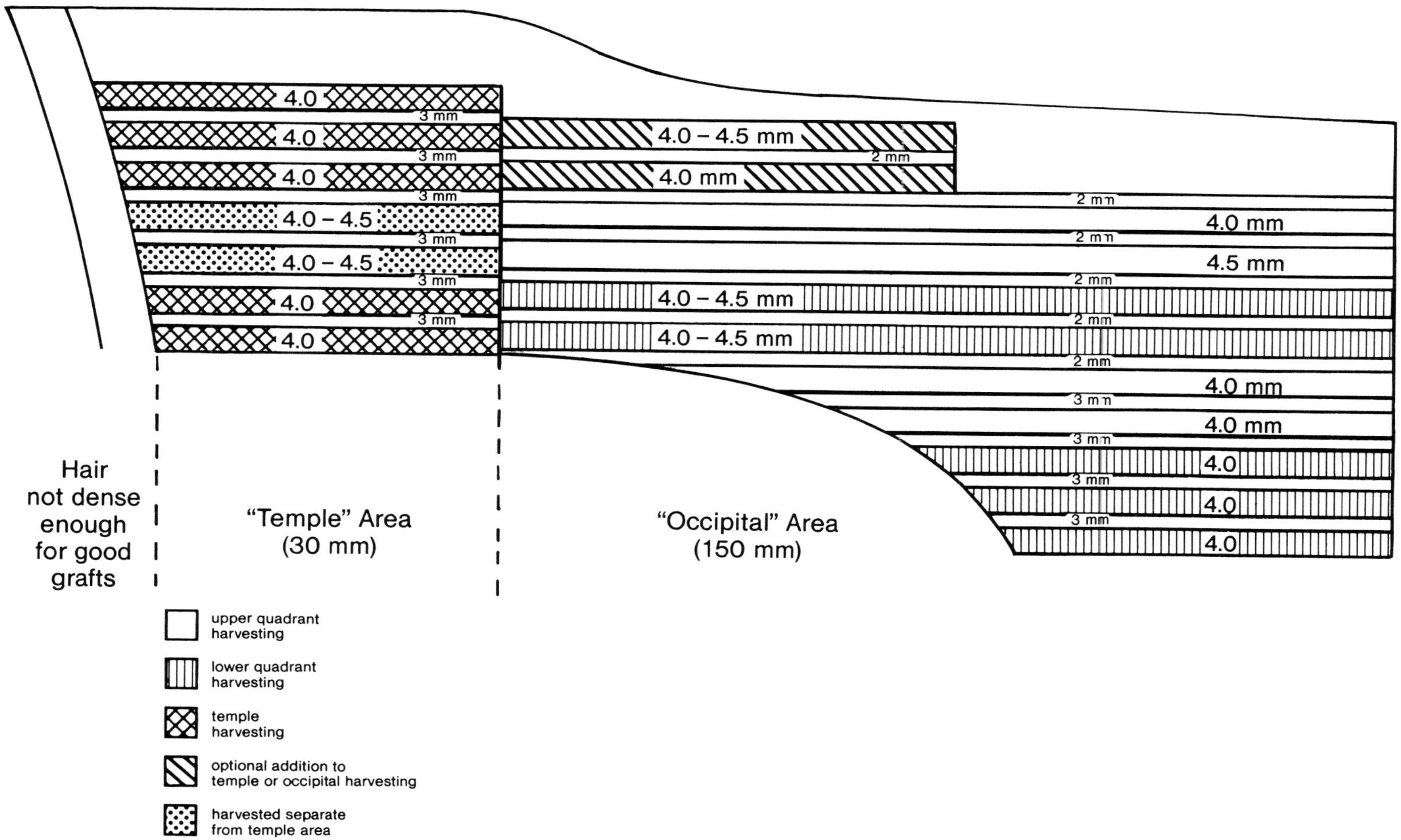

FIGURE 6
Schematic drawing of the harvesting technique employed by the author. Fewer but longer rows may be used in the temporal area or a pair of temporal rows may be harvested at the same time as the occipital area if only 2 rows are harvested where 3 normally would be taken in the inferior occipital area, in order to minimize tension there.

The Recipient Area

As noted above, the pattern I generally use in punch transplanting is U-shaped and four to five rows deep. Grafts placed during the first session start what will ultimately be rows 1, 3, 5, 7, etc., of the recipient area. The second session is carried out 6 weeks after the first, and grafts are placed into what will ultimately be rows 2, 4, 6, 8, etc. (Fig. 7). Recipient sites in the rows treated in this session should satisfy three parameters.

1. They should be exactly one recipient site hole apart from each other, that is, 3.25 to 3.5 mm, depending on which row they are on.
2. They should be off center to the rows anterior to them. That is, they should be neither directly behind the spaces between previously transplanted grafts nor directly behind the grafts.
3. They should touch the previously transplanted grafts in the row anterior as well as the row posterior to them.

The importance of these parameters is discussed elsewhere.[15] For example, because the length of row 2 in any pattern will be slightly shorter than that of row 1 and because spacing in the first session will rarely be absolutely perfect, in order to satisfy these three parameters it is usually necessary to prepare recipient sites in the second row with punches that are 3.25 to 3.5 mm in diameter and to fill such sites with grafts that are either 4 mm or 4.5 mm in diameter, respectively. The distribution of grafts in the first and second sessions apart from their location on alternate lines of the pattern is exactly the same.

FIGURE 7
In the second session, grafts are placed in alternate rows, that is, rows 2, 4, 6, 8, etc. Three parameters must be satisfied: The grafts should be one graft apart on the same row, should be offset, and should touch the grafts in the row just anterior as well as the row just posterior to them. Faint outline of grafts transplanted 6 wks earlier can be seen alternating rows of recipient holes.

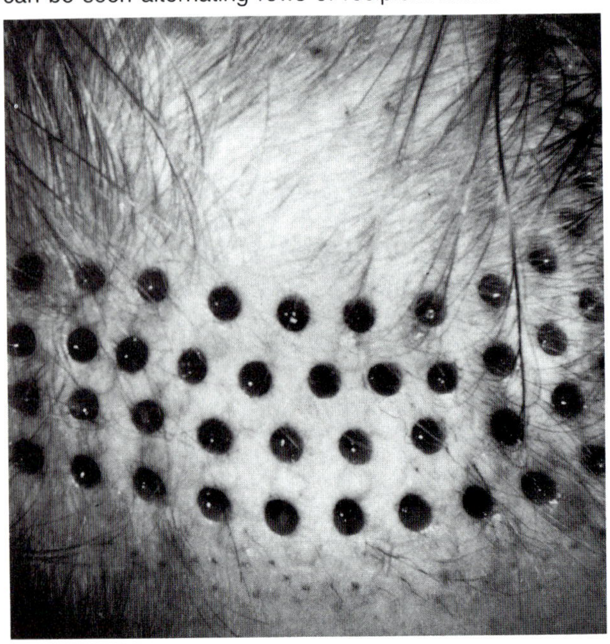

The third session is done approximately 4 months after the second. At this point, all the hair transplanted earlier is growing but hair is not dispersed evenly over the surface of each graft. Bare portions are present on some of the grafts. Waiting 4 months allows one to see these bare sections and overlap them with larger grafts while filling the space between two grafts on the same line. Similarly, there are areas where hair has grown to the edge of adjacent grafts; for example, in the first line where some allowance is made for slight overlapping, the space between these grafts may be smaller than usual, and a smaller graft would be better at that site (Fig. 8). Waiting the 4 months allows for complete filling of any remaining spaces and results in the use of several different sized grafts and a less scalloped-looking hairline.

The distribution of grafts in the recipient area during this session is somewhat different from the simple U used in the first two. Usually, three to four rows are punched out on the part side of the recipient site to just past the midline; on the nonpart side, only the first and most posterior rows are filled, with the odd graft being placed between these two rows on the nonpart side, depending on aesthetic considerations. The rest of the grafts that would have been used on the nonpart side are placed bilaterally more toward the midline. The exception to this general distribution pattern occurs when the hairstyle envisioned for the individual is to be a nonparted one, such as a short, tightly curled hairstyle. In such cases, grafts are distributed evenly bilaterally, often being put into rows, 1, 3, 7, and 9, with row 5 skipped.

The fourth session is done 4 months after the third for the same reasons that the third session is delayed. On this occasion, the distribution of grafts is primarily on the part side in rows 2, 4, and 6 and then wherever needed aesthetically. Very few

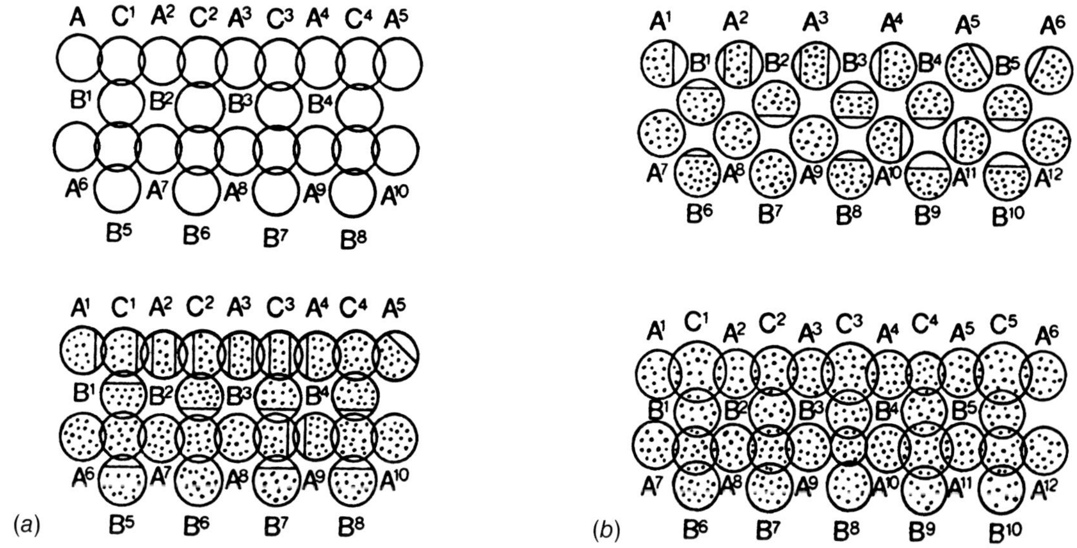

FIGURE 8

(*a*) Dots represent new hair growth. The third session (C) has been done before any hair growth has occurred in the first two sessions (upper section). When hair growth does occur (lower section), gaps can be seen between clumps of hair, as between C^3 and A^4, despite an allowance having been made by slight overlapping of grafts. (*b*) The operator has waited until hair in the first two sessions has grown in (upper section). Hairless portions of preceding grafts are clearly evident, and larger grafts can be used, as between A^1 and A^2, A^3, A^4, A^5, and A^6. When hair growth has extended to the edge of previous grafts because of allowance for slight overlapping, smaller grafts can be used, as between A^4 and A^5, A^9, and A^{10}, and so on. The use of same-sized grafts in these sites would have removed some of the hair previously transplanted.

grafts are placed into the nonpart side during this session; the bulk of them are used more posteriorly in the area started on the third session as well as occasionally in new areas toward the midline. If a short, curly hairstyle is planned, the grafts are distributed symmetrically and only in the few areas where increased hair density is necessary. Whenever grafts are placed toward the midline, room is left for alopecia reductions if their use is anticipated.

I try to angle hair in the recipient area as closely as possible to the original hair direction at that site. There is virtually always some fine hair still present that helps in this regard. Other operators change the angle somewhat to produce more overlapping or a "shingling" effect.[16] While one can debate about which approach is best for operating in an area that has no hair, it is unwise to use the latter one in an area that has hair left. In such circumstances, a physician who changes the angle from its original direction will destroy not only the hair removed from the recipient site plug but also the hairs around the periphery of that hole.

One of the most important advances in punch transplanting is the increasing use of micrografts and minigrafts containing one to several hairs. Small slices of grafts or single hairs are removed from the periphery of larger plugs. They are then inserted into recipient holes made by 16-gauge needles or No. 11 or No. 15 blades, with the cuts made perpendicular to the hairline. These hairs will grow and help blur an otherwise abrupt hairline. Quarter grafts have been described by Bradshaw,[17] and I have described our technique for single hair grafts.[18] After several years of experimenting with these various types of minigrafts, I generally use one to three hair grafts inserted into holes made by 16-gauge needles. Single hair grafts are used wherever more subtle blending is required. In my experience, quarter grafts do not produce nearly as subtle a final effect as do the two other types of minigrafts. Occasionally, however, quarter grafts and bisected (3.75-mm) grafts inserted into stab wounds made with No. 15 blades are used where slitlike hairless gaps remain in the hairline or slightly posterior to hairline grafts (Fig. 9).

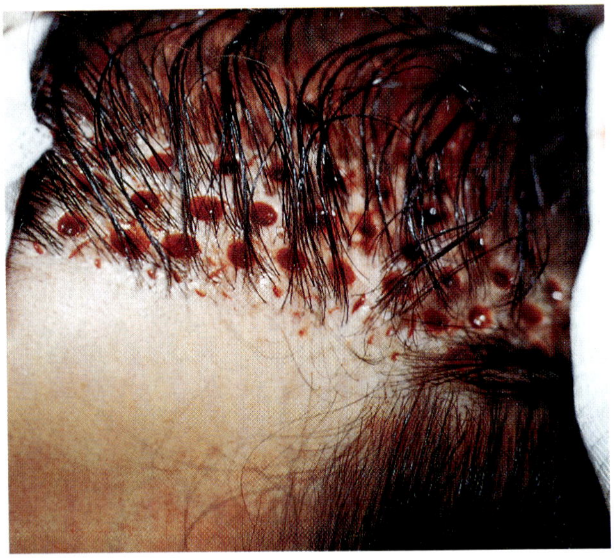

FIGURE 9
Close-up of hairline showing recipient sites made for regular grafts, micrografts, and slit incisions for quarter grafts and bisected grafts in small spaces between previously transplanted grafts.

Cleaning and Insertion of Grafts

Once the grafts have been removed from the donor area, they are placed in a dish containing a 4-in by 4-in gauze and normal saline. It is imperative that the grafts not dry out. Excess amounts of subcutaneous tissue as well as spicules of hair and hair follicles without matrices are removed carefully, using small sharp scissors and fine jeweler's forceps. The grafts are then lined up in rows in a similar dish, with the best grafts placed in the top row and the lesser ones placed in progressively lower rows. When planting is done in the recipient area, the best grafts are used in the cosmetically most important areas, and organizing them into quality rows beforehand facilitates the process. They are inserted into the recipient holes with nontoothed forceps and, as noted above, are oriented in the original hair directions. The grafts should sit flush with the scalp if they have been trimmed properly and if holes have been made deeply enough with an appropriate size recipient site punch. A standard turbanlike bandage is applied overnight. The bandage is used more to keep the grafts oriented properly and to absorb the small amount of bleeding that may occur postoperatively than to actually stop bleeding with pressure.

The morning after the operation, the bandage is removed and the area is cleansed of blood and clots with hydrogen peroxide. The hair is combed to camouflage both recipient and donor sites.[19] Patients are advised that they may begin washing their hair 2 to 3 days postoperatively. They are asked not to do any heavy exercise or anything that will cause sweating and to avoid exposure to air that may contain dirt or debris for 1 week.

The use of alkyl-2 cyanoacrylate adhesives to "glue" the grafts in place has been advocated as a way to avoid overnight bandaging.[20] Unfortunately, the glue tends to mat the surrounding hair and fixes the crusts in place, significantly delaying their shedding. Suturing of grafts in the recipient site is also not employed.[12]

For the past 5 years we have been applying a solution of 2% minoxidil in an alcohol base just after the recipient area is cleansed. In addition, patients are asked to continue twice-daily application of this solution for 5 weeks. However, patients should discontinue minoxidil 2 weeks before surgery. Most patients, though not all, note a later effluvium of hair from the transplanted grafts as well as more rapid regrowth of hair than occurred before the minoxidil solution was used. In some patients, some of the hair does not fall out of all or some of the grafts that have been transplanted. We have not used higher concentrations of minoxidil in an effort to stop effluvium entirely because of concern over the effect of the absorption of minoxidil through the incisions.

Intramuscular betamethasone sodium phosphate and betamethasone acetate 12 mg and/or a 1-week course of prednisone (30, 25, 20, 15, 10, 10, and 5 mg) are offered to patients after the first session and to patients who are anxious about postoperative edema because of previous unacceptable reactions. The usual contraindications to corticosteroid use are respected.

Postoperative Complications

Postoperative complications have been covered in detail previously.[21,22] Potential complications include mild pruritus, temporary edema, temporary discoloration, graft elevations, temporary to permanent loss of some sensation, hematomas, hypertrophic scarring, and arteriovenous fistulas. More serious complications include keloids, skin infection, osteomyelitis (one case), postoperative bleed-

ing, and poor hair growth or cosmetic effect. To put matters in perspective, all these complications are uncommon to rare when the procedure is carried out with care and skill.

ALOPECIA REDUCTION

Scalp reduction or *alopecia reduction* (AR) may be defined as the excision of an area of bald or balding scalp. The more lax the scalp and/or the more extensive the undermining, the larger the area the surgeon can excise. The resultant smaller area of alopecia can be transplanted with fewer of the limited supply of grafts that any given individual has or, alternatively, can be transplanted more densely. Other uses of AR are as follows:

To elevate the superior border of the lateral fringe of hair so that if one parts the hair through the superior part of this lateral fringe, it will be at a cosmetically appropriate level[23]

To eliminate a thinning crown in a younger patient to temporarily forestall the need for transplanting

To allow for full coverage of an extensively bald area that previously could not be covered by transplanting alone

Many patterns of AR are available (Fig. 10). The type of reduction used should be tailored to the

FIGURE 10

Basic patterns of alopecia reduction. (*a*) U-shaped AR. (*b*) Crescent-shaped AR. (*c*) Midline ellipse-shaped AR (with or without an additional transverse elliptical component). The midline ellipse is the simplest, fastest, safest, and therefore most popular pattern employed by AR surgeons. (*d*) Inverted-Y shaped AR is our favourite single pattern. It distorts hair direction in the vertex fringe the least and avoids a midline scar which would be visible if the vertex is not transplanted. (*e*) T-shaped AR is used virtually exclusively for vertex alopecia. (*f*) I-shaped advancement flap AR, for the most part replaced by serial mini-AR now.

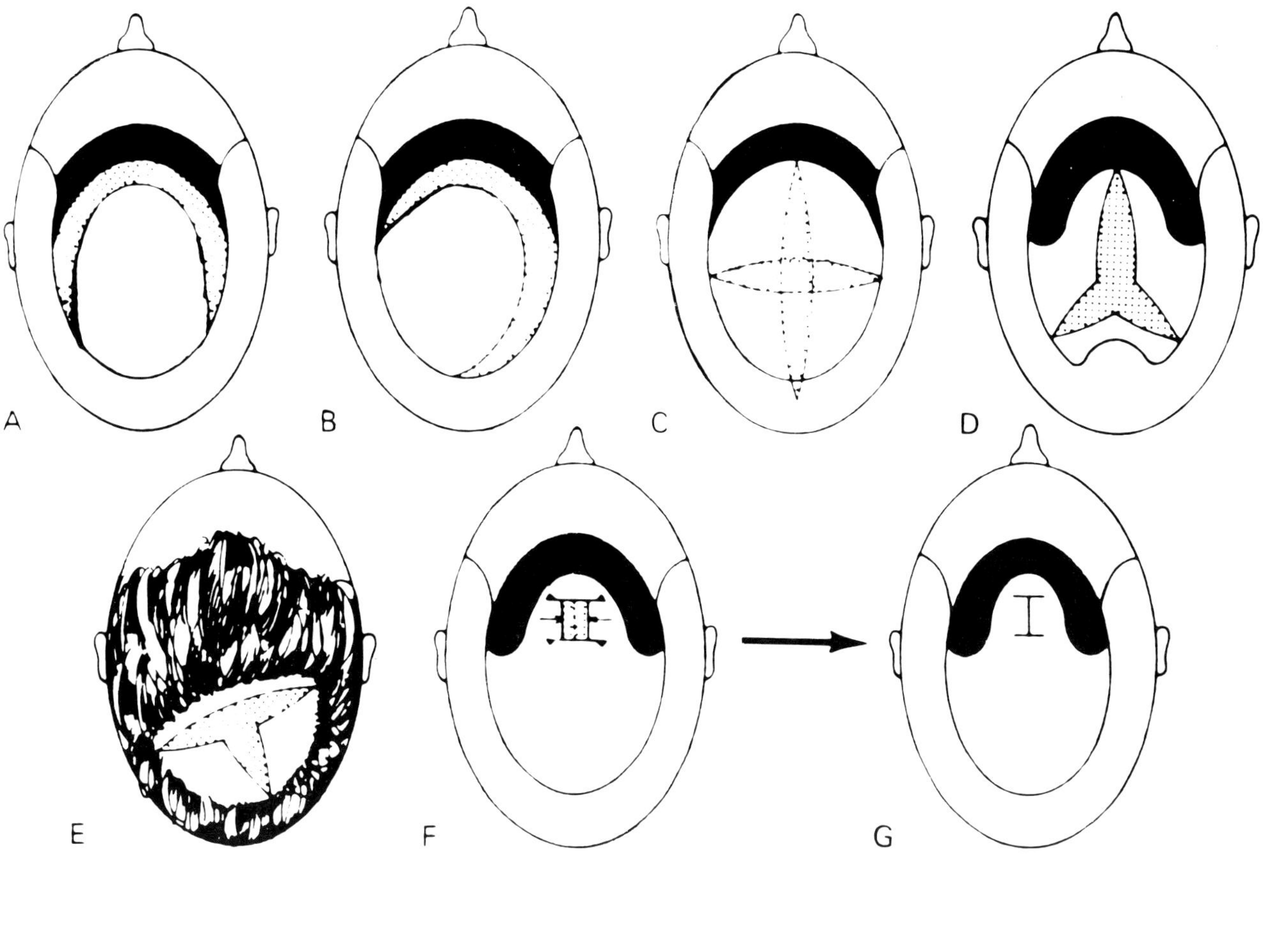

specific needs of the patient. Small or moderate-size areas of alopecia can often be excised virtually completely in one to three standard ARs spread approximately 8 to 12 weeks apart. (It is unwise to completely excise the bald site as it distorts the adjacent hair direction.) Complications have been minimal.

In most individuals, the first AR will follow the first or second punch transplanting session. An interval of 3 weeks or more is recommended between AR and punch transplant sessions. However, a midline pattern of AR can be done as close as 2 days to any punch transplanting session, as this pattern does not impair blood supply to the grafts. With large bald areas, one or two ARs may be done before punch transplantation to minimize the change such ARs may cause in the shape of a previously transplanted hairline. The pros and cons of AR before and during hair transplantation and between transplanting sessions have been discussed in detail.[23,24]

Originally, six basic patterns of alopecia reduction were described as examples of the many possible variations.[25] Other variations include the saggital midline ellipse incorporated in the original "star pattern," and the lateral crescent shape described by Alt.[26] More recently, Marzola[27] described a pattern that consists of an incision near the anterior margin of the temple hair extending posteriorly inferior to the superior border of the lateral fringe of permanent hair. Brandy[28] has done a Marzola type of reduction bilaterally in one operation instead of two. This procedure, while more effective in reducing the area of alopecia, also increases the possibility of serious complications.[29]

Surgical Technique

The surgery is performed by most physicians on an outpatient basis. Oral diazepam 15 mg is given 30 min before surgery, or 10 mg of diazepam is administered intravenously immediately before surgery. Meperidine hydrochloride 50 mg can be given intramuscularly 30 min before the operation at the physician's option. The patient is photographed, and the pattern of AR is marked on the scalp with a micropoint supermarker.

General anesthesia is used only for individuals who are unable to tolerate the procedure psychologically while awake or are unusually difficult to anesthetize with local anesthetics. Such patients constitute only a small minority.

The anesthetic of choice is 2% lidocaine with epinephrine 1:100,000, which is used to produce a field block by injecting circumferentially around the head inferior to the expected extent of undermining. Local anesthesia with epinephrine is also instilled along the lines of the proposed incision to achieve hemostasis.

Sterile surgical conditions are employed, and the patient is usually placed in a prone position with a prone pillow or bulky pillow underneath the chin. If general anesthesia is given, the patient is usually placed on the side.

The surgical area is cleansed with a chlorhexidine solution (Hibitane), and sterile drapes are applied. With most patterns (the Y and T patterns excepted), one begins by incising along the entire length of the proposed exision, down to and through the galea aponeurotica. The scalpel blade should be angled in the direction of adjacent hair follicles to avoid injuring them. A 2-mm margin of safety should be left between the incision and previously transplanted grafts. Surgical skin hooks are used to separate the wound edges, and curved Mayo scissors facilitate undermining in the loose connective tissue between the periosteum and the galea aponeurotica for at least 10 cm bilaterally. This dissection is relatively bloodless except in the vertex area, where two or more perforators may be encountered. Any transected blood vessels are cauterized.

The amount of redundant scalp tissue that can be excised can be determined in two ways. One can overlap the tissues by placing the portion of the flap to be removed on top of the other flap. Then a series of perpendicular incisions are made through the superior flap, stopping at the point where the tissues will meet. The perpendicular cuts are joined by incising along a line joining the most lateral extent of the perpendicular cuts, effectively removing redundant tissue. For more experienced physicians, a skin hook is attached to the galea, and one flap is pulled on top of the other. The staining of blood on the underlying flap can be used as a marker to show how much tissue can be removed. Hemostasis is effected with cauterization.

With Y and T patterns, the technique is somewhat similar. The physician incises along one side of the midline component of the area to be excised. Skin hooks are used, and extensive undermining is carried out. A second incision is made at the anterior margin of the lateral component on the same side, and additional undermining is done. The amount of redundant skin tissue is determined along the midline and lateral components on the same side. After blood on the underlying flap is used as a marker, redundant tissue is removed and hemostasis is achieved with cauterization. An incision is made along one side of the remaining lateral component, and further undermining is carried out before the redundant tissue is similarly excised.

Alopecia reductions should always be closed in two layers. The galea aponeurotica is sutured with 2-0 Dexon or Vicryl interrupted sutures placed approximately 1.5 cm apart. With Y and T patterns, the lateral components are usually closed prior to the midline component. The most medial suture of each lateral component is placed very close to the junction where the three flaps meet, while the most posterior suture of the vertical component is 0.5 cm from this junction.

The skin is closed using a running 4-0 chromic catgut suture. In patterns where three flaps meet at the junction, a single interrupted corner suture is used first, and then each component is closed with a separate running suture.

Three or four layers of gauze are placed over the area treated, and a piece of six-inch stockinette is modified to form a cap to hold the gauze in place. The patient removes this dressing the following morning and may comb any hair present over the incision in order to camouflage it. The hair may be washed 3 days postoperatively.

It is always best to excise slightly less tissue than to produce too much tension at the suture line. Interrupted sutures are preferable to running sutures, and the more extensive the undermining at the time of surgery, the better.

Galeotomies are not routinely used but may be employed if one has been slightly too aggressive in estimating the amount of tissue that can be safely excised so that there would be undue tension at the suture line if galeotomies were not carried out. In addition, galeotomies may be used to maximize raising of the hairline on the part side more superiorly.[30]

The more tension utilized in closure of the galea and skin, the greater any subsequent stretchback will be. Nordström[31] reported up to 50 percent stretchback occurring postoperatively. This is considerably in excess of what we have encountered using a policy of removing only redundant scalp tissue and thus minimizing tension at closure.

ARs may be repeated every 3 to 8 weeks. Our preference is for 8 weeks as the minimum interval. While AR can be carried out at the same time punch grafting is done, the additional trauma, time, and local anesthetic make this impractical in most instances unless these are minireductions (see below).

A Shaw knife ("hot" knife) or a CO_2 laser may be used for scalp reductions and will considerably shorten the operating time. The use of these instruments in such surgery will probably increase significantly over the next several years.

Minireductions

Minireductions are small, usually midline ARs carried out during punch transplanting sessions. In most cases, a hand or power punch is used to excise a line or small ellipse composed of punched-out holes. The defects are sutured closed instead of being filled with punch grafts. Such small reductions can be carried out with minimal tension on the suture line in a very short time. Over a period of four or five operations it is not unusual to save 100 or more grafts with this technique.[32] It is also particularly useful in repair cases where one is running out of available grafts.

Major Reductions

At the other end of the scale from minireductions are the *major alopecia reductions* first proposed by Marzola[33] and then elaborated upon by Brandy.[34,35] In these procedures, virtually the entire hair-bearing portion of the scalp is undermined after an incision is made just posterior to the anterior hairline of the temple region and extended just inferior to the superior border of the lateral fringe, traversing the contralateral side in a similar fashion. During the undermining, the anterior branch of the superficial temporal artery and veins, the occipital arteries and veins, and the posterior auricular arteries and veins are divided. In addition, the greater occipital nerve and the third occipital nerve are cut; on occasion, the mastoid emissary vein is also severed.

The result of such massive underminings are ARs of impressive size. As one would expect from such extensive undermining and damage of the arterial and venous circulation, the potential for postoperative complications is much higher than that seen with regular ARs. Significant complications include necrosis, wound dehiscence, and sensory nerve deficits. In the opinion of most physicians, this added potential danger is rarely

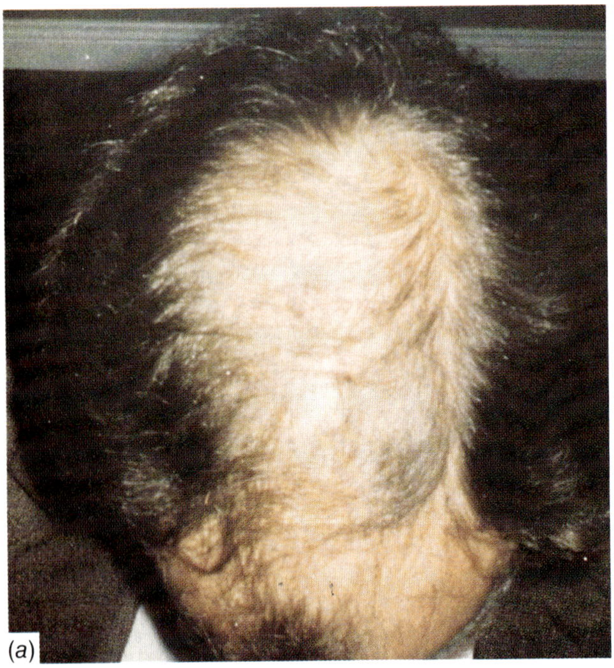

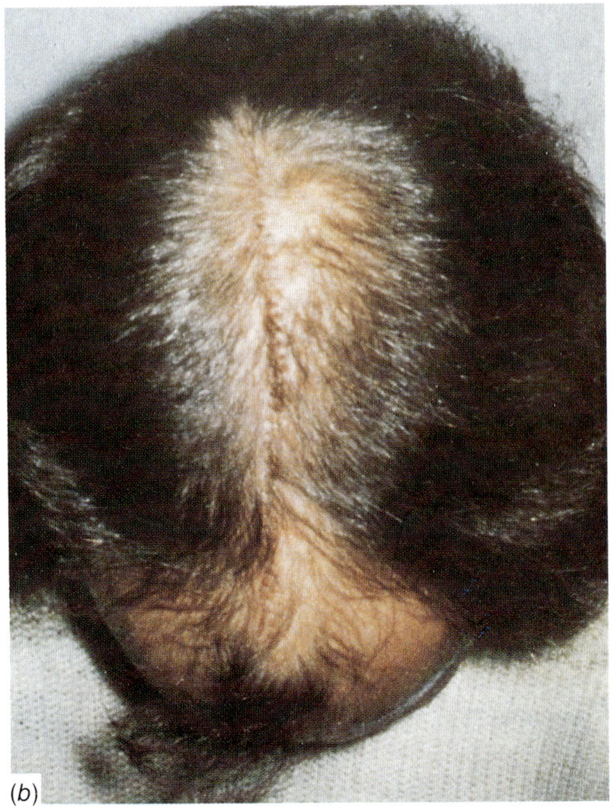

FIGURE 11
(*a*) Preoperative view of an area of alopecia. (*b*) Postoperative result of a modified major reduction utilizing a sagittal midline elliptical pattern. (*Photos courtesy of Martin Unger, M.D.*)

warranted (W. Bradshaw, personal communication). A compromise modified major reduction has been described by Unger and basically consists of a more routine type of AR, but with very extensive undermining which stops short of severing the major blood vessels to the scalp.[36] While it takes two modified major ARs to accomplish the same results as those achieved with a major AR, the added margin of safety makes the modified procedure worthwhile (Fig. 11).

Tissue Expanders

The concept of tissue expansion before the excision of a portion of skin was formulated by Radovan.[37] Initially, tissue expanders were used for the expansion of chest tissue as part of postmastectomy reconstruction.[37] They are now applied to scalp surgery, most frequently to remove large areas of cicatricial alopecia or posttraumatic defects.[38,39] While this method can be used in the treatment of male pattern baldness, in most cases the patient will not tolerate the temporary cosmetic disability that is necessary.

SCALP FLAPS

A variety of *scalp flaps* have been used for male pattern baldness (MPB).[40] The most common type of transposition scalp flap consists of a flap inferior to but running parallel to the permanent fringe of hair on the side of the scalp. It is designed to have a base approximately 3 cm wide. As the flap moves posteriorly within the permanent hair-bearing rim, it is tapered to approximately 2.25 cm in width and usually is 12 to 15 cm long (Fig. 12).

The advantage of such flaps is immediate hair growth with excellent hair density. The disadvantages include hair being directed posteriorly instead of in the normal anterior direction and an abrupt, dense hairline. Partial loss of the rotated flap and poor healing in the donor area are other potential drawbacks.

Technique

The procedure begins with locating the superficial temporal artery by palpation or a Doppler flowmeter and marking its course. The pedicle should be designed so that the vessel enters the center of its base. The flap should be approximately 4 cm wide and long enough to completely traverse the area of alopecia. The flap begins in the temporal area and runs through the parietal zone before moving inferiorly into the occipital region. It does not cross the midline. Its length can be varied by designing it with greater or lesser curvature of the flap. "Dog ears" can be minimized by beginning it as superiorly as possible on the parietal scalp. One should also try to anticipate the eventual superior border of the permanent hair rim in order to keep the superior border of the flap inferior to that level.

Two delays are normally employed. For the first surgery, patients are told to let the hair grow a little longer than usual to help camouflage the surgery postoperatively. The flap is designed, and the hair is clipped short along the proposed borders. The hair within the flap can be braided and/or taped out of the way. Lidocaine 1% with epinephrine 1:100,000 is injected along the proposed incision lines. Incisions are made, cutting parallel to the hair shafts and without raising the bed. These lines are subsequently closed with a running 3-0 nylon or prolene suture. This procedure can be carried out in the physician's office with or without the use of diazepam preoperatively.

The posterior 6 cm of flap is incised and elevated 1 week after the first session. Occipital vessels are cauterized or ligated, and the incision lines are sutured as noted above. These two delays help establish an autonomous vascular supply to the flap.

The entire flap is raised and transposed to the recipient site 1 week after the second delay. A beveled incision is made along the proposed hairline, and the anterior scalp is undermined. Beveling of the incision results in hair growing through the anterior border scar of the flap. The donor area is then closed, and the amount of glabrous skin that must be removed to allow easy placement of the flap is excised. Extensive undermining of both the recipient area and the retroauricular area should result in closure with minimal tension on the suture lines. Closure is carried out on two levels: aponeurosis and skin. For the galea aponeurotica, 3-0 interrupted buried Dexon sutures are used and 5-0 interrupted nylon sutures or prolene sutures are used for the skin. Suturing is started from the proximal end of the defect.

The entire procedure is carried out under general

FIGURE 12

(*a*) Closure of the donor area following undermining. (*b*) Resection of the glabrous frontal zone. (*c*) Placing and suturing of the flap. (*Reprinted with permission of Marcel Dekker, Inc., New York.*)

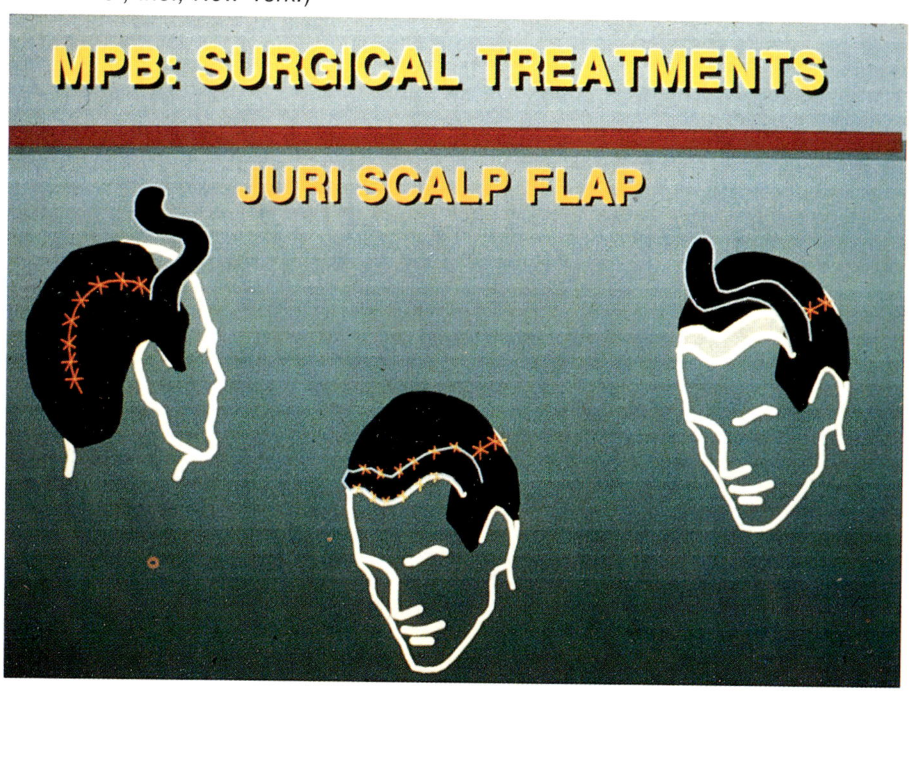

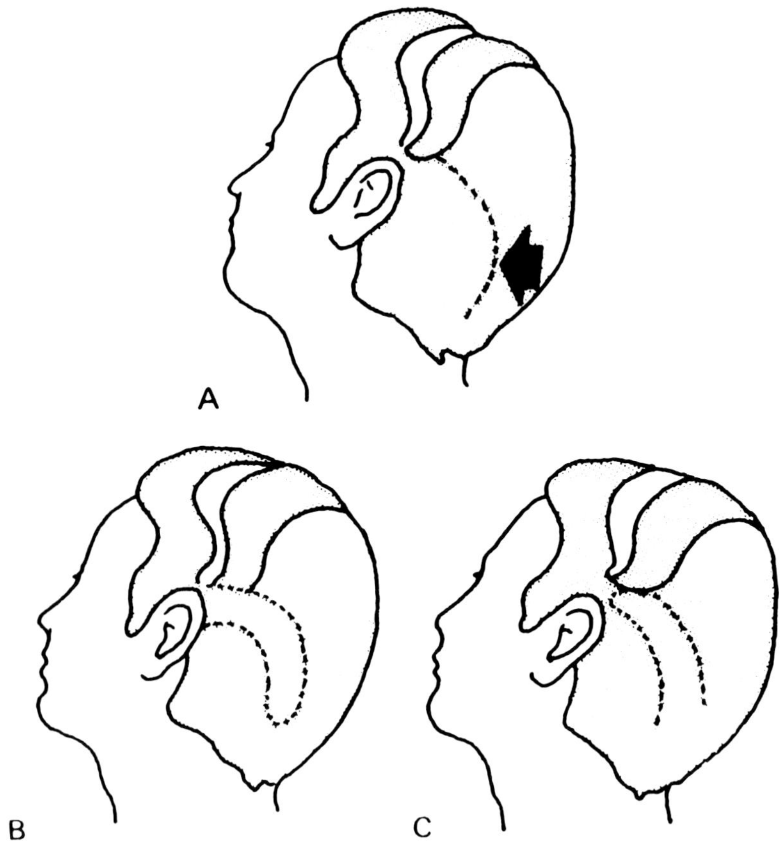

FIGURE 13
(*a*) Two flaps have been rotated for temporoparietal baldness. The residual donor scar on one side is seen (arrow). (*b*) The design of a third flap with a retroauricular pedicle. (*c*) The design of a third flap with an occipital pedicle. (*Reprinted with permission of Juri J: Use of rotation scalp grafts for treatment of occipital baldness. Plast Reconstr Surg. 1978; 61:23–26.*)

anesthesia, but lidocaine 1% with adrenaline 1:000,000 is used along the lines of incision to minimize bleeding. A second flap from the contralateral side of the scalp may be carried out 1 month later (Fig. 13). It is placed posteriorly to the first one and may be adjacent to the first flap or 3 cm or more posterior to it. In the latter case, the hairless gap may be excised several months later.

REFERENCES

1. Unger WP, Nordström RE. Hair Transplantation 2d ed. New York: Marcel Dekker: 1988.
2. Norwood OT, Shiell RC. Hair Transplant Surgery 2d ed. Springfield, IL: Charles C Thomas: 1984.
3. Orentreich N, Orentreich D. J Dermatol Surg Oncol. 1985; 10:970–971.
4. Unger WP. A study of some innovations in hair transplanting. J Dermatol Surg Oncol. 1977;3:536–538.
5. Unger WP, Nordström RE. Hair Transplantation 2d ed. New York: Marcel Dekker, 1988: Appendix E.
6. Unger WP. Punch transplantation in "early" androgenetic alopecia. J Dermatol Surg Oncol. 1988;10:12.
7. Unger WP, Nordström RE. Hair Transplantation 2d ed. New York: Marcel Dekker, 1988:285–295.
8. Ibid:295–300.
9. Unger WP. Hair replacement surgery in the black male and female, in Pierce HE (ed) Plastic Surgery in Non-White Patients. New York: Grune & Stratton, 1982:51–69.
10. Unger WP, Nordström RE. Hair Transplantation 2d ed. New York: Marcel Dekker, 1988:105–128.

11. Ibid:133–144.
12. Unger WP. A new method of donor site harvesting. J Dermatol Surg Oncol. 1984;10:7.
13. Unger WP, Nordström RE. Hair Transplantation 2d ed. New York: Marcel Dekker, 1988:145–210.
14. Hill TG. Closure of the donor site in hair transplantation by a cluster technique. J Dermatol Surg Oncol. 1980;6:190–191.
15. Unger WP. Punch hair transplantation. Dermatol Clin. 1984,2:303 317.
16. Stegman S, Tromovich T. Cosmetic Dermatologic Surgery. Chicago: Year Book, 1984:87–92.
17. Bradshaw W. Quarter-grafts: A technique for minigrafts, in Unger WP, Nordström RE. Hair Transplantation 2d ed. New York: Marcel Dekker, 1988:333–351.
18. Unger WP, Nordström RE. Hair Transplantation 2d ed. New York: Marcel Dekker, 1988:284–285.
19. Ibid:375–380.
20. Wilkinson TS, et al. Tissue adhesives and an adjunct in hair transplantation. South Med J. 1974;67:1408–1410.
21. Tromovich T, Stegman S, Glogau R. Sequelea and complications of hair transplantation, in Unger WP, Nordström RE. Hair Transplantation 2d ed. New York: Marcel Dekker, 1988:399–408.
22. Unger WP. Hair Transplantation. New York: Marcel Dekker, 1979:131–136.
23. Unger WP, Marritt E. General principles of recipient site organization and planning, in Unger WP, Nordström RE. Hair Transplantation 2d ed. New York: Marcel Dekker, 1988:105–128.
24. Unger WP, Unger MG. In Epstein E (ed), Alopecia Reduction in Skin Surgery 5th ed. Springfield. IL: Charles C Thomas, 1982:530–545.
25. Unger MG, Unger WP. Management of alopecia of the scalp by a combination of excisions and transplantations. J Dermatol Surg Oncol. 1978;4:9.
26. Alt TH. Scalp reduction as an adjunct to hair transplantation: Review of relevant literature, presentation of an improved technique. J Dermatol Surg Oncol. 1980;6:1011–1018.
27. Marzola M. An alternative hair replacement method, in Norwood OT (ed) Hair Transplant Surgery 2d ed. Springfield, IL: Charles C Thomas, 1984:315–324.
28. Brandy DA. The bilateral occipito-parietal flap. J Dermatol Surg Oncol. 1986;12:1062–1066.
29. Unger MG. Counterpoint: The risk of the bilateral lateral scalp reduction. J Dermatol Surg Oncol. 1988;14:353–354.
30. Unger MG. Alopecia reduction, in Unger WP, Nordström RE. Hair Transplantation 2d ed. New York: Marcel Dekker, 1988:435–518
31. Nordström RE. Stretchback in scalp reductions for male pattern baldness. Plast Reconstr Surg. 1984;73:422–426.
32. Unger WP. Concomitant mini-reductions in punch hair transplanting. J Dermatol Surg Oncol. 1983;9:388–392.
33. Marzola M. The Marzola scalp reduction. Presented at the Fifth National Symposium on Hair Replacement Surgery, Miami, FL, 1983.
34. Brandy DA. The Brandy bitemporal flap. Cosmetic Surg. 1986;3:11–15.
35. Brandy DA. A six-step approach for the treatment of extensive baldness. J Dermatol Surg Oncol. 1987;13:519–525.
36. Unger MG. The modified major scalp reduction. J Dermatol Surg Oncol. 1988;14:80–84.
37. Radovan CG. Adjacent flap development using expandable silastic implant. American Society of Plastic and Reconstructive Surgery Forum, Boston, Sept. 30, 1976.
38. Argenta L, Anderson R. Tissue expansion, in Unger WP, Nordström RE. Hair Transplantation 2d ed. New York: Marcel Dekker, 1988:519–551.
39. Nordström RE. The Nordström system, in Unger WP, Nordström RE. Hair Transplantation 2d ed. New York: Marcel Dekker, 1988:551–560.
40. Kabaker S. Lateral scalp flaps in surgery for male pattern baldness, in Unger WP, Nordström RE. Hair Transplantation 2d ed. New York: Marcel Dekker, 1988:621–634.
41. Fleming R, Mayer T. Punch grafts versus flaps: A role for each, in Unger WP, Nordström RE. Hair Transplantation 2d ed. New York: Marcel Dekker, 1988:603–620.
42. Ohmori K. Hair transplantation with microsurgical free flaps. J Dermatol Surg Oncol. 1984;10:974–978.

CHAPTER

24

Nails: Cosmetic Details

SUSAN C. TAYLOR
RICHARD K. SCHER

The physical appearance of the nail is universally important to both men and women. In oriental societies where the nail was a reflection of social and economic status, nail guards were applied over the nail and the distal aspect of the finger for protection from breakage. In our society attractive nails may impart a sense of well-being and confidence to members of both sexes. For men, well-groomed and trimmed nails are indicative of good personal hygiene and provide a meticulous appearance. Long, skillfully manicured nails are a reflection of beauty for many women.

The nail unit also serves a structural and functional role. Nails provide a protective covering for the fingertips, augment the sensation of fine touch, and assist in manual dexterity. The ability to scratch is utilized for physical defense and the relief of itching. The importance of these functions is often overshadowed by the quest for a cosmetically attractive nail. This chapter reviews the currently available cosmetic nail preparations, the purposes for which they are used, adverse reactions to them, and their application to improve the appearance of abnormal nails.

A wide range of cosmetics, accessories, and instruments are used to enhance the appearance of structurally normal nails and to camouflage defects in diseased nails. Several categories of cosmetic preparations for nails exist. Manicuring implements are durable mechanical aids that are used to alter the nail plate or cuticle. They include the nail file, emery board, orangewood stick, cuticle nippers and scissors, cuticle pusher, nail brush, and nail buffer. Nail accessories consist of gems and decorative metal jewelry which are affixed to the nail plate. Appliqués may be attached to the nail to produce elaborate designs and patterns.

Cosmetic products applied to the nail are quite varied. Nail enamels, top coats, and base coats are the most commonly used cosmetic nail preparations. Nail hardeners as well as conditioners and silk and paper nail wrappings are said to protect and promote the growth of nails. Artificial nails and sculptured nails, which are applied over the natural nail, may be used to conceal broken nails and improve the appearance of short or deformed nails.

Adverse reactions and damage to the nail may occur as a result of the use of nail preparations and implements. The reactions may involve the nail unit and periungual area or other sites that come into contact with the nail. They range from irritant or allergic eczematous reactions to paronychia, nail discoloration, and onycholysis. Hence, preparations or implements that are thought to improve the appearance of the nails may result in damage to previously cosmetically acceptable nails.

NAIL IMPLEMENTS

Mechanical aids for the nails are divided into those that are used to shape, file, clean, or shine the nail plate and those that adjust or trim the cuticle. The following implements are commonly used by manicurists.

Nail files are long, thin, flexible steel instruments used to shape and smooth the free edge of the nail plate. *Emery boards* file the nail plate down and shape the free edge with the coarse side and bevel the surface with the fine side (Fig. 1). *Nail brushes* cleanse the nail and fingertips with the aid of a soap and water solution. *Nail buffers* polish and buff the surface of the nail plate (Fig. 2). *Orangewood sticks* loosen the cuticle and are used for applying substances to the nail and cuticle. *Cuticle pushers* loosen the cuticle and push it back from the nail plate (Fig. 3). *Cuticle nippers* or *scissors* trim the cuticle (Fig. 4).

FIGURE 1
Application of an emery board to shape the nail plate.

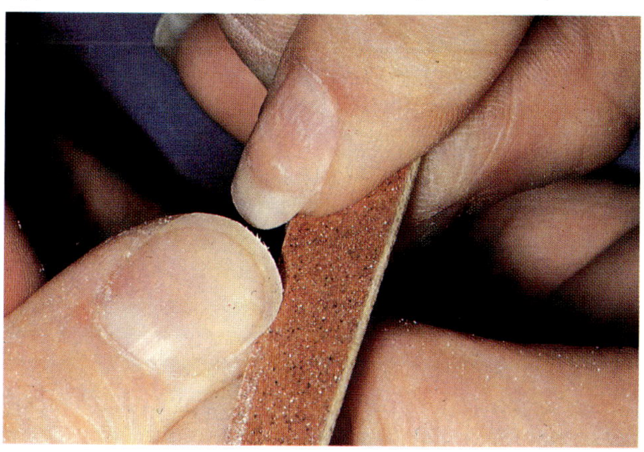

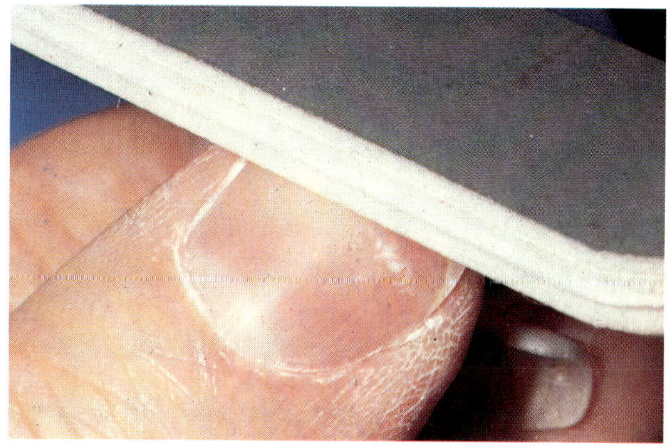

FIGURE 2
A nail buffer used to polish and shine the surface of the nail plate.

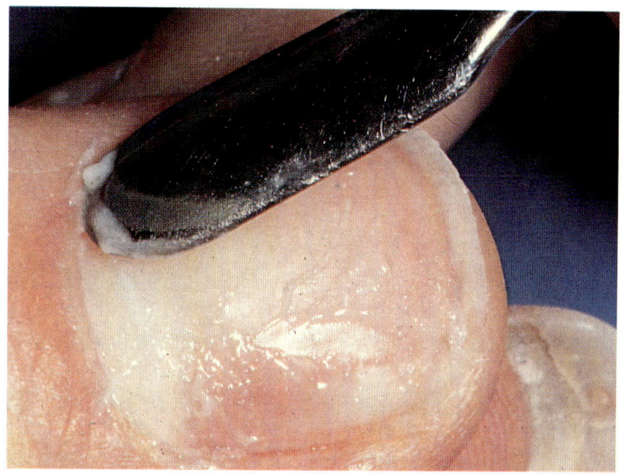

FIGURE 3
A cuticle pusher used to loosen the cuticle and push it back from the nail plate.

FIGURE 4
Cuticle nippers clipping the cuticle.

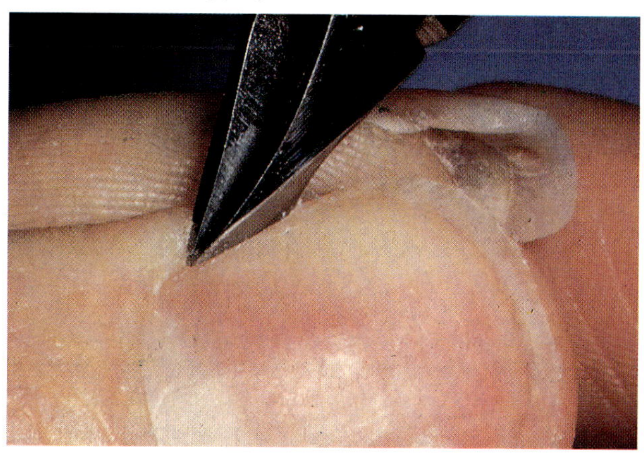

Overzealous use of nail files, emery boards, orangewood sticks, or cuticle pushers or excessive manipulation of the cuticular area may result in injury to the nail matrix or cuticle. Paronychia, longitudinal or transverse furrows, and leukonychia may occur.[1]

NAIL ACCESSORIES

Jewelry of various types is used to adorn the nail. Gold, silver, and other metals as well as gemstones ranging from rhinestones to diamonds are affixed to the nail plate. The jewelry may be glued onto the nail surface. If the jewel is mounted on a post, a hole is drilled into the distal nail plate and the post is placed through the opening much as a pierced earring is placed through the earlobe (Fig. 5).

Appliqués in a wide range of designs or patterns may be glued onto the nail plate to enhance the appearance of the nail. Alternatively, designs may be hand painted onto the surface of the nail with an acrylic water paint.

COSMETIC PREPARATIONS

Nail enamels, top coats, and base coats are composed of varying amounts of five basic components. *Nail enamel* is used to color or gloss the nail plate. The enamel may produce discoloration of the nail plate which is not eradicated with enamel remover.[2] The *base coat,* which is colorless, is applied before the nail enamel to a clean nail surface. The base coat enhances the adherence of the nail enamel to the nail surface and forms a protective layer over the nail plate to prevent the color in the nail polish from staining the nail. It also prevents chipping, cracking, and peeling of the enamel. The *top coat,* which is applied over the nail enamel, protects the enamel, provides gloss and sheen, prevents chipping, and prolongs the wearing time of the enamel.

FIGURE 5
Posterior aspect of the nail showing jewelry mounted through the nail plate.

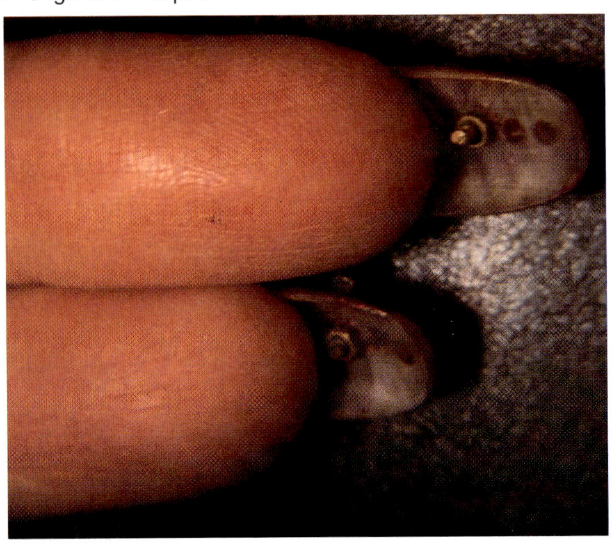

The five components of the enamel, base coat, and top coat include a nitrocellulose film former, a toluene sulfonamide formaldehyde resin, a plasticizer, a volatile solvent, and a pigment colorizer (Table 1).[3,4] The base coat has increased amounts of resin, and the top coat has increased amounts of nitrocellulose film formers and plasticizers. Among these components, the most common sensitizer is the toluene sulfonamide formaldehyde resin. Dermatitis may develop on the eyelids and about the face and neck. Allergic contact sensitization occurs while the resin is in a liquid state. Patients who are allergic to the resin may safely wear the enamel since the solid resin is nonsensitizing. Care must be taken while applying the liquid to the nail in these patients to prevent contact with distant sites or the periungual area. An alternative for allergic individuals is the use of a hypoallergenic alkyl polyester; however, these products contain resins which are less durable than the toluene sulfonamide formaldehyde resin.[3,5] The solvent extenders are nonsensitizers, but they may produce local irritation as a result of their dehydrating properties.

Nail hardeners are composed of polyesters, acrylics, and polyamides. They serve to strengthen fragile or very flexible nail plates.[4] Those that contain free formaldehyde, even in the low 1 to 2% concentration permitted by the U.S. Food and Drug Administration, may cause allergic eczematous contact dermatitis as well as onycholysis.

Nail conditioners contain proteins and lipids which form an oil in water emulsion. They retard dehydration of the nail plate in brittle nails and fill in imperfections on the nail plate surface.

Buffing creams consist of waxes and pumice. They smooth and enhance the luster of the natural nail. Buffing creams are usually nonsensitizing.[11]

Preformed plastic nails are composed of small pieces of plastic in the shape of the nail or nail tip which are glued on top of the natural nail (Fig. 6).

TABLE 1
CONSTITUENTS OF NAIL ENAMEL, TOP COATS, AND BASECOATS

Ingredient	Chemical Component	Function
Bentonites	Natural clay modified by the addition of quaternary ammonium compounds	Allows enamel flow and suspension of pigment after shaking
Film Former	Composed of nitrocellulose	Provides hardness and waterproof quality
Resin	Toluene sulfonamide formaldehyde resin	Improves gloss, adhesion, hardness, and flow
Plasticizers	Dibutyl phthalate and camphor	Improves adhesion, flexibility, and wearability; minimizes shrinking
Solvents	Toluene, butyl or ethyl acetate, isopropyl alcohol	Improves flow, maintains other components in a liquid state
Pigment Colors		
Frosts	Crystalline guanine, natural pearl essence, bismuth oxychloride, and titanium dioxide–coated mica (synthetics)	Provides frosted appearance
Colorants	Lithiol Rubin B, tartrazine yellow, Alizurol Purple	Provides color
Fluorescents	Eosin, fluorescein, rhodamine B	Provides color

Source: From Scher.[4] Modified with permission.

FIGURE 6
Preformed plastic nail tips glued on top of the natural nail to add length.

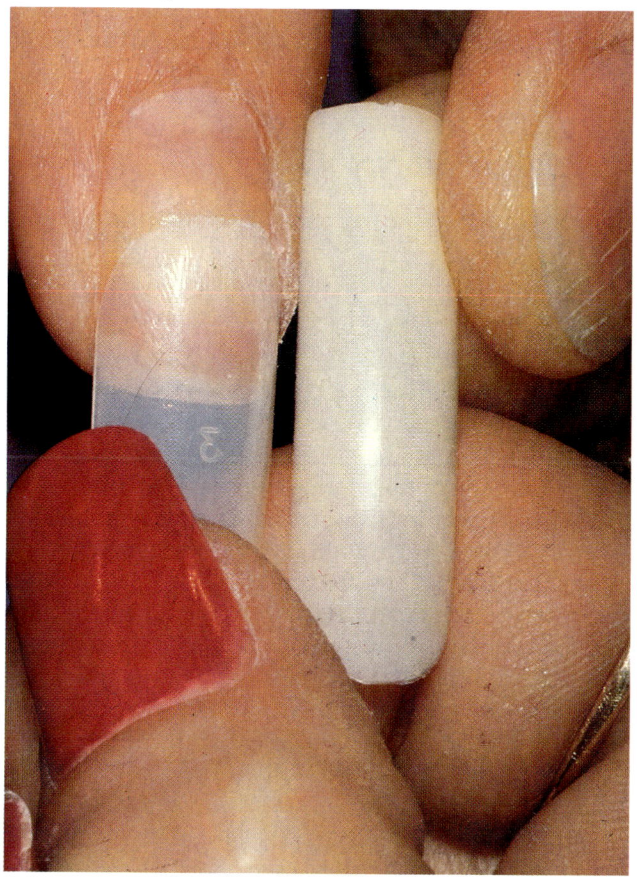

Plastic nails are used by persons with abnormal or short nails and may cover the entire nail plate or just extend the tip of the nail. The nail is held in place by an acrylic glue, which may be sensitizing.[6] Furthermore, peeling and splitting of the nail may result from the trauma of removing the artificial nail.[7]

Sculptured nails are prosthetic devices made by combining a liquid methyl, ethyl, or isobutyl methacrylate monomer with a powdered polymethyl methacrylate polymer. After polymerization and in the presence of an accelerator (benzoyl peroxide), the acrylic nail is shaped over the natural nail (Fig. 7). The acrylic nail produces a long cosmetically attractive nail. Methyl methacrylate is a potent sensitizing agent that is no longer used in the United States.[8,9] Ethyl and isobutyl methacrylate monomers have been substituted. These monomers are sensitizing as well, and cross-reactions between the monomers occur.[10] The polymer has a mild sensitizing ability. The adverse reactions that may result include onychia, paronychia, onycholysis, eyelid and distal site dermatitis, and paresthesia of the fingertips. Permanent nail destruction has also been reported.[11]

Ultraviolet light may be used to cure sculptured nails, allowing easier application and faster drying. The end result has been found to be less cosmetically acceptable and not as durable or strong. Photosensitivity may also occur.

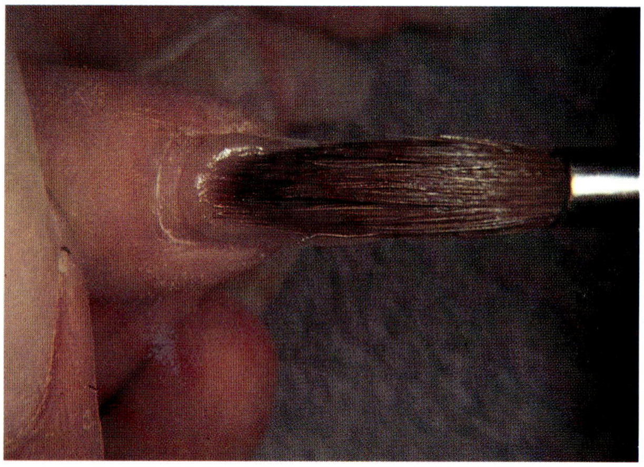

FIGURE 7
An acrylic sculptured nail being formed by molding the methacrylate monomer and polymer over the natural nail.

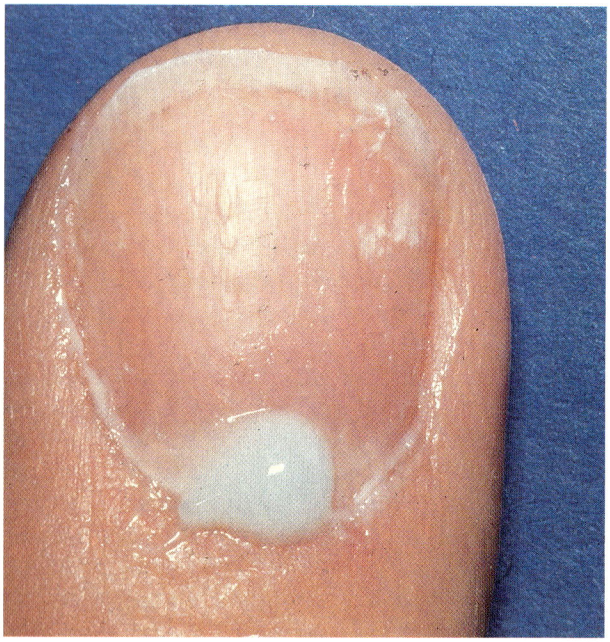

FIGURE 8
A cuticle remover used to soften and remove the cuticle.

Nail wrapping consists of tissue paper, cotton, wool, or silk which is applied to the free edge of the nail to repair a fractured nail plate or strengthen the free edge of the nail. The wrapping is glued with nail enamel or acrylic glues, which may be sensitizing.[11]

Nail enamel removers contain organic solvents such as ethyl acetate and acetone that remove the enamel.[12] These removers are dehydrating and hence may be primary irritants. Oils may be added to decrease the drying effects.

Cuticle removers are composed of 2 to 5% sodium hydroxide or potassium hydroxide. After application of the hydroxide, the cuticle is softened, allowing easier removal. Cuticle removers may be primary irritants (Fig. 8).

TESTING FOR SENSITIVITY TO NAIL COSMETICS

If sensitivity to a cosmetic preparation is suspected, patch testing to the sensitizing components may yield valuable information. The toluene sulfonamide formaldehyde resin is the most sensitizing component of nail enamel. A closed patch test of 10% toluene sulfonamide formaldehyde in petrolatum can be used.[13] A positive patch test indicates sensitization. Nail enamels should be avoided in this case, especially in the liquid state. Sculptured nail patch testing is used to determine sensitization to methyl methacrylate, ethyl methacrylate, and isobutyl methacrylate. The closed patches contain 1 to 5% of the monomer in petrolatum, olive oil, or ethyl alcohol. Primary irritants such as nail enamel removers and cuticle removers should not be used for closed patch testing.

COSMETIC THERAPY FOR ABNORMAL NAILS

Many abnormal or diseased nails can be effectively treated or camouflaged with currently available nail cosmetic preparations (Fig. 9). The abnormal nail, however, may be more susceptible to some of the adverse reactions known to occur from these cosmetic products. Therefore, utmost care must be taken not to contact the periungual area or other areas when applying the cosmetic preparation. In addition, close monitoring for signs of sensitization is important. Commonly encountered nail abnormalities involve the nail surface, consistency, configuration, or color.

Conditions producing modifications of the nail surface which are amenable to cosmetic therapy include the following.

Beau's lines are transverse grooves which occur weeks after illness, with the longitudinal width representing the duration of the illness. Similar horizontal depressions may result from injury or trauma to the nail matrix or plate. The transverse grooves may be made less pronounced with the aid

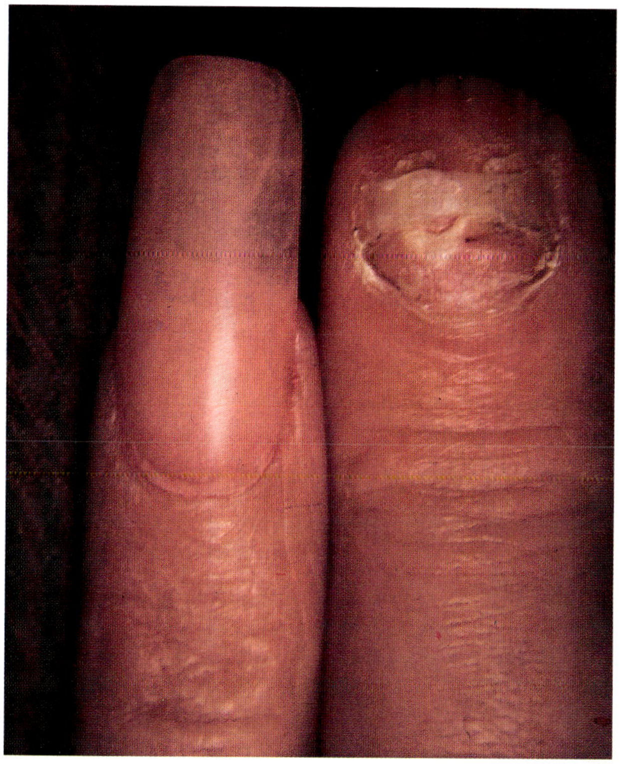

FIGURE 9
A diseased nail effectively camouflaged by the application of a preformed plastic nail to the nail plate, resulting in a cosmetically acceptable nail.

of a pumice-containing buffing cream used in conjunction with a nail buffer. The grooves can be camouflaged by the application of preformed plastic nails or acrylic sculptured nails placed over the abnormal nail surface.

Longitudinal grooves are parallel shallow furrows of the nail plate. They are attributed to trauma to the nail or the process of aging. Therapy is similar to that for transverse grooves and includes buffing the nails with pumice powder and applying preformed plastic nails or acrylic to fill in the defects or to form a complete sculptured nail. Nail wrapping is also beneficial.

Nail pits are small punctate depressions in the nail plate secondary to parakeratosis of the proximal nail matrix. Nail pits are observed in patients with psoriasis, alopecia areata, eczema, pityriasis rosea, and secondary syphilis and in those who have sustained trauma.[14] The pits may be camouflaged with several coats of base coat and nail enamel. The entire nail plate may be covered with preformed or sculptured nails. Therapy designed for the parakeratosis of the proximal nail matrix which produces nail pitting consists of intralesional corticosteroid injections to the proximal nail fold.

Rough nails may be congenital or idiopathic in origin, or they may be caused by psoriasis, alopecia areata, ichthyosis, lichen planus, or chemicals. The nail surface is rough and brittle with gray opacities. Splits occur readily at the free edge. Nail conditioners which contain proteins and lipids may be used to treat the brittleness. Nail buffers smooth the roughness. Finally, wrapping of the nail tip repairs the splitting and fortifies the brittle nail.

Longitudinal splitting of the distal aspect of the nail may be secondary to dehydration or trauma such as careless filing. Palliative therapy consists of nail wrapping or the application of an acrylic to fill in the nail surface defect.

Onychoschizia, or splitting of the nails horizontally into layers, is related to constant dehydration and rehydration of the nail. Small pieces of the nail may flake. Nail enamel, base coat, and top coat may cover the abnormality on the nail surface. Nail acrylic may be used to fill in the defect and thicken the nail tip.

Modifications in the consistency of the nail include hard nails, soft nails, and brittle nails. *Hard nails* are seen in pachyonychia congenita. The nails must be soaked in warm water prior to cutting with professional nail clippers. *Soft nails* are less than 0.5 mm thick, bend easily, and split at the free edge. Nail hardeners may be used to strengthen the nail plate. The nail may be fortified with nail wrapping. Alternatively, the nail may be thickened with an acrylic nail. *Brittle nails* occur when the nail plate, which normally contains 18% water, becomes dehydrated. They commonly occur in homemakers whose hands are immersed in water and subsequently dry out. Other causes include impaired peripheral circulation and iron deficiency. Therapy is designed to decrease the loss of water by decreasing the surface area exposed to the atmosphere.[15] Cutting the nail is recommended, along with the application of nail enamel, base coat, or top coat to trap the moisture. The nail enamel should be applied to the undersurface of the nail as well. The nail should be filed with the enamel in order to protect the nail and minimize tearing and splitting. Preparations such as Lac Hydrin are also of considerable benefit.

Modifications of the nail configuration include koilonychia and onychogryphosis. *Koilonychia* involves nails that are concave with everted edges.

TABLE 2
NAIL DYSCHROMIA

Color	Cause	Site
Induced by external agents		
Brown	Anthralin	Nail plate
	Formaldehyde	Nail plate
	Nail enamel	Nail plate
	Nicotine	Nail plate
	Pecans	Nail plate
Black	Photographic developer	Nail plate
	Silver nitrate	Nail plate
	Red wine	Nail plate
Yellow	Amphotericin	Nail plate
	Fluorescein	Nail plate
Induced by systemic drugs		
Gray	Phenolphthalein	Lunula
	Argyria	Nail bed or lunula
	Minocycline	Nail bed or plate
Brown	Tetracycline	Nail bed or plate
	Phenothiazines	Nail bed
	Bleomycin	Nail plate
	Busulfan	Nail plate or lunula
	Hydroxyurea	Nail plate or bed
Induced by fungi or bacteria		
Green	*Pseudomonas*	Nail plate
Black	*Proteus*	Nail plate
White	*Trichophyton*	Nail plate
Secondary to dermatoses		
Brown	Acanthosis	Nail plate
	Vitiligo	Nail bed
	Psoriasis	Nail plate
Secondary to systemic disorders		
Blue	Wilson's disease	Nail plate
Brown	Adrenal insufficiency	Nail plate
	Chronic renal failure	Nail plate
	Hemochromatosis	Nail plate
	Hyperthyroidism	Nail plate

Source: From Daniel and Osment.[17] Modified with permission.

The nail is normal, thinned, or thickened. This disease is associated with iron deficiency anemia, hemochromatosis, trauma, and avitaminosis. The defect is often corrected when the iron deficiency is reversed. The concave depression may be filled in with acrylic. Such nails may be camouflaged with plastic nails applied to the nail surface. *Onychogryphosis* is an abnormality of the nail configuration produced by trauma. The nail is thickened and laterally curved. Therapy is directed at mechanically trimming the nail with scissors, clippers, or a drill. After paring, nail enamel may be applied. On occasion permanent nail avulsion followed by matricectomy may be required.

Modification of nail color may occur at various locations in the nail unit. If the color is in the nail bed, it will disappear with transillumination of the bed. Superficial nail plate dyschromia may be removed after the application of a solvent or by scraping the nail plate. Deeper nail plate dyschromia cannot be removed with a solvent or with scraping. External agents, systemic drugs, fungi and bacteria, dermatoses, and systemic disorders may produce nail dyschromias (Table 2).[16–19] Most nail dyschromias can be camouflaged with colored nail enamels. Many colorless enamels have a yellow or pink tint that may provide some coverage for men.

CONCLUSIONS

Americans spend $200 million per year on nail cosmetics. There is a close relationship between nail appearance and beauty, personal hygiene, and good grooming. Cosmetic nail preparations are used by persons with diseased nails as well as those with normal nails to enhance nail appearance. Adverse effects from these products range from primary irritation to allergic sensitization. Overall, the incidence of reactions is low, and many sensitizers such as formaldehyde and methyl methacrylate have been removed or minimized in concentration. If used properly, nail cosmetics may be of benefit for many patients.

REFERENCES

1. Brauer E. Cosmetics: The care and adornment of the nail, in Baren R, Dawber RPR (eds) Diseases of the Nails and Their Management. Oxford: Blackwell, 1984:289–301.
2. Fisher AA. Contact Dermatitis. Philadelphia: Lea & Febiger, 1986:95.
3. Fisher AA. Contact Dermatitis. Philadelphia: Lea & Febiger, 1986:383.
4. Scher RK. Cosmetics and ancillary preparations for the care of the nails. J Am Acad Dermatol. 1982;6:523–528.

5. Schlossman, ML. Nail enamel resins. Cosmet Technol. 1979;1:53–55.
6. Burrows D, Rycroft RJG. Contact dermatitis from PTBP resin and tricresyl ethyl phthalate in a plastic nail adhesive. Contact Dermatitis. 1981;7:336.
7. Baden HP. Diseases of the Hair and Nails. Chicago: Year Book, 1986.
8. Fisher AA, Franks A, Glicks H. Allergic sensitization of the skin and nails to acrylic plastic nails. J Allergy Clin lmununol. 1957,28:84 89.
9. Food and Drug Administration Seizure Action. FDA Consumer. 1974;8:37.
10. Marks JG, Bishop ME, Willis WF. Allergic contact dermatitis to sculptured nails. Arch Dermatol. 1979;115:100–103.
11. Fisher AA. Contact Dermatitis. Philadelphia: Lea & Febiger, 1986:384.
12. Wilkinson JB, Moore RJ. Harry's Cosmetology. New York: Chemical Publishing, 1982:27–30.
13. Cronin E. Contact Dermatitis. New York: Churchill Livingstone, 1980:361–363.
14. Baran R, Dawber RPR. Diseases of the Nails and Their Management. Oxford: Blackwell, 1984:25–79.
15. Samman PD, Fenton DA. The Nails in Disease. Chicago, Year Book, 1986:89–101.
16. Jeanmougin M, Civatte J. Nail dyschromia. Int J Dermatol. 1983;22:279–290.
17. Daniel CR, Osment LS. Nail pigmentation abnormalities. Cutis. 1982;30:348–359.
18. Daniel CR, Scher RK. Nail changes caused by systemic drugs or ingestants. Dermatol Clin. 1985;3:491–500.
19. Daniel CR, Scher RK: Nail changes secondary to systemic drugs or ingestants. J Am Acad Dermatol. 1984;10: 250–258.

CHAPTER

25

Nails: Surgical Aspects

ECKART HANEKE
ROBERT BARAN

The nail is often an eye-catcher, especially in people with vivid gestures. Therefore, even minor changes may cause considerable embarrassment. Unfortunately, the results of topical treatment of disfiguring nail changes are generally poor, and surgical therapy may be indicated in these cases. Fungal infections of the nails may require up to 18 months of oral griseofulvin or ketoconazole, while intralesional steroid injections into the nail bed for psoriasis are not only painful but also inconsistent in results. Apart from onychomycosis and psoriasis of the nails, the most frequent nail deformities are due to habits such as picking, biting, fiddling, manipulation of the cuticle, and exaggerated manicure. These habits are not amenable to surgical treatment.

DEVELOPMENT AND STRUCTURE OF THE NORMAL NAIL

The nail is a hard horny plate covering the dorsal aspect of the tip of the digits. Its appearance depends on the integrity of the terminal bony phalanx, periungual tissues, nail bed, and matrix (Fig. 1).

The *nail plate,* formed by the matrix, grows out from a pocketlike invagination of the skin, and adheres firmly to both the *nail bed* and the undersurface of the *proximal nail fold*; the *nail pocket* is sealed by the cuticule.

The nail plate is smooth, convex, and pink. The most distal part of the matrix, the *lunula,* is not covered by the proximal nail fold and is white. Size, form, growth, and structure vary considerably

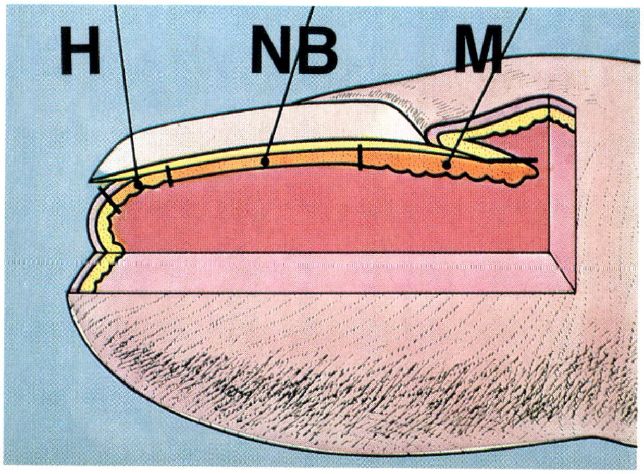

FIGURE 1
Anatomy of the nail. H = hyponychium; NB = nail bed; M = nail matrix. The base of the nail plate lies beneath the proximal nail fold.

according to location (finger or toe), age, professional activity, frequency and intensity of manicure, general health, etc.

The objectives of nail surgery in the framework of aesthetic medicine are to correct deformities.

ANESTHESIA

Our preference among anesthetics is the digital ring block. We use 1% or 2% lidocaine (Xylocaine) without adrenaline.

A thin short needle is inserted on the radial and ulnar aspect of the digit, opposite and just proximal to the volar flexion crease at the base of the proximal phalanx, tangential to the sides of the phalanx, as far as the lateral sides of the flexor tendon.

When one is dealing with the toes, where the digital nerves lie on the plantar side of the coronal plane, anesthesia should be supplemented with a small amount of anesthetic across the dorsal aspect. Using this technique, complete anesthesia is achieved after 10 to 15 min and is maintained for 1 h.

HEMOSTASIS

Hemostasis is accomplished by simple pressure on the lateral aspect of the digit with the thumb and index finger of the free hand.

When a bloodless field is required (e.g., for phenol matricectomy), a wide Penrose drain is placed around the base of the digit as a tourniquet and is secured with a hemostat. It should not be left in place more than 15 min.

CHRONIC PARONYCHIA

Paronychia is manifested as a red and painful swelling of the perionychial tissue. After a period of months, the cuticle disappears and the nail plate separates from the the undersurface of the proximal nail fold, leading to a progressive retraction of the perionychial tissue.

The etiology of this condition has not been clearly defined. *Candida ablicans* has been implicated, and it is often cultured with intestinal bacteria and streptococci from perionychial swabs.

Specific reactivity of the tissue to chemicals contained in everyday food items is an interesting etiological hypothesis. Foreign bodies such as hair, bristles, wood splinters, and vegetables may also be responsible.

Lack of response to medical therapy (local steroids, either topical or intralesional, and anticandidal agents) in a patient avoiding wet work (cotton gloves beneath rubber gloves) is an indication for surgical therapy (Fig. 2).[1] A crescent-shaped full-thickness piece of the proximal nail fold (PNF) that is 5 mm at its greatest width and extends from one

FIGURE 2
Excision of a crescent-shaped full-thickness piece of the proximal nail fold in a patient with chronic paronychia.

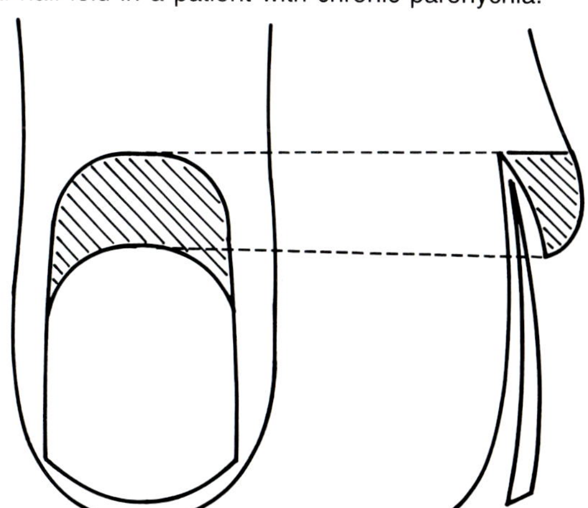

lateral nail fold to the other is excised. The excision includes the entire swollen portion of the PNF. Complete healing by secondary intention takes about 2 months, leaving a nail plate with a more visible lunula.

RE-CREATION OF THE PROXIMAL NAIL FOLD

When the PNF is partially torn, after fingertip injury, the remaining portion is excised in a uniformly crescent-shaped section (Fig. 3).

FIGURE 3
Re-creation of the crescent shape of the proximal nail fold.

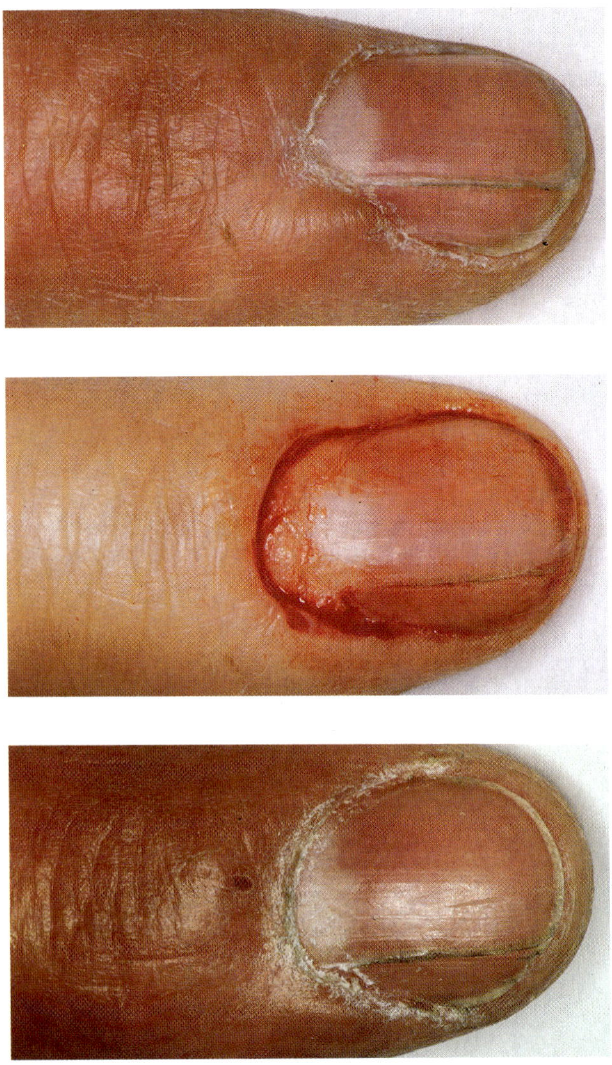

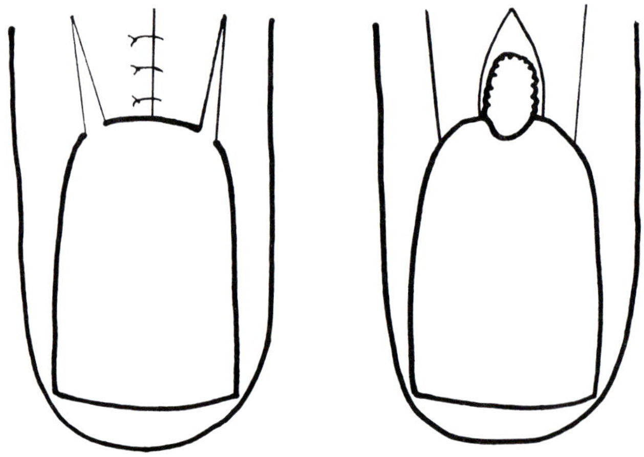

FIGURE 4
Treatment for median tumors of the proximal nail fold.

TUMORS OF THE PROXIMAL NAIL FOLD

Some tumors, such as fibrokeratoma and paronychial mucoid cyst involving only the distal portion of the proximal nail fold, may be treated with the same crescent section technique used for chronic paronychia. Tumors of the proximal nail fold in a median position which have a longitudinal diameter greater than 3 to 5 mm are too large to be removed by excision of the PNF. They can be excised with a wedge of the PNF whose base is located at the free margin and whose apex points proximally. Two lateral incisions of the PNF then allow suturing of the wedge-shaped defect after the undersurface of the PNF has been released from the nail plate (Fig. 4). The resulting symmetrical narrow defects at both sides heal rapidly by secondary intention, and the cosmetic and functional results are excellent.

PERIUNGUAL TISSUE

Myxoid pseudocysts (dorsal finger cysts, mucinous degeneration cysts) are seen mostly in elderly persons. They are commonly located in the PNF and may give rise to deep longitudinal grooves in the nail plate subsequent to prolonged permanent pressure to the matrix region. Cysts may rupture and discharge a yellowish viscous substance; however, if the cysts ruptures into the nail pocket, wavelike irregularities develop in the nail groove. Cysts are often associated with degenerative osteoarthritis of the distal interphalangeal joint, adding to the disfigurement of the finger. Of the many treatment modalities described in the literature, two approaches have proven to be successful.

Careful cryotherapy has been shown to be highly efficacious without injuring the matrix; a single freeze of the cyst and its potential tract to the joint appears to be sufficient.[2] The surgical technique utilizes intraarticular methylene blue injection to visualize the extent of the pseudocyst (Fig. 5). The skin over the pseudocyst is incised, and the lesion is carefully dissected from the surrounding connective tissue, which is not stained by methylene blue. A small rotation flap is raised to cover the defect. The lesion often extends farther in all directions, and all stained tissue should be removed. The small defect from the flap rapidly heals by secondary intention.[3] Both functional and cosmetic results are excellent, and no recurrences have been observed.

LATERAL NAIL FOLD

When the lateral nail fold is inflamed and accompanied by protuberant granulation tissue, it becomes grossly hypertrophic. This is usually due to an ingrown toenail of long duration. A simple fusiform excision taken from the lateral aspect of the

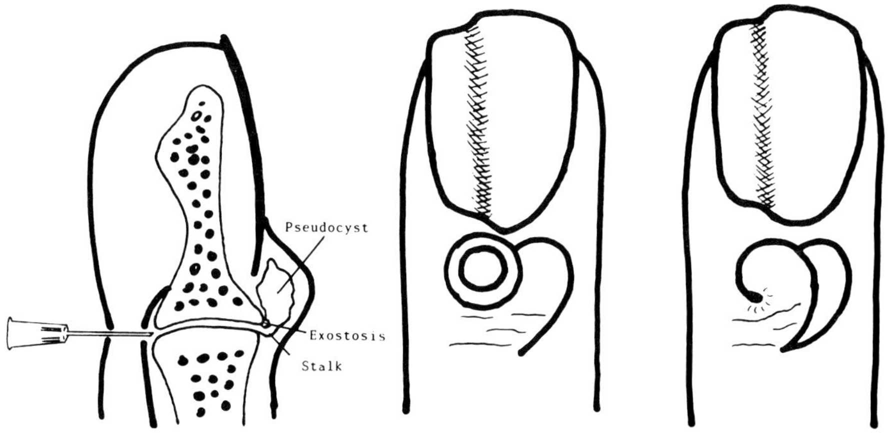

(a) (b) (c)

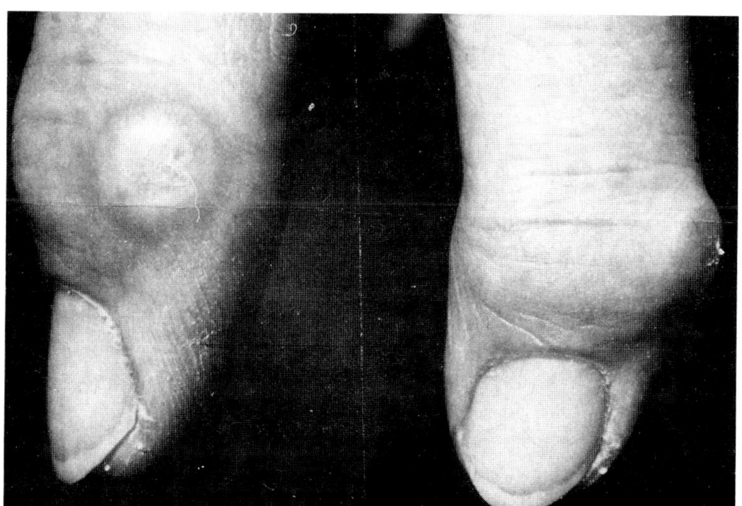

(d)

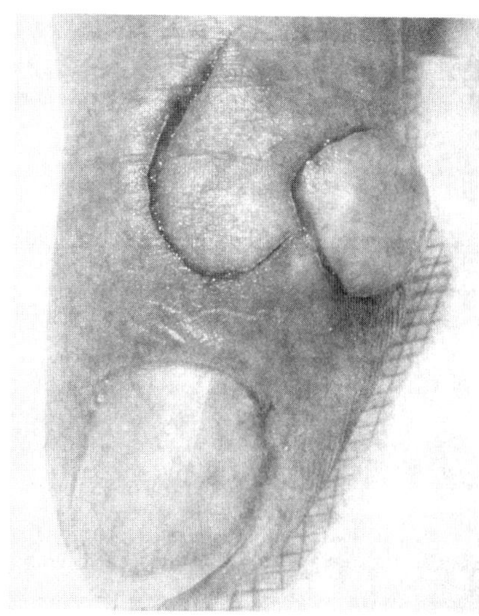

(e)

FIGURE 5
Dorsal myxoid pseudocyst. (*a*, *b*, and *c*). The intraarticular methylene blue injection visualizes the extent of the pseudocyst. (*d*) Before the operation. (*e*) The start of the operation. (*f*) The lesion is removed, and flaps are raised to show the methylene blue. (*g*) Stained connections with the joint (arrow). (*h*) Completion of the operation 1 year postoperatively.

(*continued*)

FIGURE 5 (*Continued*)

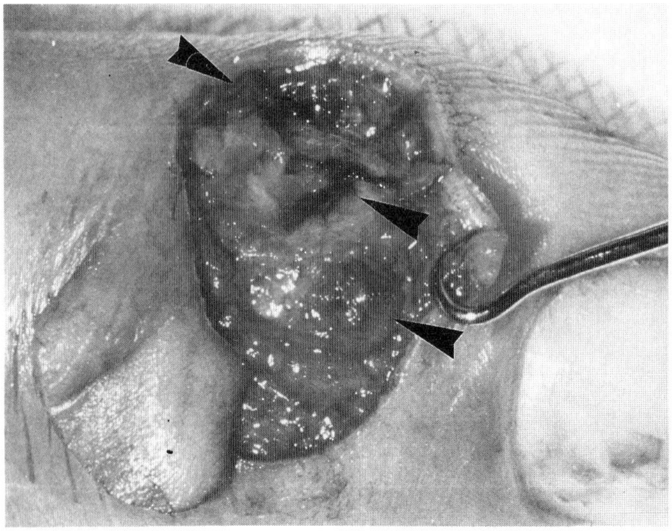

(*f*)

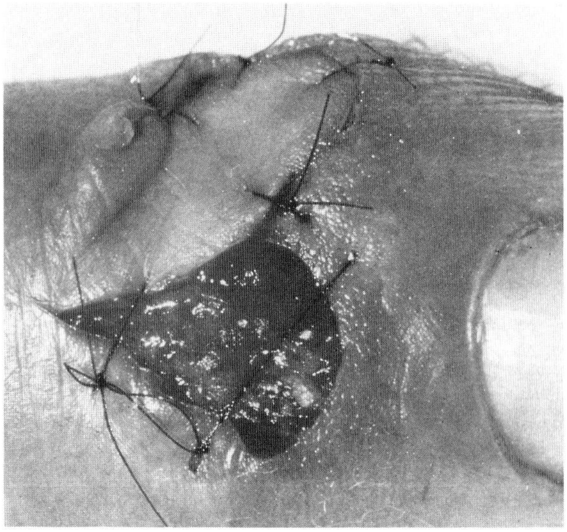

(*g*)

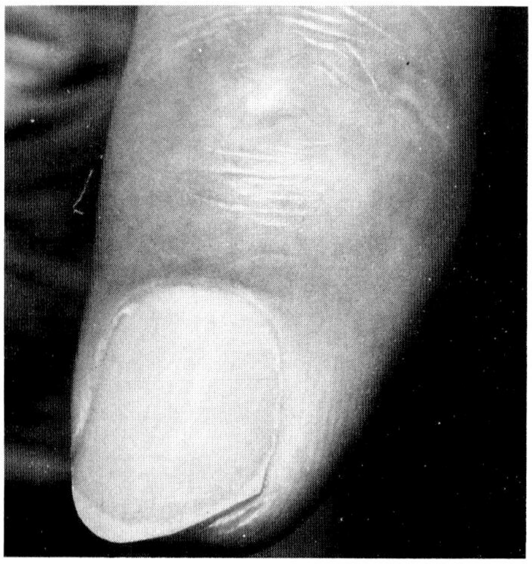

(*h*)

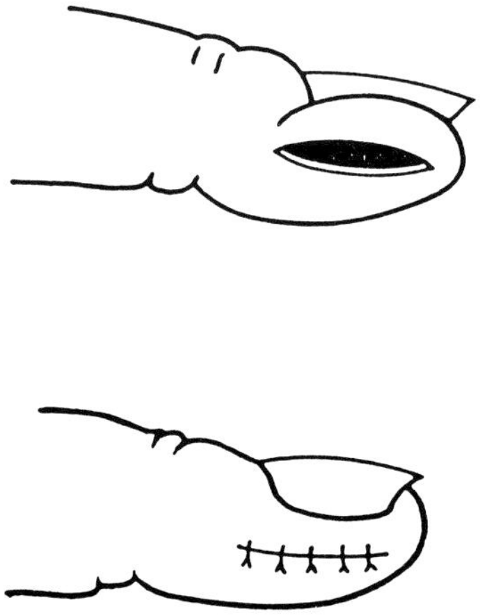

FIGURE 6
Fusiform excision of the lateral nail wall.

toe usually reduces the bulky lateral nail fold and, under optimal conditions, pulls the lateral nail sulcus away from the offending lateral nail plate margin (Fig. 6). The cosmetic results are usually acceptable.

WARTS

Warts may be periungual and/or subungual. *Periungual warts* are unsightly benign tumors with a rough keratotic surface. They are common in nail biters and may involve several fingers. Sometimes periungual warts become fissured and may cause pain and infection.

The treatment of periungual warts is frustrating, and we do not advocate surgery for such lesions. "Magic" approaches in children, who sometimes respond to therapeutic suggestion, should be attempted. Cryotherapy is unsuitable for children because of pain (the subungual tissue at that age is prone to swell) and secondary damage to the matrix.

Carbon dioxide laser treatment has been used with success but is not harmless, since it can be followed by nail dystrophies. Small amounts of bleomycin (15 mg diluted in 100 ml of saline) injected strictly intralesionally constitute a useful treatment but may be followed by dystrophy.

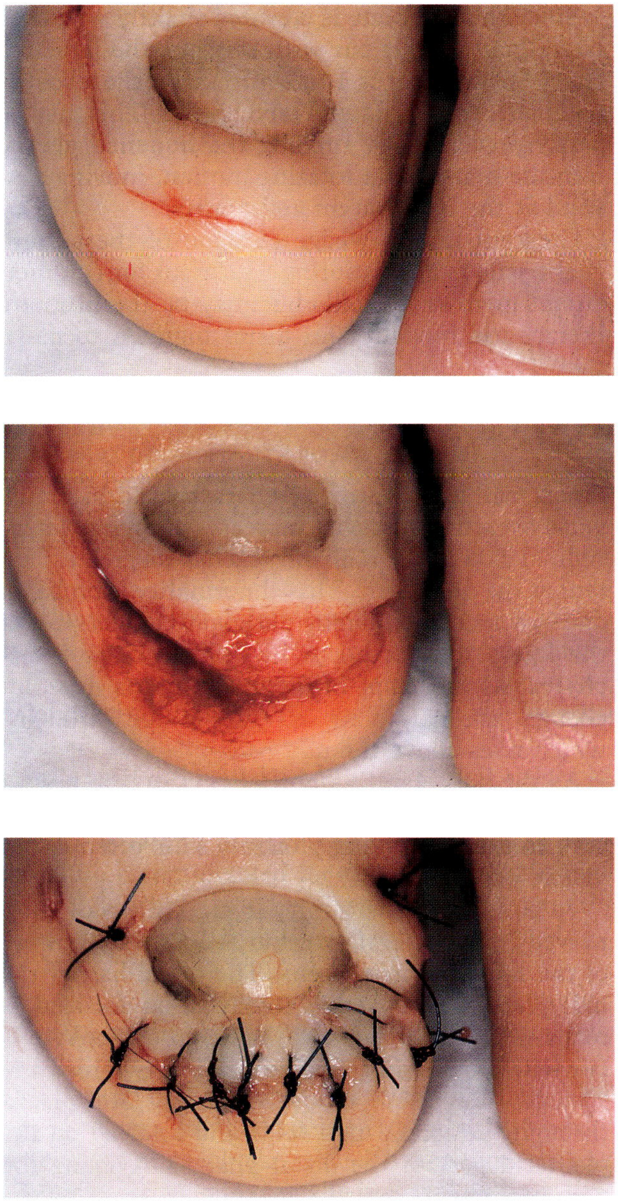

FIGURE 7
Distal nail wall.

Subungual warts can be treated with the same cytotoxic drug or by curettage. If surgery is chosen, removal of a large portion of the nail protecting the wart is essential to obtain the best results.

Repeated aggressive keratolytic treatment using salicylic acid, lactic acid collodion, and 30% salicylic acid plaster under occlusion for 24 to 48 h, followed by a hot bath in salt water, often allows successful atraumatic removal of the macerated horny masses.

DISTAL NAIL WALL

Repeated avulsion of the hallux nail often results in a distortion of the tip of the toe. The nail plate in its normal position counteracts the forces that are exerted during walking; without the nail, the pulp is gradually distorted dorsally, giving rise to a distal nail wall. The terminal phalanx looks shorter, and the nail plate may cut into the tissue when regrowing. Occasionally persistent massage of the distal nail wall in a distal-plantar direction enables the nail to overgrow the wall, eventually resulting in a normal toe. However, when this procedure is not effective, a crescent-shaped wedge excision becomes necessary (Fig. 7). A fish-mouth incision is carried parallel to the former hyponychium around the tip of the toe, starting and ending 3 to 5 mm proximal to the end of the lateral nail fold. A second incision is then done to yield a spindle of 3 to 8 mm in greatest width, depending on the height of the distal nail wall.[4]

INGROWN TOENAIL

Ingrown toenails occur very frequently and may cause both pain and disfigurement. A wealth of treatment modalities are advocated in the medical, surgical, and podiatric literature. Many of these modalities carry an extreme risk of recurrence, induce long-standing morbidity, or mutilate the toe. We have found that the selective lateral matrix excision (Fig. 8) not only prevents recurrences but gives the best cosmetic results.

FIGURE 8
Selective lateral matrix excision. S = nail spike digging into toe; IN = ingrown lateral nail margin; MH = matrix horn. Excision of the dashed area.

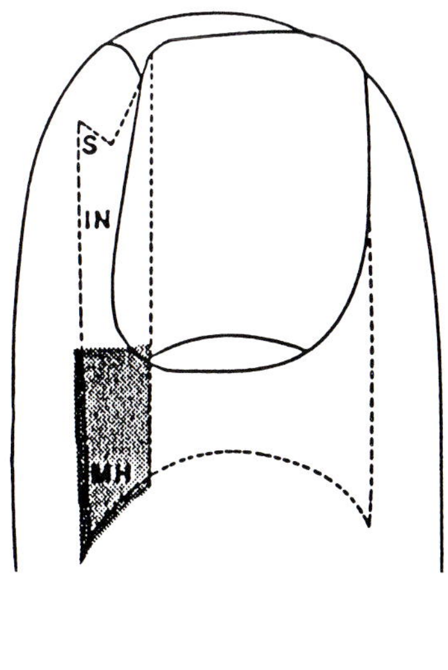

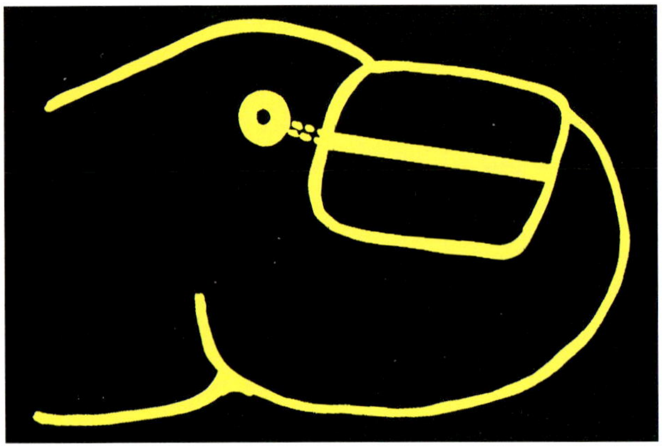

FIGURE 10
Longitudinal melanonychia. Punch biopsy at the beginning of the pigmented band.

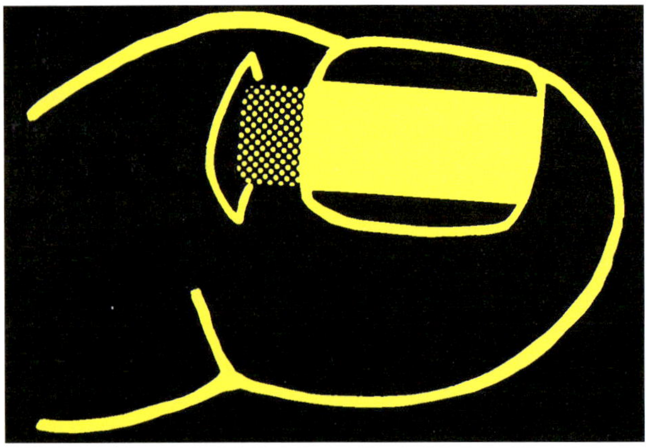

FIGURE 11
Longitudinal melanonychia. Transverse matrix biopsy.

of the band in the nail plate, and the width of the linear pigmentation.

The anatomic site of the matrix affected is inferred from the level of the melanin pigment identified with Fontana's silver stain of the nail clipping obtained from the distal free edge.[6]

If the pigment is located within the ventral portion of the nail plate, one must choose the proper biopsy procedure to be used according to the width of the band. A punch biopsy should be performed when the width of the band is less than 3 mm (Fig. 10). Removal of the base of the nail plate allows the specimen to be released more easily and above all to check the integrity of the region distal to the biopsied matrix area. A transverse matrix biopsy is required for a band wider than 3 mm (Fig. 11).

If the pigment involves the upper portion of the nail, it is obviously difficult to use these two procedures to remove the source of melanin pigment because of anatomic reasons and the risk of secondary dystrophy, at least if the band is wider than 3 mm.

A rectangular block of tissue is excised, using two parallel incisions down to the bone. An L-shaped incision is carried back along the lateral nail wall, freeing this flap. The lateral section may then be rotated medially and approximated to the remaining nail segment (Fig. 12). If the band is wider than 6 mm or if the whole thickness of the

FIGURE 12
Longitudinal melanonychia. Rectangular monoblock excision associated with total nail flap permitted by L-shaped incision of the lateral nail wall.

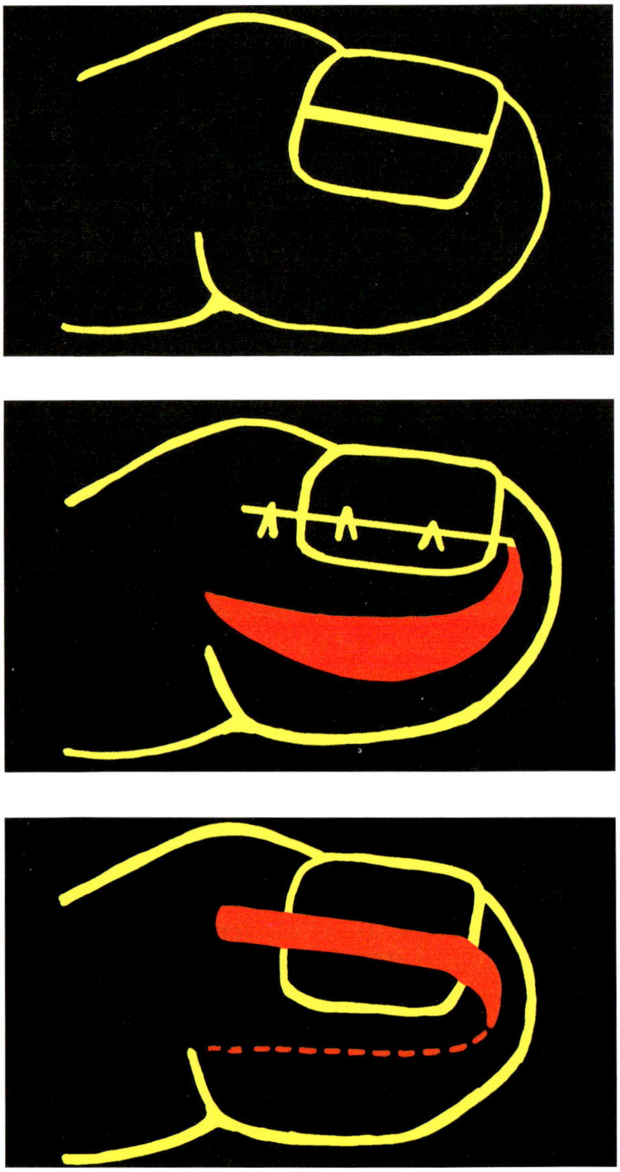

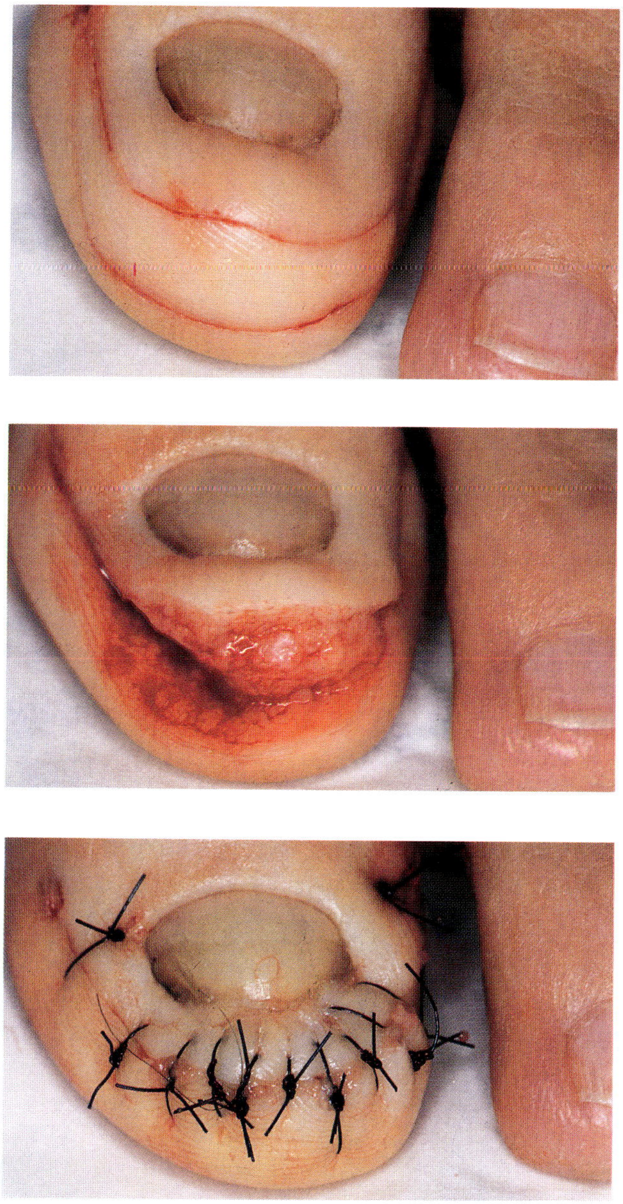

FIGURE 7
Distal nail wall.

Subungual warts can be treated with the same cytotoxic drug or by curettage. If surgery is chosen, removal of a large portion of the nail protecting the wart is essential to obtain the best results.

Repeated aggressive keratolytic treatment using salicylic acid, lactic acid collodion, and 30% salicylic acid plaster under occlusion for 24 to 48 h, followed by a hot bath in salt water, often allows successful atraumatic removal of the macerated horny masses.

DISTAL NAIL WALL

Repeated avulsion of the hallux nail often results in a distortion of the tip of the toe. The nail plate in its normal position counteracts the forces that are exerted during walking; without the nail, the pulp is gradually distorted dorsally, giving rise to a distal nail wall. The terminal phalanx looks shorter, and the nail plate may cut into the tissue when regrowing. Occasionally persistent massage of the distal nail wall in a distal-plantar direction enables the nail to overgrow the wall, eventually resulting in a normal toe. However, when this procedure is not effective, a crescent-shaped wedge excision becomes necessary (Fig. 7). A fish-mouth incision is carried parallel to the former hyponychium around the tip of the toe, starting and ending 3 to 5 mm proximal to the end of the lateral nail fold. A second incision is then done to yield a spindle of 3 to 8 mm in greatest width, depending on the height of the distal nail wall.[4]

INGROWN TOENAIL

Ingrown toenails occur very frequently and may cause both pain and disfigurement. A wealth of treatment modalities are advocated in the medical, surgical, and podiatric literature. Many of these modalities carry an extreme risk of recurrence, induce long-standing morbidity, or mutilate the toe. We have found that the selective lateral matrix excision (Fig. 8) not only prevents recurrences but gives the best cosmetic results.

FIGURE 8
Selective lateral matrix excision. S = nail spike digging into toe; IN = ingrown lateral nail margin; MH = matrix horn. Excision of the dashed area.

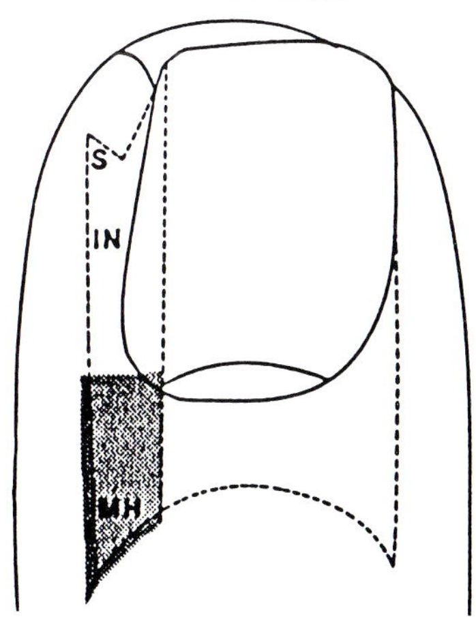

The lateral portion of the proximal nail plate is freed from the overlying PNF with a blunt instrument and the PNF is incised in an angle of about 110 degrees at both sides. The incision is opened with fine hooks. The ingrown nail plate strips are cut, released from the nail bed, and removed, exposing the lateral matrix horn, which has to be carefully dissected and excised from the base of the terminal phalanx bone. No matrix remnants must be left in place in order to avoid nail spicules and cyst formation. The resulting wound cavity is filled with antibiotic pellets that prevent wound infection and allow blood and serous exudate to escape. The incision is closed with sterile tape (e.g., steristrips) or with 5-0 monofilament sutures. Nonadherent tulle grass and a thick layer of an antimicrobial ointment (e.g., povidone-iodine) are applied before a bulky dressing is applied. The dressing is changed after 24 to 48 h to remove bloodstained gauze that can lead to bacterial infections. The second dressing is left in place for about a week. Postoperative pain is minimal, and healing is rapid.

Phenol cautery of the lateral matrix horn is a simple alternative.[5] The ingrown lateral nail strips are freed from the nail bed and the undersurface of the PNF, cut longitudinally and pulled out, and extracted with a lateral rotational force to aid removal of the lateral horn. An applicator with a cotton tip dipped into liquefied phenol (88 to 90% phenol) is rubbed vigorously into the lateral nail pocket in a completely bloodless field. Any liquefied phenol spilling over the PNF or the lateral nail fold is wiped off immediately with a gauze pad moistened with 70% alcohol. The phenol has to be rubbed onto the matrix epithelium for at least 3 min to ensure complete cautery of the matrix. The wound is filled with tapered antibiotic pellets; abundant antimicrobial ointment and a bulky padded dressing are applied after the tourniquet is released. Because of the local anesthetic action of phenol, there is virtually no postoperative pain. The antibacterial effect of phenol also helps prevent wound infections.

The dressing is removed after 24 h, and a foot bath with an antiseptic soap is applied. Clotted blood and serous crusts are easily removed with either 3% hydrogen peroxide or chloramine-7. This procedure is repeated every day. Though there is no incision, healing takes about 3 to 6 weeks until the chemonecrosis has been sloughed off and oozing stops.

Since the nail plate is elevated slightly when the lateral nail strip is cut with scissors, the liquefied phenol usually seeps 1 to 2 mm under the adjacent nail plate, causing lateral onycholysis. This may be partly prevented by rubbing the liquefied phenol into the matrix in a rotating motion, moving outward at the nail margin and matrix.

Crescent-shaped wedge excision of the periungual tissue is not a routine treatment for common lateral ingrown toenails but may be the ultimate therapeutic modality for distal ingrown toenails.

PINCER NAILS

Pincer nail is a dystrophy characterized by transverse overcurvature that increases along the longitudinal axis of the nail and reaches its greatest extent at the distal part. This abnormality is probably due to selective widening of the proximal aspect of the lateral matrix horns by juxtaarticular osteophytes. As the shape of the distal matrix does not change, the nail plate assumes a conical shape which rises above the nail bed.

As the nail plate is tightly bound to the periosteum, it lifts a traction osteophyte from the dorsum of the underlying phalanx. This often is not visible on radiography.

To correct this deformity (Fig. 9), the nail is removed by a bilateral excision followed by cautery of the lateral matrix horns. The distal half of the nail plate is removed, a longitudinal incision is made in the nail bed, and the distal osteophyte is cut with a bone rongeur; the nail bed is spread and sutured. Reversed tie-over sutures are placed through the lateral nail folds and knotted on the plantar aspect of the distal phalanx, keeping the nail bed tissue spread. To avoid cutting of the threads through the tissue, small rubber tubes or plastic gutters may be placed into the lateral nail sulci around which the sutures have to be carried. These sutures are left for 2 to 3 weeks to allow firm healing of the readapted nail bed.

SPLIT-NAIL DEFORMITY

Wounds running vertically through the matrix and/or nail bed as well as tumors of these regions (e.g., glomus tumor) may cause a split in the nail. Treatment is aimed at narrowing the scarring to such an extent that normal nail growth will result. To cor-

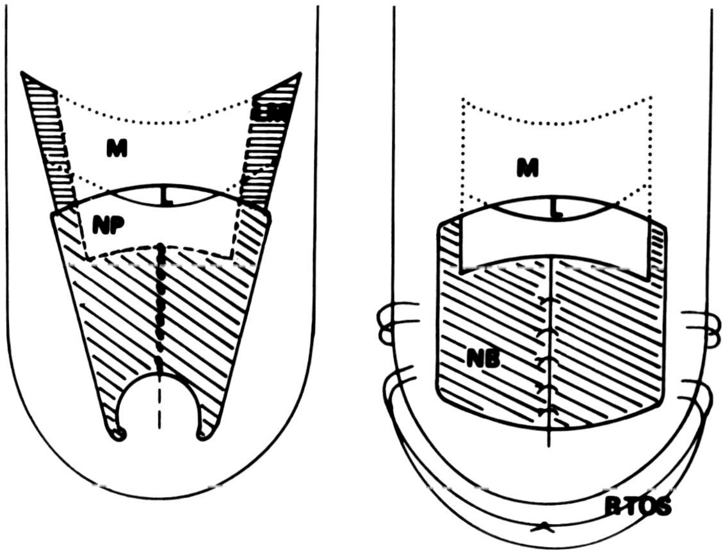

FIGURE 9
Correction of pincer nail. L = lunula; LM = lateral matrix horn; M = matrix; NB = nail bed; NP = nail plate; DT = dorsal tuft of distal phalanx; RTOS = reversed tie-over sutures.

rect this unsightly deformity, different procedures are available. The type of surgery selected depends on the history (e.g., previous trauma), the location of the longitudinal split in the nail, and the length of the split.[4]

If the split is located within the lateral third of either portion of the nail, especially when it is close to its lateral margin, the best method is the technique recommended for the lateral-longitudinal nail biopsy, i.e., the removal of the lateral portion of the nail with the defect. (Look ahead to Fig. 13.)

An elliptical excision is made on the segment of the nail and the corresponding PNF delineated by the split margin and the lateral margin of the plate in the lateral nail groove. The incisions which parallel the lateral edge of the nail segment to be removed have to reach the bone. This ensures that a full-thickness fragment of the nail bed and matrix with its lateral horn is removed, allowing primary wound closure. Iris scissors are useful for dissecting the tissue from the bone. The lateral wound margin is mobilized to allow the re-creation of the lateral nail fold using back stitches.

If the split is located in the middle region of the nail and involves its whole length, the PNF is obliquely incised at both sides, carefully freed from the underlying nail plate, and reflected to expose the whole matrix area. The nail plate along the split is cautiously cut as a rectangular block about 1 mm wider than the scar which has to be excised. The nail bed and matrix of the defective tissue are dissected from the bone to allow an exact approximation of the remaining bed and matrix, which are sutured with 6-0 monofilament resorbable sutures. To prevent cutting of these stitches, 3-0 sutures are put through the nail plate. When these threads are knotted firmly, the matrix and nail bed are further approximated, relaxing the 6-0 sutures.

If the scar is too wide to allow primary closure of the defect, relaxing longitudinal incisions along the lateral nail sulci down to the bone usually permit suturing. An alternative approach is the formation of a nail bed-matrix flap with an L-shaped incision of the lateral aspect of the finger. The secondary defect of the distal lateral nail fold heals readily by secondary intention.

In distal fissuring of the nail, removal of the distal two-thirds of the nail plate is essential. It may be therapeutic by itself or may permit visualization and evaluation of a subungual lesion. It is then possible to undertake the appropriate surgical measures, such as 3- to 4-mm punch biopsy in the nail bed, longitudinal elliptical excision, or curettage.

LONGITUDINAL MELANONYCHIA

Longitudinal melanonychia (LM) is a linear pigmentation of the nail plate or nail bed due to melanin. The development of LM in white people or the darkening of a preexisting band in blacks is likely to be a feature of melanoma. Therefore, complete excisional biopsy is crucial for both diagnosis and therapy. The type of biopsy selected depends on the site of the matrix melanin production, the location

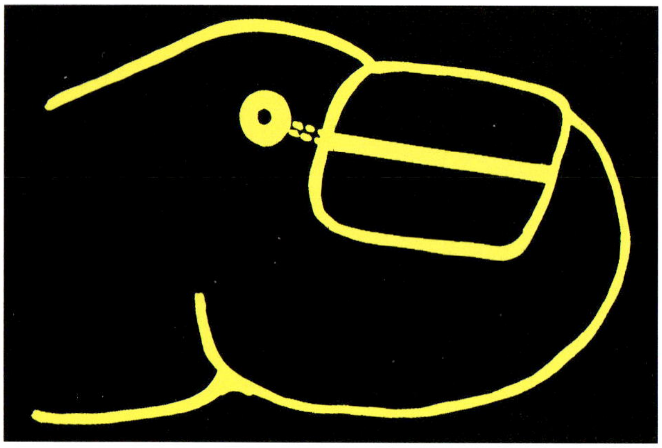

FIGURE 10
Longitudinal melanonychia. Punch biopsy at the beginning of the pigmented band.

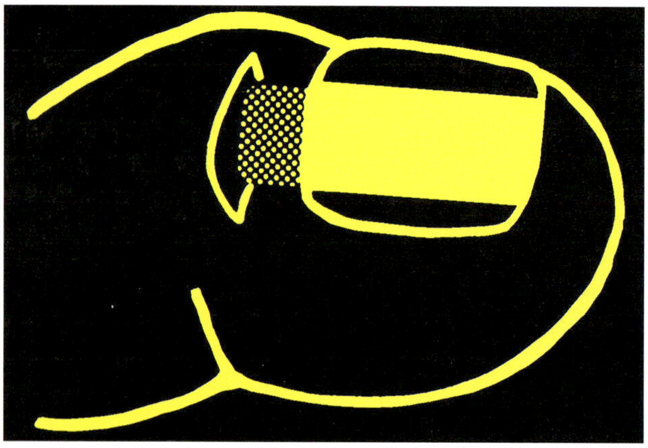

FIGURE 11
Longitudinal melanonychia. Transverse matrix biopsy.

of the band in the nail plate, and the width of the linear pigmentation.

The anatomic site of the matrix affected is inferred from the level of the melanin pigment identified with Fontana's silver stain of the nail clipping obtained from the distal free edge.[6]

If the pigment is located within the ventral portion of the nail plate, one must choose the proper biopsy procedure to be used according to the width of the band. A punch biopsy should be performed when the width of the band is less than 3 mm (Fig. 10). Removal of the base of the nail plate allows the specimen to be released more easily and above all to check the integrity of the region distal to the biopsied matrix area. A transverse matrix biopsy is required for a band wider than 3 mm (Fig. 11).

If the pigment involves the upper portion of the nail, it is obviously difficult to use these two procedures to remove the source of melanin pigment because of anatomic reasons and the risk of secondary dystrophy, at least if the band is wider than 3 mm.

A rectangular block of tissue is excised, using two parallel incisions down to the bone. An L-shaped incision is carried back along the lateral nail wall, freeing this flap. The lateral section may then be rotated medially and approximated to the remaining nail segment (Fig. 12). If the band is wider than 6 mm or if the whole thickness of the

FIGURE 12
Longitudinal melanonychia. Rectangular monoblock excision associated with total nail flap permitted by L-shaped incision of the lateral nail wall.

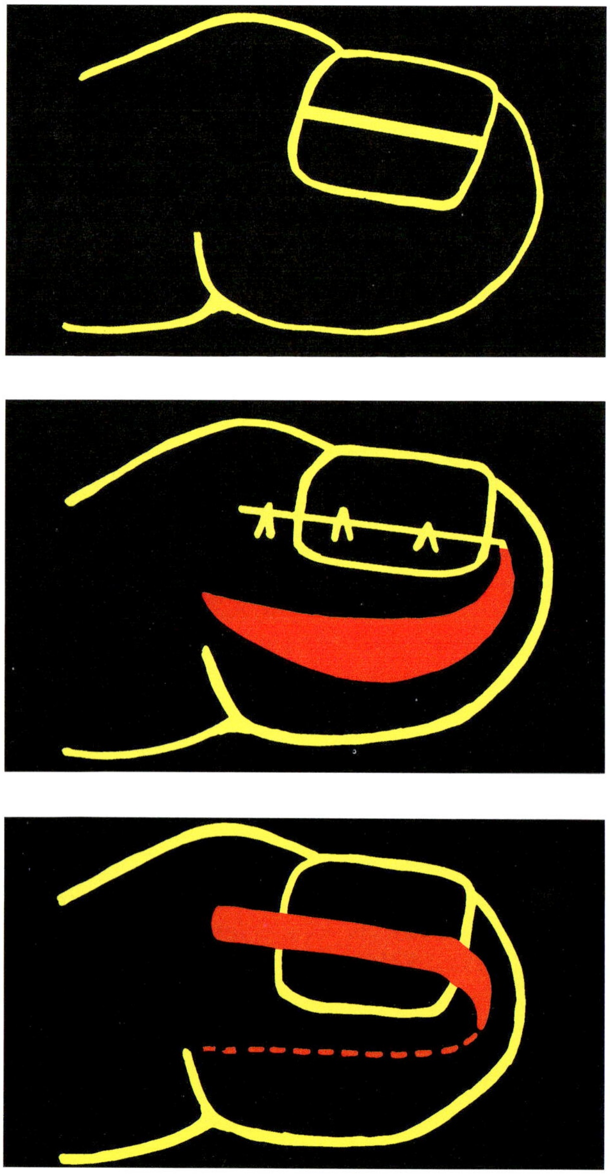

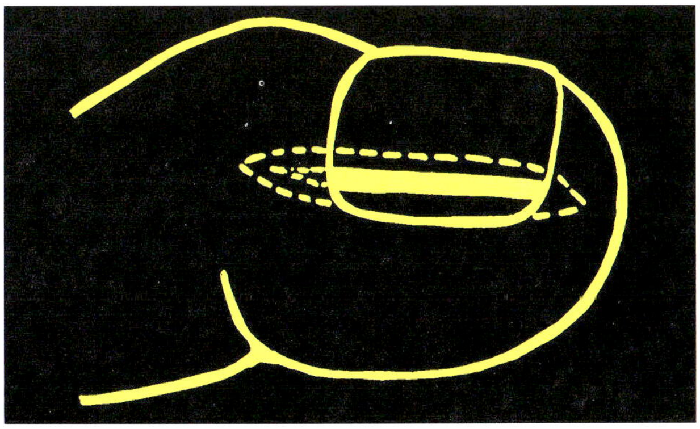

FIGURE 13
Longitudinal melanonychia. Lateral-longitudinal biopsy.

nail plate is involved by the pigment, surgical removal of the entire nail apparatus is the most logical method. If LM is accompanied by periungual pigmentation, removal of the entire nail apparatus is essential when pseudo-Hutchinson signs can be ruled out.

If the pigmented streak is located within the lateral third of either portion of the nail, a lateral-longitudinal biopsy is performed (Fig. 13).

SUBUNGUAL EXOSTOSIS

Subungual exostoses are mostly due to repeated trauma and are usually found on the big toe, although they may occur on any digit. They are painful and cause the nail to become heaped up and deformed. Treatment depends on the location and size.

Before the operation, a radiograph is mandatory, though this usually does not show the true extent of the exostosis since the lesion usually has a fibrocartilaginous cap. If necessary, the nail plate over the exostosis is partially removed and the skin is incised and dissected from the lesion, which is then removed with a bone rongeur or a chisel. Any excess of overstretched volar skin is removed before wound closure, but nail bed and matrix tissue is not excised (Fig. 14).

FIGURE 14
Subungual exostosis. (*a*) Before the operation. (*b*) Exostosis removed with a bone rongeur. (*c*) Wound closure. (*d*) Four months postoperatively.

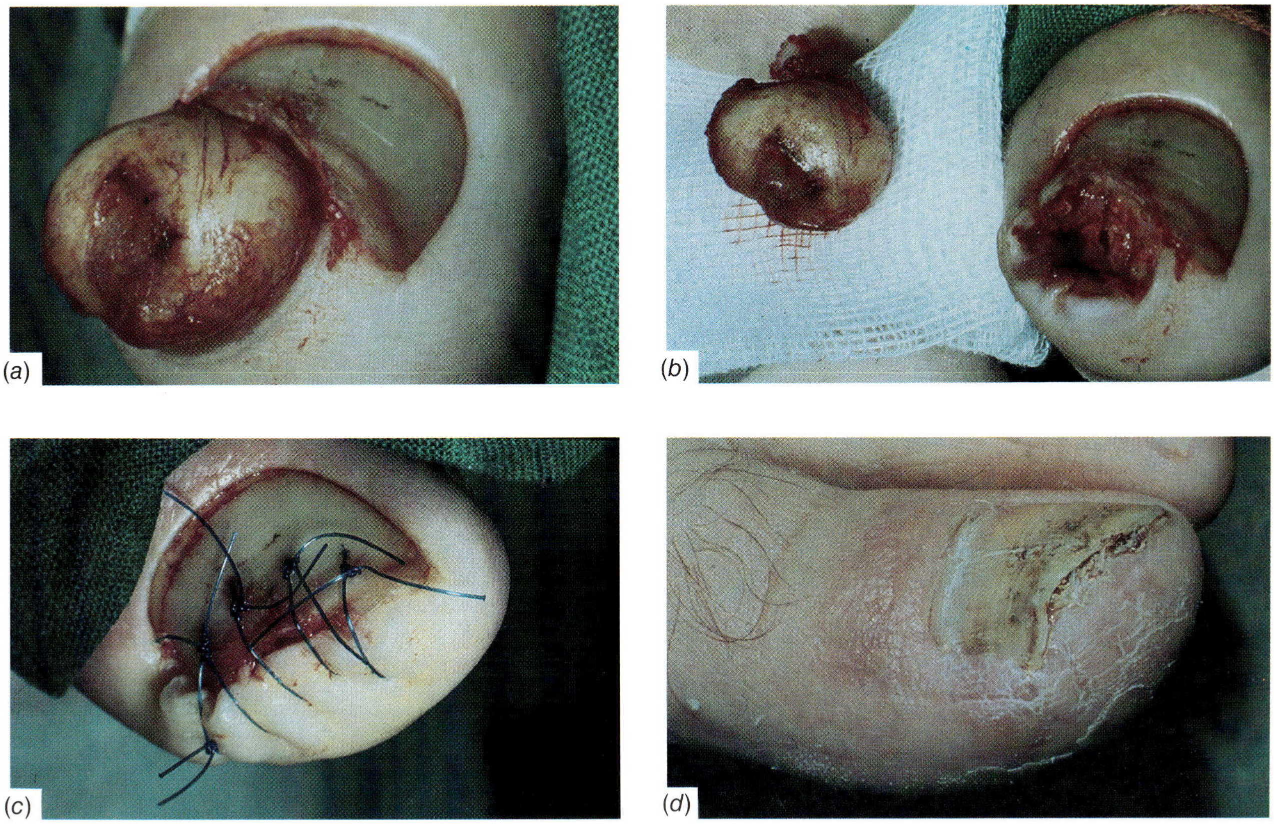

ONYCHOGRYPHOSIS

Onychogryphosis is seen mostly in elderly patients with foot deformities. However, it may develop in children, most often as a consequence of neglected malalignment of the hallux nails (Fig. 15). Onychogryphosis is usually associated with an enlarged matrix field and a tendency to vertical instead of horizontal nail growth so that the nail plate loses its cohesion with the nail bed. The nail bed in turn shrinks and undergoes epidermal metaplasia so that the nail plate never adheres again. Since attempts at decreasing the size of the matrix cannot reestablish normal nail growth, the nail has to be reduced in volume by repeated trimming and filing or be permanently eradicated. Nail trimming is greatly facilitated by softening the nail with 40% urea ointment under occlusion for about 48 h. Permanent nail eradication is best achieved by avulsion followed by cautery of the nail matrix, using liquefied phenol for at least 3 min in a completely bloodless field.

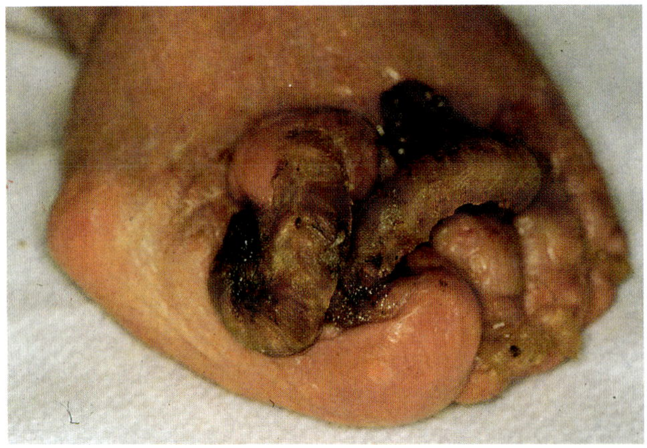

FIGURE 15
Onychogryphosis.

PACHYONYCHIA CONGENITA

This inherited malformation complex involves extremely thick, discolored, slow-growing nails on all digits. No conservative treatment is available. If treatment is sought, complete obliteration of the matrices is the only successful approach. We have found that phenol cautery is the simplest and most effective technique.

RACKET THUMBNAIL

A short, broad terminal phalanx of the thumb results in a short and wide nail plate that usually lacks lateral nail folds. The aesthetic appearance may be improved by narrowing the nail plate and creating lateral nail folds (Fig. 16).

Lateral-longitudinal nail biopsies are performed on both sides of the thumbnail. The lateral soft aspects of the distal phalanx are dissected from the bone, and back stitches are used to create lateral nail folds. The needle is run into the lateral aspect about 2 to 3 mm volar to the plane of the nail bed–bone interface, through the nail bed and plate, and back again through the lateral thumb skin, which

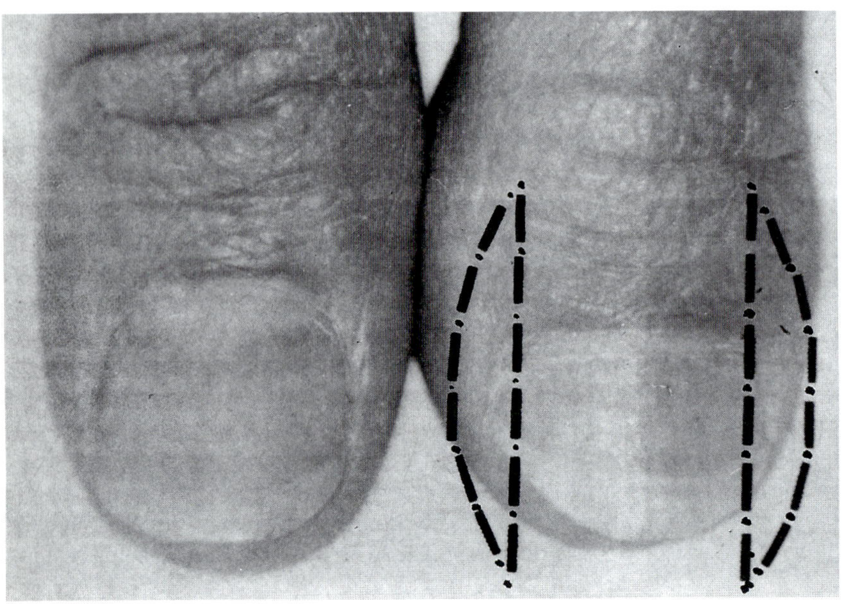

FIGURE 16
Racket thumbnail.

upon knotting will be elevated, thus forming a lateral nail wall. Sulcus epithelium develops by secondary intention.

CONCLUSIONS

Treatment of nail disease is important to many individuals because the hands are readily visible, and disfiguring nail changes will attract immediate notice, especially in individuals who use their hands for emphasis while speaking. Surgical therapy may be the most effective method of treatment for disfiguring nail changes. In most cases, the affected nail or nail component can be excised, leading to complete eradication of disease and excellent cosmetic results. Surgery is not effective in the treatment of disorders that arise because of biting or picking the nails or cuticles.

REFERENCES

1. Baran R, Dawber RPR. Guide médico-chirurgical des onychopathies. Paris: Arnette, 1990.
2. Dawber RPR, Sonnex T, Leonard J, et al. Myxoid cyst of the finger: Treatment by liquid nitrogen spray cryosurgery. Clin Exp Dermatol. 1983;8:153–155.
3. Haneke E, Baran R, Bureau H. Tumours of the nail apparatus and adjacent tissues, in Baran J, Dawber RPR (eds). Diseases of the Nails and Their Management. Oxford: Blackwell, 1984:403–452.
4. Bureau H, Baran R, Haneke E. Nail surgery and traumatic abnormalities, in Baran J, Dawber RPR (eds). Diseases of the Nails and Their Management. Oxford: Blackwell, 1984: 347–402.
5. Morkane AJ, Robertson RW, Inglis GS. Segmented phenolization of ingrowing toenails: A randomized controlled study. Br J Surg. 1984;71:526–527.
6. Baran R, Haneke E. Diagnostik und Therapie der streifenförmigen Nagel pigmentierung. Hautarzt. 1984;35:359–365.

PART

V

TISSUE INCREASES AND DECREASES

CHAPTER 26

Gelatin Matrix Implant and Collagen

JOHN M. YARBOROUGH
LARRY E. MILLIKAN

Not every scar needs surgical intervention. Irregularities that do not warrant such intervention can be reduced and the smoothness of minor residual defects can be enhanced by augmentation. In the past, peanut oil, paraffin, and olive oil were injected into the site to augment soft tissue, but intense local inflammation, granuloma formation, and even occasional systemic toxicity thwarted the continuing use of these agents. Silicone is effective, but its use has been limited by the relative inaccessibility and often unpredictable quality of the injectable material (see Chap. 27).

Approval by the U.S. Food and Drug Administration of purified reconstituted bovine fibrillar collagen (Zyderm I and II and Zyplast) in recent years and a gelatin matrix implant (Fibrel) in 1986 has led to the use of two relatively natural types of injectable materials that are biologically compatible with most human dermis. Both products are used to augment diminished or altered native collagen secondary to wrinkles and scars. Because each device "ages," as does the tissue into which it is implanted, periodic maintenance injections are necessary to sustain correction. Therefore, disproportionate disfigurement will not develop as the skin loses elasticity.

PURIFIED RECONSTITUTED BOVINE COLLAGEN

Three formulations of sterile injectable collagen—Zyderm Collagen Implants I and II (ZCI I and ZCI II) and Zyplast (ZI)—are currently in widespread clinical use. All three products are derived from solubilized purified bovine collagen whose antigenic telopeptide linkages have been enzymatically digested. In the final preparation, the reconstituted fibrils are suspended in neutralized phosphate-buffered saline containing 0.3% lidocaine. ZCI I and ZCI II differ only in their concentrations of collagen, with the former containing 35 mg/ml and the latter 65 mg/ml. The collagen content of Zyplast is the same as that of ZCI I except that the fibrils have been cross-linked by the addition of 0.0075% glutaraldehyde, theoretically reducing immunogenicity and increasing resistance to proteolytic degradation. All three formulations, which closely resemble human collagen, are supplied in tuberculin syringes, require refrigerated storage, and can be extruded intradermally through 30-gauge needles during outpatient visits.[1–4]

Injectable collagen therapy is not indicated for all lesions, and not all individuals are eligible for treatment with this material. Sharply marginated, punched-out ice-pick or pox scars are not amenable to correction with injectable filling agents, and collagen should not be implanted into sites of inflammation, induration, or infection. Patients with autoimmune disease, severe allergies, and sensitivity to lidocaine or bovine collagen should not be treated with injectable collagen. The safety of implantation during pregnancy and the suitability for use in infants and children have not been determined, and these products should not be used in immunosuppressed patients.

CHARACTERISTICS

Because bovine collagen implants were found to be immunogenic in approximately 3 percent of human recipients in the Zyderm clinical verification trials, a skin test of 0.1 ml of ZCI I is recommended. It is implanted into the volar aspect of the forearm 4 weeks before treatment with either formulation. Positive test responses may be local (2.4 percent) or local and systemic (0.4 percent), and 70 percent occur during the first 72 h. Localized reactions are characterized by erythema, induration, and infrequently pruritus (Fig. 1). Systemic symptoms include myalgia, arthralgia, and urticaria.[5–7] Since 1.3 percent of patients have had immune responses after the initial negative test dose and only 0.6 percent of patients have reacted after two negative skin tests, some physicians elect to perform two skin tests before the start of treatment (Table 1). Patients should be alerted, however, that 1 person in 100 will develop self-limited allergic reactions at sites of implantation during maintenance therapy (Figs. 2 and 3). Among those having localized hypersensitivity reactions, 90 percent have circulating antibodies against bovine collagen. The antibody response is species-specific and does not cross-react with other animal or

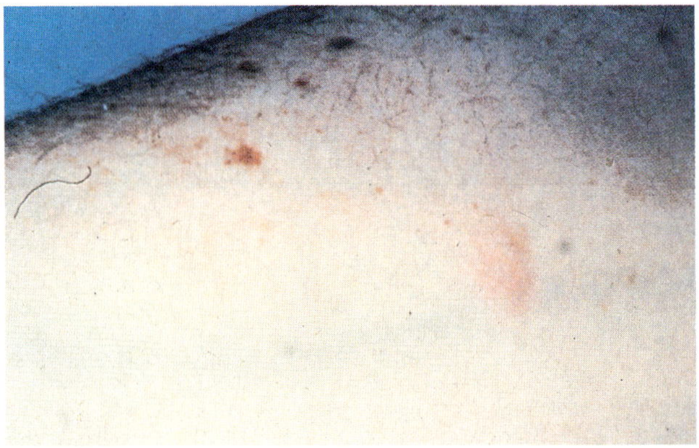

FIGURE 1
Erythema and induration as a local positive response to a skin test.

TABLE 1
ZYDERM COLLAGEN IMPLANT: INCIDENCE OF IMMUNE TYPE REACTIONS BY NUMBER OF EXPOSURES TO ZYDERM COLLAGEN IMPLANT

Exposure	Number	% of Those Reacting
First	284	90.1
Second	16	9.0
Third	7	0.4
Subsequent	8	0.5
Total	315	100.0

FIGURE 2
Improved contour and more youthful appearance 4 months after implantation of ZCI II and ZCI I.

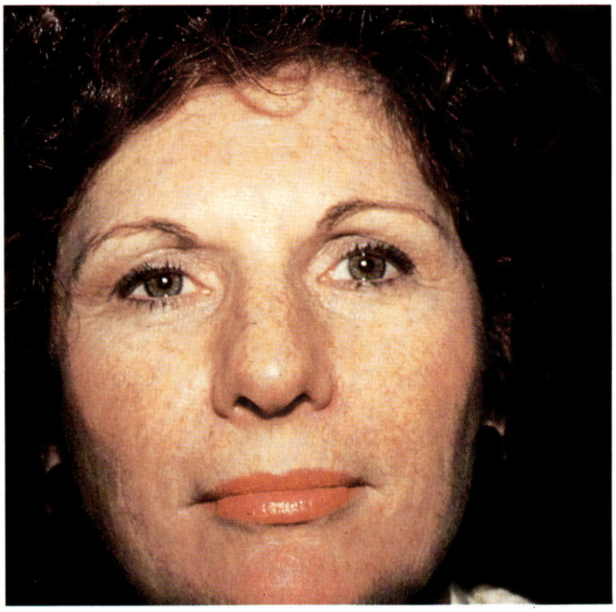

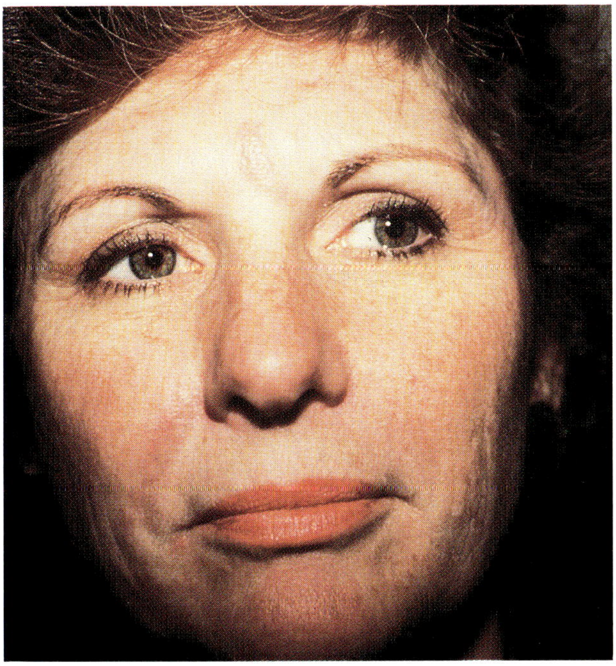

FIGURE 3
Erythematous, indurated ridges of 16 months' duration at sites of implants after the third series of injections.

human collagen. Patients who have systemic symptoms without local reactions show no evidence or circulating antibodies, and there is no correlation between the cumulative volume of injected collagen and the incidence of immune reactions (Table 2).

Certain adverse reactions at treatment sites are related to physical or mechanical rather than immunologic factors. Transient erythema secondary to multiple punctures often follows injection and subsides within several hours. Overcorrection with ZCI II or ZI usually causes persistent ridging or beading. Bruising and ecchymosis of several days' duration may result from trauma to superficial vasculature. Rarely, exercise, exposure to the sun, alcohol ingestion, and other causes of vasodilatation may precipitate transient, intermittent erythematous induration at implant sites that may recur for several months. Obstruction or laceration of a small vessel is the assumed cause of infrequent superficial ulceration and subsequent scar formation at the site of injection. A single case of unilateral blindness secondary to arterial occlusion is the only known systemic complication associated with injectable collagen.[8] No other reproducible statistically significant systemic complication, including various complaints of myalgia, arthralgia, and urticaria, has been verified to be caused by collagen implants.

TABLE 2
ZYDERM COLLAGEN IMPLANT: INCIDENCE OF IMMUNE TYPE REACTIONS BY VOLUME OF ZYDERM COLLAGEN IMPLANT

Volume Implanted cc's	Number	% of Those Reacting
⟨0.1⟩	284	90.1
⟨0.1–0.5⟩	2	0.7
⟨0.5–1.0⟩	8	2.3
⟨1.0–2.0⟩	10	3.3
⟨2.0⟩	11	3.5
Total	315	99.9

Persistence of correction depends on the type, degree, and location of the defect; the choice of material; the technique of injection; and the skill of the physician in the proper placement of the material.[8,9] Tissues in regions of greater mechanical stress, such as the glabellar and perioral areas, do not sustain correction as well as do scars on the middle to lateral cheeks, temples, and nose, where muscle movement is less.[10] Although ZCI I affords greater finesse in injection, it is modestly more transient than ZCI II and ZI. Regardless of the choice of device, maintenance will be necessary for between 4 months and 2 years. The "tunneling" technique that is sometimes used for the injection of silicone lacks the necessary sensitivity of multiple punctures to correctly place collagen. Physicians who lack the patience to master correct intradermal implantation will not appreciate the potential of this material in augmenting soft tissue and "fine-tuning" postoperative results. When the concept of maintenance is comprehended by patients, they regard the usefulness of injectable collagen therapy with the same appreciation that they have for the benefits of recurrent visits to beauty parlors or barbershops.

GELATIN MATRIX IMPLANT

The newest implant is Fibrel. Initial studies have been very promising for this new agent, which provides further flexibility for the dermatologic surgeon in selecting the most appropriate agent to use as a dermal filler. The product has been approved for the treatment of depressed cutaneous scars. Studies of this agent in the treatment of wrinkles have been done at many centers, but final approval for this indication has not yet been obtained from the U.S. Food and Drug Administration.

Historically, this agent was developed from original work with the use of fibrin foam. Fibrin foam has been available for many years as a hemostatic agent marketed under the trade name of Gelfoam (gelatin).[11] The powder form of this agent was used by Spangler as one of the original dermal fillers in 1957. It was mixed with pooled patients' plasma, preservatives, and thrombin at the Massachusetts General Hospital, Boston, and Spangler[12] reported good results injecting this material after local anesthetization. The implant technique was interesting in that the needle entry sites were the points of entry of an undermining lancet to free fibrous constricting bands in the depressed area, and the material was then injected into these spaces, elevating the depressed scars.

In 1975, Spangler reported the results of 17 years' experience.[13] This seemed to be a safe and effective technique with good to excellent results in 89 percent of the ungulating type of scars. There seemed to be minimal side reactions, which perhaps could have been anticipated from the long history of tolerance and safety with the use of Gelfoam.

The main impediment to the wider use of this product was the necessity of mixing the material and the fact that in its early use the correction apparently was short-lived. This product stimulated work with other collagens, ultimately resulting in the introduction of Zyderm in 1981, 6 years later. In the interim, Gottlieb,[14] who had learned the technique from Spangler, further modified and improved this fibrin foam implant and formulated the new name GAP. GAP repair technique evolved from 1975 to its ultimate final modification into Fibrel.[15]

Fibrel, or the gelatin matrix implant, consists of three major portions modified from the original GAP:

G = gelatin (Gelfoam), which provides a matrix for the interposition of clotting factors and ultimately neocollagen deposition

A = ϵ-aminocaproic acid, which is important in the clotting mechanism because it inhibits the formation of fibrinolysins and thereby allows a more permanent deposition of clot and subsequent collagen

P = patients' plasma, which provides an appropriate amount of fibrinogen

What happens in the space where this material is injected is a repetition of the normal clotting and wound-healing process, that is, deposition of clotting factors, formation of a fibrinogen clot, and proliferation of fibroblasts with subsequent deposition of neocollagen in the defect. It is thought by some that this rapid formation of native collagen assures the more permanent result that has been reported in the initial studies of this agent. The safety of this product seems very great when one considers that Spangler in 17 years of experience treating 7493 scars in 573 patients saw no allergic reactions and Gottlieb in 11 years of use of the modified GAP repair technique reported no allergic manifestations.

The recently approved Fibrel Gelatin Matrix Implant similarly has had a very low incidence of reaction. It comes in a kit which consists of a lyophilized mixture of 100 mg of absorbable gelatin powder, 125 mg of ϵ-aminocaproic acid (EACA), a vial of 0.9% NaCl, and syringes and tubes to obtain the patient's plasma. The gelatin EACA mixture is mixed with 0.05 ml of the patient's plasma and 0.05 ml of 0.09% NaCl. It is thoroughly mixed and homogenized and then used as the implant.

The multicenter study of the treatment of depressed scars with the gelatin matrix implant summarized the results from 22 centers from widely differing geographic areas that treated 288 patients with a total of 840 scars. Perhaps the most significant attribute of this product is its long-standing retention of scar correction. Using a standard technique nearly identical to that used with Zyderm II collagen, half the treated scars were shown within the limits of the study design to have an improvement of greater than 65 percent; most importantly, scar correction was maintained for 1 year. After 2 years the amount of correction still was very high.[16] The original study had limitations in that it allowed only two injections of the scar, minimizing the flexibility of correction by the dermatologic surgeon. Perhaps the most meaningful information derived from this study is the fact that this appears to be a very long lasting correction. This finding may constitute a major reason for its use in certain patients.

TECHNIQUE OF IMPLANT INJECTION

Collagen

Of all forms of injectable collagen, ZCI I affords the greatest finesse. Its versatility permits sensitive correction of tiny wrinkles, expression lines, crevices, areas of steroid atrophy, and distensible scars with smooth borders, whether derived from disease-induced, surgical, or accidental trauma (Figs. 4–10). Except for "crows-feet," which should be injected only to a normal contour, persistent elevation, lumpiness, and beading, which are predictable with superficial dermal placement of ZCI II or ZI, rarely occur after treatment with ZCI I. ZCI II and ZI are appropriate for augmentation of more prominent defects such as glabellar creases, nasolabial folds, oral commissures, and wider, deeper scars in which less than satisfactory correction can be achieved with ZCI I (Figs. 11 through 14). Like ZCI I, ZCI II, although more concentrated (65 mg/ml versus 35 mg/ml), disperses among host collagen.

After syneresis, the fibrils of ZCI I and ZCI II augment dermal deficiencies. As a lattice network, ZI is deposited in boluses that do not condense, and superficial placement produces obvious milia-like beading. With deeper dermal implantation of either ZCI II or ZI, ZCI I can be layered over to enhance finesse.

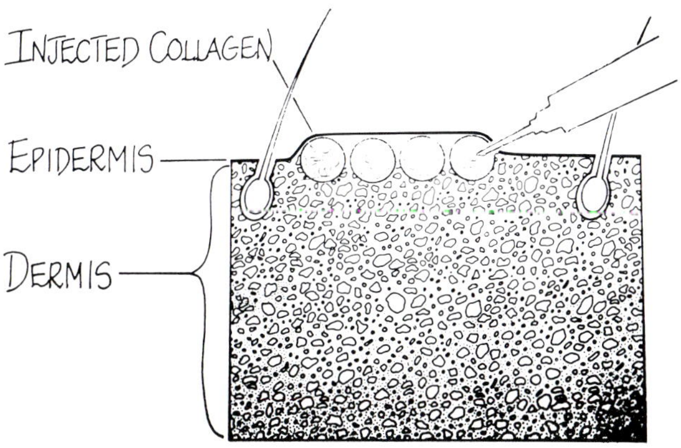

FIGURE 4
For continuity of "flow," collagen should be injected in serial but overlapping punctures with the bevel of the needle down.

FIGURE 5
Wrinkles and expression lines of the glabella; deep nasolabial folds secondary to aging.

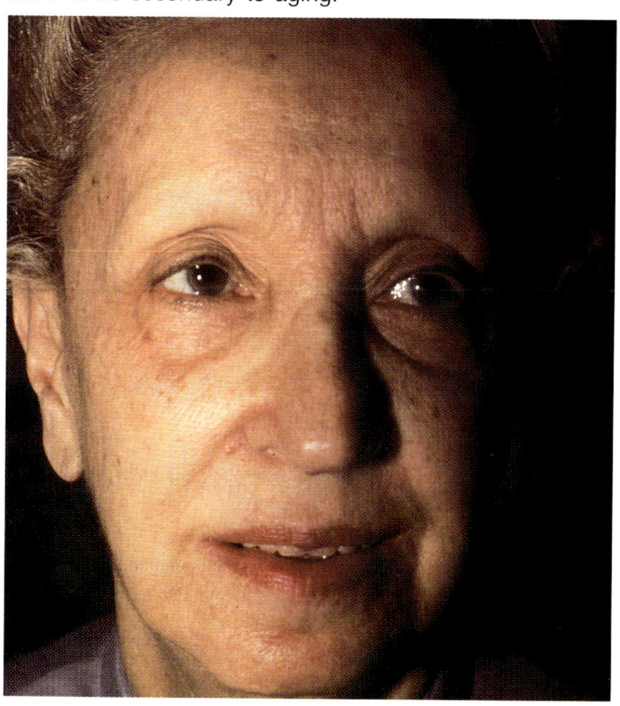

FIGURE 6
Smoother contours and more youthful appearance after the implantation of ZCI I.

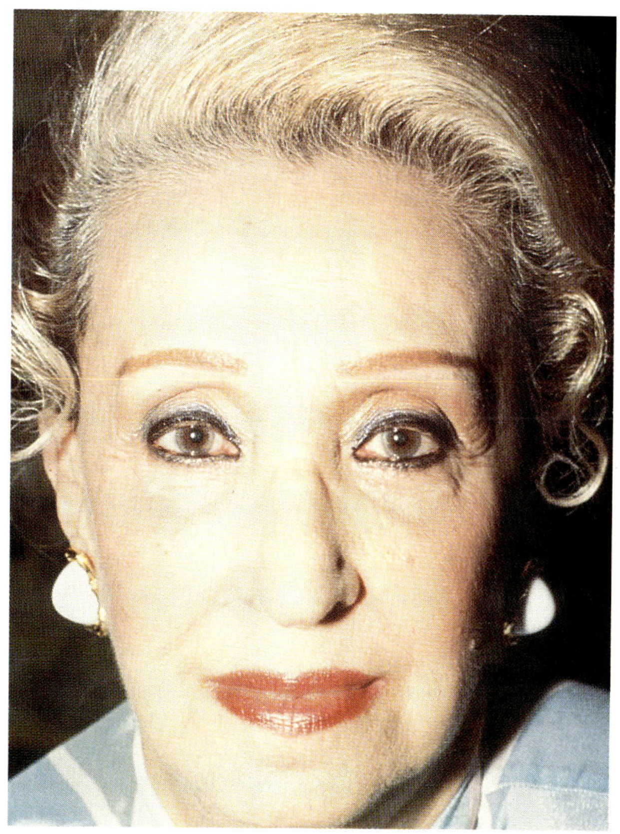

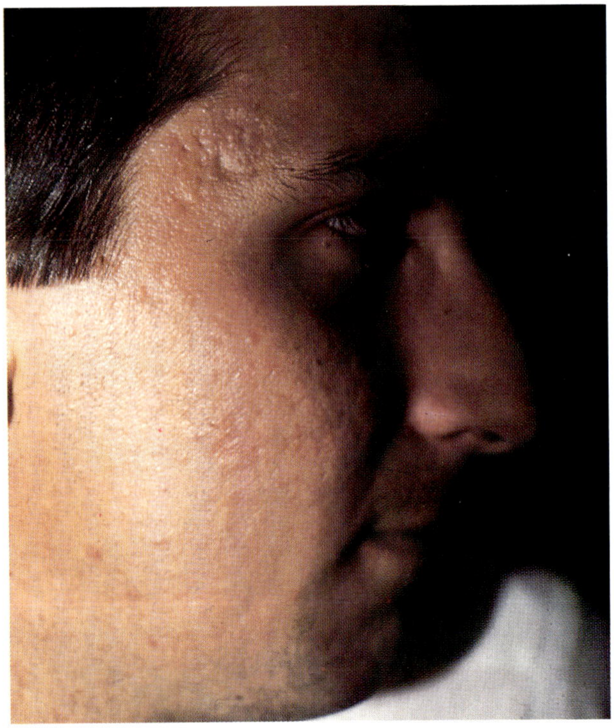

FIGURE 7
Prominent, distensible soft scars on the temple and cheek after acne.

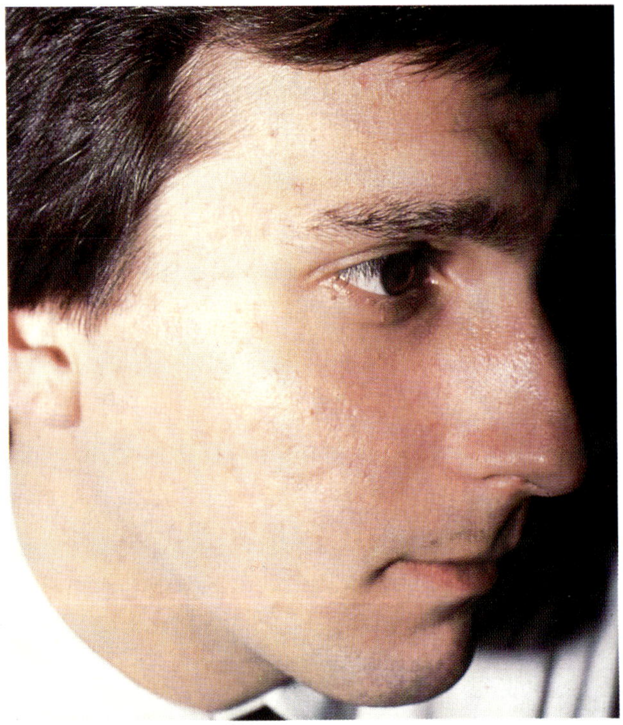

FIGURE 9
Improved contour of scars 1 year after the injection of ZCI I.

FIGURE 8
Transient erythema, which subsides after several hours, often follows multiple punctures. Note overcorrection with ZCI I.

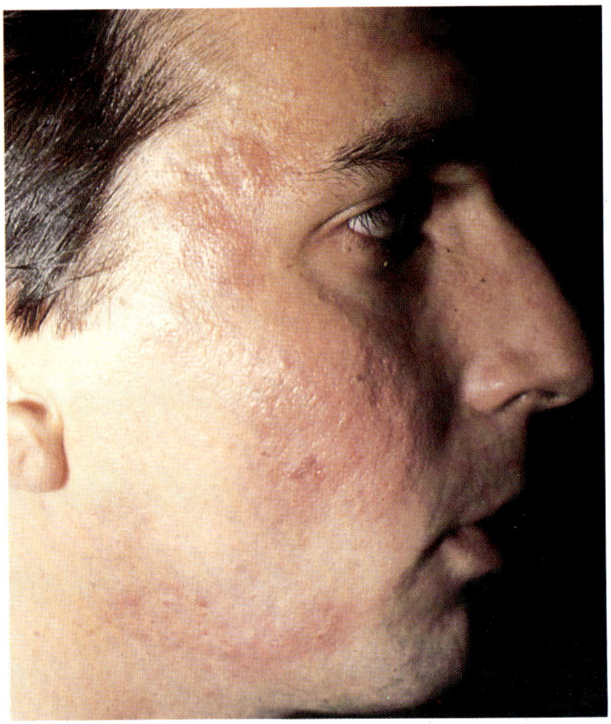

FIGURE 10
Redundant perioral folds of skin after rhytidectomy.

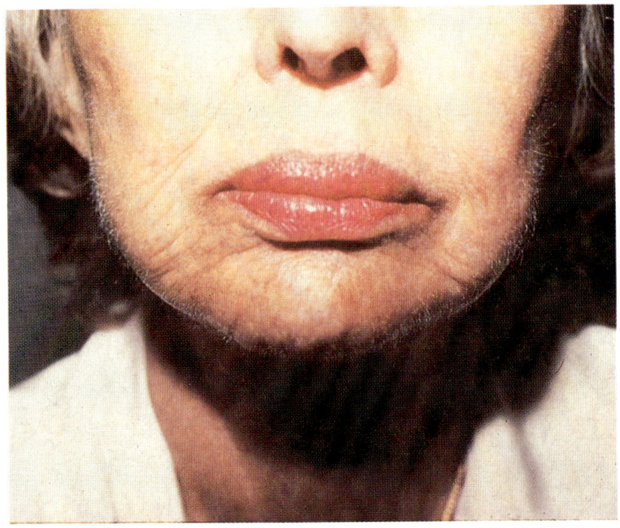

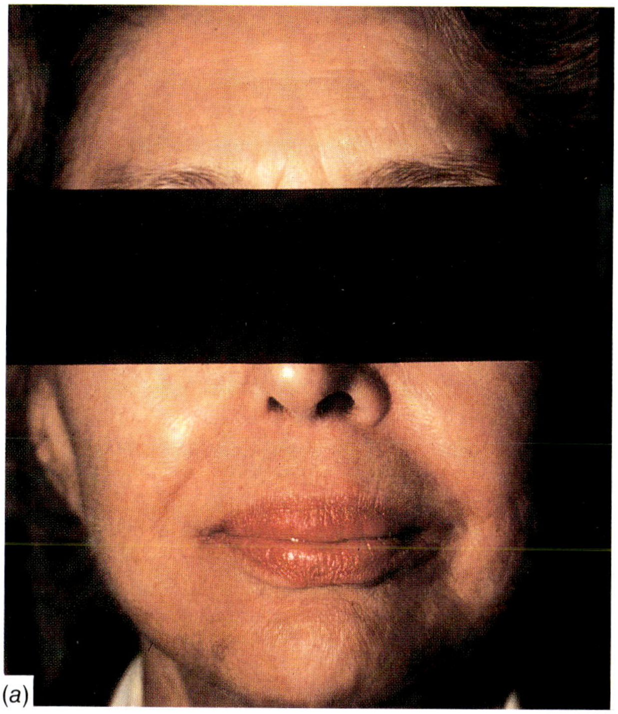

(a)

FIGURE 11
Sustained improvement 6 months after the implantation of ZCI I over ZCI II (*a–c*).

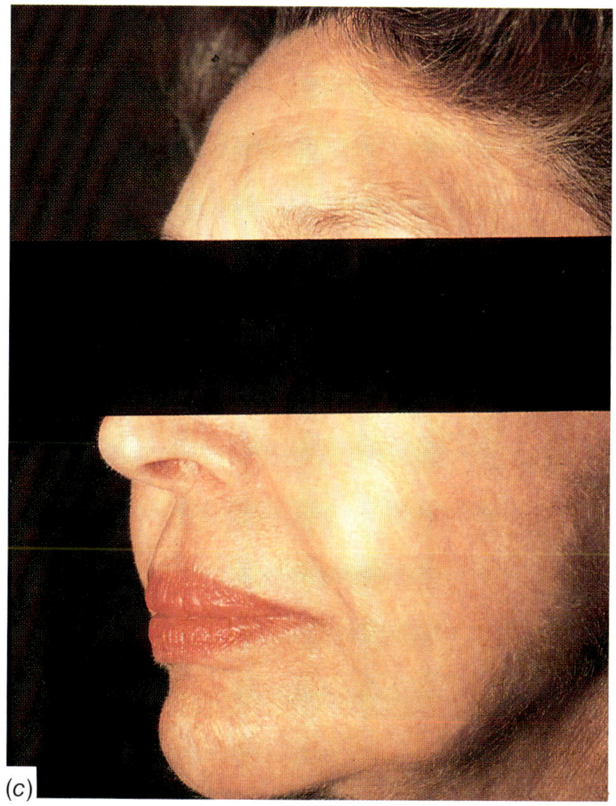

(c)

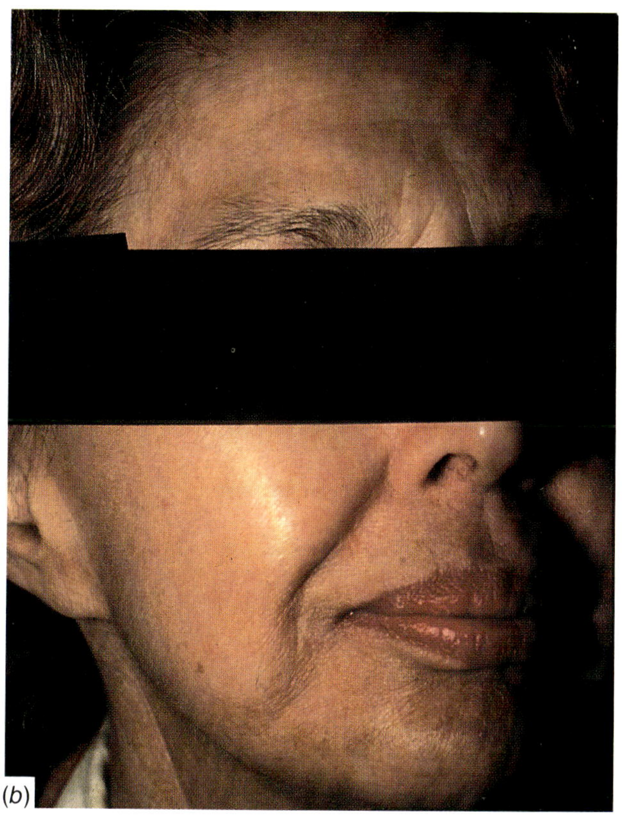

(b)

FIGURE 12
Full-face dermabrasion enhances texture and improves the facial surface contour in the border of a large scar which is not abraded.

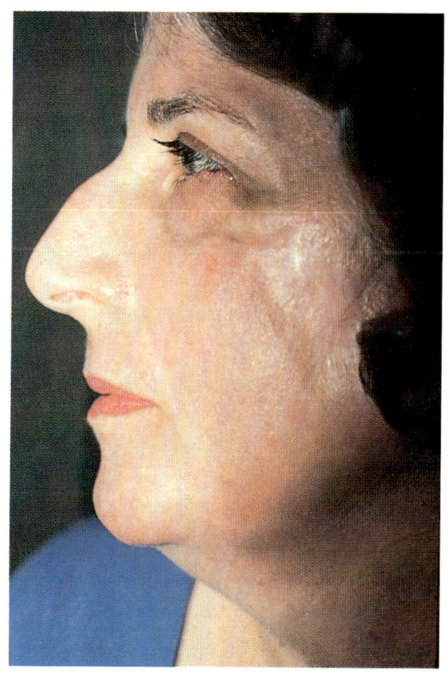

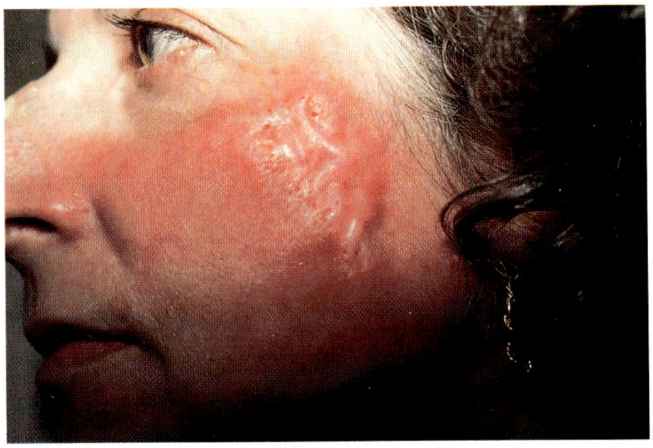

FIGURE 13
ZCI II is more appropriate for the augmentation of wider, deeper scars in which less than satisfactory correction can be maintained with ZCI I. Note transient erythema induced by injection.

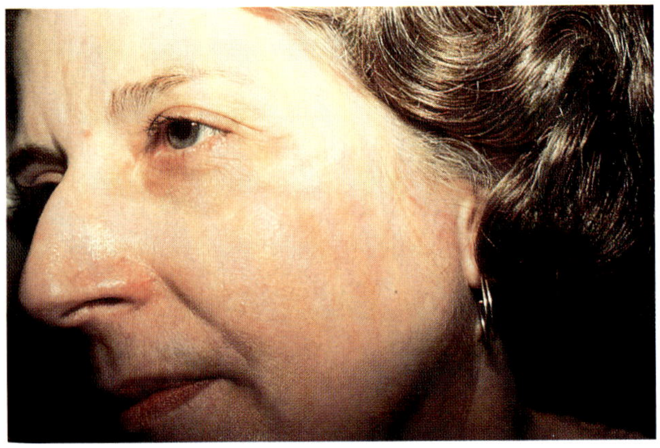

FIGURE 14
Sustained enhancement of facial contour after augmentation with ZCI II.

For continuity of placement, experienced physicians inject the material in serial but overlapping punctures with the bevel of the needle held downward. With the bevel up, an inordinate amount of collagen is extruded through the pores onto the skin during implantation. For optimal correction, ZCI I should be implanted very superficially in the dermis. Proper placement, which is characterized by simultaneous creation of blanche and wheal, is achieved by insertion of the needle at a 30-degree angle no deeper than the length of the bevel. Except in periorbital lines, overcorrection is essential with ZCI I to compensate for the saline, which is quickly absorbed.

ZCI II should be implanted in the mid to deep reticular demis with little or no overcorrection. ZI should be placed intradermally near the dermal-subdermal juncture with no overcorrection to avoid unsightly beading and persistent ridging. With each device a slight blanche and modest resistance during injection characterize dermal placement. For stabilization during implantation, the skin should be stretched or pinched by the free thumb and index finger.

Fibrel

The technique of injection essentially is the same as that used for ZCI II. The deeper injection site used for Zyplast generally is not the preferred one for the gelatin matrix implant. The depth of position of the collagen, however, can be varied somewhat depending on unique injection sites and the preferences of the dermatologic surgeon using the gelatin matrix implant. Within the Fibrel kit is a "custom needle" which we have found to be extremely useful as an undermining tool. This is a larger-gauge needle with a broad knifelike tip that allows dissection of some of the fibrous bands in the scar. This enables one to free the depressed epidermis more and to create a broader pocket for deposition of the implant.

Patients who have developed a sensitivity to bovine collagen may be able to use the gelatin matrix implant, which is primarily a porcine-based product. There have been no signs of potential problems with the use of the gelatin matrix implant in patients with collagen vascular disease, but one certainly would need to use extreme caution in treating patients with this type of history of immunologic hypersensitivity.

The ultimate place for Fibrel in the therapeutic armamentarium has not been determined. It may very well provide an alternative for patients who have proved to be sensitive to bovine collagen. It should be used in such patients with great caution. More important, the greater permanence of the correction may provide an important indication for its use.

PATIENT SELECTION

In choosing patients for injectable collagen therapy, the physician initially must assess the extent to which aging or scarring has occurred. Individuals whose facial wrinkles are expressed as generalized redundant folds will be improved optimally by a combination of surgical procedures such as rhytidectomy, blepharoplasty, dermabrasion, and chemical peeling. If necessary, minor residual flaws may then be enhanced with a modest volume of collagenous filling material. If expression lines, pronounced nasolabial folds, glabellar grooves, and perioral rhytids are superimposed on a setting of relatively elastic skin, augmentation with injectable collagen can often produce the desired improvement.

Most physicians who are experienced in the proper placement of collagen believe that nearly total correction of these wrinkles and furrows can be attained with the proper technique. Faces that are marred by profusions of deep undulating scars or multitudes of soft distensible scars with rounded margins and low width/depth ratios should be dermabraded, sometimes more than once, before collagen is offered for maximal enhancement. Patients who present with modest regional scars that hardly justify full-face dermabrasion may be improved by augmentation alone. Surgical scars, particularly those secondary to Mohs chemosurgical extirpation and repair of harelip and those which become depressed after excision of neoplasms are optimally improved if they are abraded before they become organized approximately 8 weeks after injury. Older scars, however, can be improved, although to a lesser degree.

Other contour defects not associated with age or scars may be amenable to correction by injections of collagen. Sunken cheeks may be enhanced remarkably, and lips whose vermilions are barely perceptible with the mouth closed can be given improved substance and definition with collagenous implants (Fig. 15).

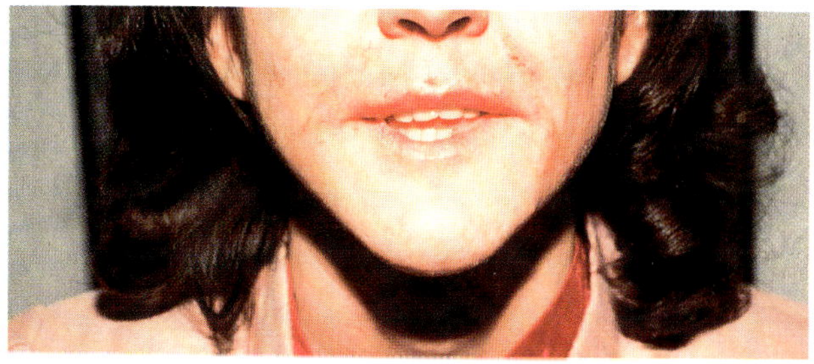

FIGURE 15
Upper vermilion with improved substance and definition after ZCI II.

CONCLUSIONS

Patients who request injectable collagen therapy must be counseled about the relative safety, precautions, and contradictions of the material; realistic expectations; the need for pretreatment skin tests and the statistical potential for later immunologic reactivity; longevity of effect; necessity for maintenance therapy to sustain correction; and economic considerations of probable cost.

Because treatment is entirely cosmetic, it should be rendered only if and when the deficiency or deformity is a problem to the patient, but the physician should inform the patient of its availability. As more surgeons become familiar with this agent, its final role in therapeutics will undoubtedly become clearer.

Bovine collagen implants are effective agents whose minimal toxicity is rare, local, and temporary. No associated systemic problems have been identified after years of extensive intercontinental use. The major concern with current formulations is the rate of degradation after placement in tissue. The development of analogs that afford greater longevity of correction will be welcome.

REFERENCES

1. Yarborough JM. The treatment of soft tissue defects with injectable collagen. Am J Med Sci. 1985;290:28–31.
2. Stegman SJ. Current status of zyderm collagen implants, in Callen JP, et al. (eds) Current Issues in Dermatology. Boston: GK Hall, 1983:255–268.
3. Klein AW. Implantation techniques for injectable collagen: Two-and-one-half years of personal clinical experience. J Am Acad Dermatol. 1983;9:224–228.
4. Parish LC, Witkowski JA. Collagen implants: Soft tissue augmentation. Int J Dermatol. 1985;24:499–504.
5. Swanson NA, Stoner JG, Siegle RJ, et al. Treatment site reactions to Zyderm collagen implantation. J Dermatol Surg Oncol. 1983;9:377–380.
6. Cooperman L, Michaeli D. The immunogenicity of injectable collagen: II. A retrospective review of seventy-two tested and treated patients. J Am Acad Dermatol. 1984;10:648–651.
7. Siegle R, McCoy J, Shade W, et al. Intradermal implantation of bovine collagen. Humoral response associated with clinical reactions. Arch Dermatol. 1984;120:183–187.

8. Written communication, Collagen Corporation.
9. Knapp TR, Vistnes LM. The augmentation of soft tissue with injectable collagen. Clin Plast Surg. 1985;12:221–225.
10. Nicolle FV. Correction of age- and disease-related contour deficiencies of the face. Aesthetic Plast Surg. 1985;9:159–162.
11. Bailey OT, Ingraham FD. Chemical, clinical and immunologic studies on the products of human plasma fractionation: XXI. The use of fibrin foam as a hemostatic agent in neurosurgery: Clinical and pathological studies. J Clin Invest. 1944;23:591–596.
12. Spangler AS. New treatment for pitted scars: Preliminary report. Arch Dermatol. 1957;76:708–711.
13. Spangler AS. Treatment of depressed scars by fibrin foam injection. Acta Derm Venereol. (Stockh) 1957;suppl. II:526–530.
14. Gottlieb SK. Soft tissue augmentation: The search for implantation materials and techniques, in Millikan LE (ed) Clin Dermatol. 1987;5:(4)128–134.
15. Millikan LE, Rosen T, Monheit G, et al. Treatment of depressed cutaneous scars with gelatin matrix implant: A multicenter study. J Am Acad Dermatol. 1987;16:1155–1162.
16. Millikan LE, et al. Long term safety and efficacy with Fibrel in the treatment of cutaneous scars: Results of a multicenter study. J Dermatol Surg Oncol. 1989;15:837–842.

CHAPTER

27

Silicone

DAVID M. DUFFY

The term *silicone* was coined to describe a large family of polymers which contain the element silicon. These polymers, whose viscosity is a function of their degree of polymerization, exist as solids, gels, and even liquids. Silicones are generally considered to be biologically inert and structurally unaltered by exposure to a wide range of environmental conditions.

Silicones are utilized for a number of medical purposes. As lubricants, they coat hypodermic needles and line intravenous tubing. As antiflatulants, they are ingested as components of proprietary antacids. Fluid silicone is injected into the human eye for the treatment of some ophthalmologic disease.[1] Solid silicones are routinely implanted in the human body as orthopedic prostheses or nonantigenic envelopes for breast implants, which also may be filled with silicone gel.

The use of *liquid* silicone for soft tissue augmentation has provoked a prolonged, fervent, and profoundly emotional debate. Proponents of liquid silicone feel certain that pure liquid silicone, properly used in small volumes, is intrinsically safe and effective. They state that the misuse of silicone in high volumes containing adulterants, particularly in breast augmentation, has created a negative impression. Opponents of silicone use are equally certain that liquid silicone is intrinsically unsafe and have cited news stories that support their opinions. They also suspect that the advocates of silicones are not telling the whole truth.

UNDERSTANDING SILICONE REACTIONS

Lost in the passion of debate is the fact that not all silicone implants are used in the same way. The responses of biological systems to implanted foreign materials is subject to a legion of variables, including the following:

1. The surface area, volume, mass, and anatomical location of the implant.[1–3]
2. The surface and near surface atomic structure of

the implant and the outcome of the "race" between bacteria and host tissue cells to colonize "dangling bonds" on the same surface.[4]

3. The presence or absence of immunoreactive small molecules measuring 10 to 60 μm.[3]
4. The ability of the implant or its degradation products (silicone-silica)[3] to act as haptenes or adjuvants after host immunologic "processing" to produce immune disease, particularly in subjects with hereditary or environmental risk factors. Further complicating an understanding of the behavior of various implants is the fact that the histologic response to silicone elastomers is different from that for silicone liquid or gels; this difference has not been explained.[3]
5. An appreciation of the almost boundless complexity of implant bioreactivity mandates that each type of implant be individually evaluated in a *specific application* and *host*. An analysis of the behavior of one type of implant in one application will not necessarily be applicable to the behavior of other implants.

TYPES OF SILICONE IMPLANTS

Silicone breast implant shells contain 2, 3-dimercapto-1-propane sulfonic acid (DMPS) polymer and 30% silicone dioxide filler. The shedding of particles of the filler has been implicated in autoimmune phenomena and in phagocytosis and capsular contraction.[3]

Silicone Gels

These materials used in breast implants contain "troublesome impurities"[5] that may be involved in the production of capsular constrictures. Small quantities of the gel may "bleed" through intact envelopes or may cause autoimmune phenomena when massive volumes spill from ruptured implants with subsequent phagocytosis and dissemination throughout the reticuloendothelial and other systems.

Solid Silicone Implants

Elastomers, which are used in joint prostheses, also contain fillers and catalysts. The shedding of particulate matter from these devices has produced a newly described condition—*small particle synovitis*—characterized by inflammatory and erosive bone lesions following silicone arthoplasty.[3]

Pure Liquid Silicone

Pure liquid silicone, which consists solely of glucose-linked simethicone (dimethyl polysiloxane) DMPS polymer chains used in small volumes, is theoretically the least antigenic material for implantation. Several forms of this fluid are discussed below.

MDX 4-0411, used in extensive studies involving 1,400 patients followed for over 20 years, was developed for soft tissue augmentation by Dow Corning. Norman Orentreich coined the term *injectable-grade silicone* to describe a sterile DMPS fluid essentially of his own manufacture which appears to be the equivalent of MDX 4-0411.

Dow Corning medical grade 360 liquid silicone is a fluid that was never intended or authorized for soft tissue augmentation; however, it was sold in large quantities, unsterilized and often contaminated. It was used for soft tissue augmentation in human and animal studies as well as (occasionally in large volumes) for hemiatrophy without significant problems.[3,6] Several adverse reactions probably occurred following its use for breast and facial injections. The shedding or spallation of this fluid from hemodialysis pump tubing is known to cause severe hepatitis and pancytopenia, when large volumes of silicone particles engulfed by macrophages accumulate throughout the reticuloendothelial system.[7–9]

Dirty Silicone Fluids

A wide range of silicone fluids of differing viscosities were injected indiscriminately in large volumes into soft tissue, particularly the breasts.[1] Sudden death by intravascular embolization occurred in some cases. Delayed consequences, including massive necrosis, nodule formation, and ulceration secondary to pressure-induced vascular lymphatic compromise or migration of fluid to sites distant from the areas originally injected, occurred after months to years.[1]

Many adulterated silicones were created; for example, the Sakarai formula contained 1% olive oil. Many other materials masquerading as silicone or containing liquid silicone along with contaminants and adulterants were also implanted. Orentreich compiled lists of these substances, which include linseed oil, flax oil, and fatty acids.[1]

Paraffins have been used to loosen tight scalps. Months to years after use, nodules, plaques, and ulcerations have developed in sites where the paraffin was injected.

GUIDELINES TO UNDERSTANDING LIQUID SILICONE

Background

When evaluating reports dealing with silicones, one should disregard those in which "high volumes" or silicones of unknown purities were used. Reports in which Dow Corning 360 medical grade silicones were implanted also should be disregarded, along with reports by "authorized investigators" who injected the breasts. (No one was authorized to inject the breast during a 20-year FDA-monitored study.)

One must again remember that an understanding of the behavior of solid implants or silicone gels or membranes in specific applications will not necessarily be applicable to the behavior of silicone liquid in different and equally specific applications.

The following questions should be asked.

1. How many patients have been treated with liquid silicone using the Orentreich protocol, and what were the benefits? How many documented adverse reports are available, and how were they explained.
2. Why do adverse reports involving silicone seem to be so much more numerous, dramatic, and memorable than beneficial reports?
3. Is there evidence that advocates of liquid silicone use are concealing the truth? Why has liquid silicone not been released for private use?

The answers to these questions are as follows:

1. Over 1400 patients were monitored by the FDA in a 20-year study involving a number of authorized investigators using Dow Corning MDX 4-0411. In that study, only two documented serious adverse reactions were reported (one case of migration and one case of necrosis). In another recent review[10] involving over 100,000 patients, no serious reactions were reported, although several reports[1,2] have suggested that adverse reaction "granulomas" and "idiosyncratic reactions" have occurred in at least 1 of 10,000 patients treated.[1]
2. Bad news sells newspapers and provides memorable reading. A careful review of the literature reveals only a handful of credible scientific or lay reports in adverse reactions.[2,11] If one eliminates reports in which clear improprieties occurred involving the use of liquid silicone, one must agree with Orentreich's characterization of silicone as "the safest material I have used in the treatment of over 100,000 patients."[10]
3. Certain theoretical considerations and evidence appearing in newspapers, FDA reports, and meetings suggest that the uncritical belief that pure DMPS cannot produce immunologically mediated events is not entirely correct. The fact that "no antibodies have ever been reported to pure silicone"[1] does not take into account more recent immunological knowledge. A certain vagueness can be seen in reports in which advocates discuss rare reactions.[1,2] In brief, DMPS is not perfect but appears to be very safe. Liquid silicone has not been released because the Dow Corning Corporation "could not effectively prevent its misuse,"[10] although it was found to be safe and effective.[12]

Patient Evaluation

Patients must understand that silicone is not perfect, it has not been approved by the U.S. Food and Drug Administration (FDA), and rare side effects consisting of lumps, granulomas, color changes, and intermittent swelling can occur, sometimes years after use. Patients who have recurrent or chronic systemic or localized infections and those with a personal or family history of immune disorders may be at greater risk for such side effects. Patients also should be told that multiple treatments will be necessary and that only small volumes of silicone can or should be employed slowly, usually at 6- to 8-week intervals (minimum 2 weeks). Patients should be told that silicone lasts forever but that as they age, the tissue around the silicone may shrivel, leaving small lumps. Accordingly, complete correction is not attempted.

The most suitable areas for correction of wrinkles are the nasolabial and glabellar creases; however, a patient who has a large, sagging cheek adjacent to the groove is not an ideal candidate for treatment. Horizontal forehead grooves that result from constant lifting of the brows are also usually unsuitable. Ridges commonly occur lateral to the injected area. Periorbital tissue ("crows' feet"), is often a poor choice because it is too distensible. It is often appropriate to use Zyderm several months before silicone to determine the patient's response.

METHOD OF IMPLANTING LIQUID SILICONE

After explaining the procedure to the patient and cautioning the patient that no aesthetic method is a cure-all, the physician cleans the area with alcohol. Anesthesia can be provided by local infiltration, nerve blocks, or topical freezing. Required equipment includes a Luer-lock syringe and a 30-gauge needle for the injection.

Three methods of deposition are recommended. In the *fanning* technique, the needle is injected subcutaneously and then rotated to be parallel to the skin surface. Minute amounts of silicone are deposited. Overcorrection should be avoided. The interval between treatments is generally 4 to 6 weeks, with touch-ups recommended every 6 to 12 months. The *microdroplet* technique involves subdermal deposition. The needle is held almost perpendicular to the surface, and the material is injected at close intervals. Finally, the silicone can be *tattooed* in by rapid puncturing of the skin.

Personal Experience with Implantable Liquid Silicone

During a 6-year period, I treated over 2,000 patients with injectable silicone, following the criteria for its use outlined by established authorities. To date, my experiences have mirrored the results presented by other advocates of its use. Over 95 percent of all patients were satisfied with the results, and some, particularly those with atrophic scarring, were very pleased. Those who were not pleased were generally impatient with the rate of improvement.

Areas Treated

Excellent results, as shown in Figs. 1–3, were obtained with saucer-shaped, pliable depressions the base of which could be elevated flush with the cutaneous surface by the application of gentle traction, i.e., groove-like scars and nasolabial and glabellar creases. Treatment of deep oral commissures and reduced salivary incontinence has also been successful. The results were much less satisfactory with fibrotic or varicelliform scars, and overcorrection or beading (i.e., a lump was substituted for a depression) occurred when silicone was injected into tissue that was tightly attached to muscle or bone, particularly on the forehead or nose. In these areas, silicone must be used with great caution.

Adverse Reactions

Transient erythema, edema, and bruising are common reactions; occasionally the bruising is persistent. Four patients noted overcorrection involving the rhytid of the upper lip, which responded satis-

FIGURE 1
(*a*) A middle-aged woman had plastic surgery following trauma. (*b*) Twenty months later, her appearance significantly improved as a result of silicone augmentation.

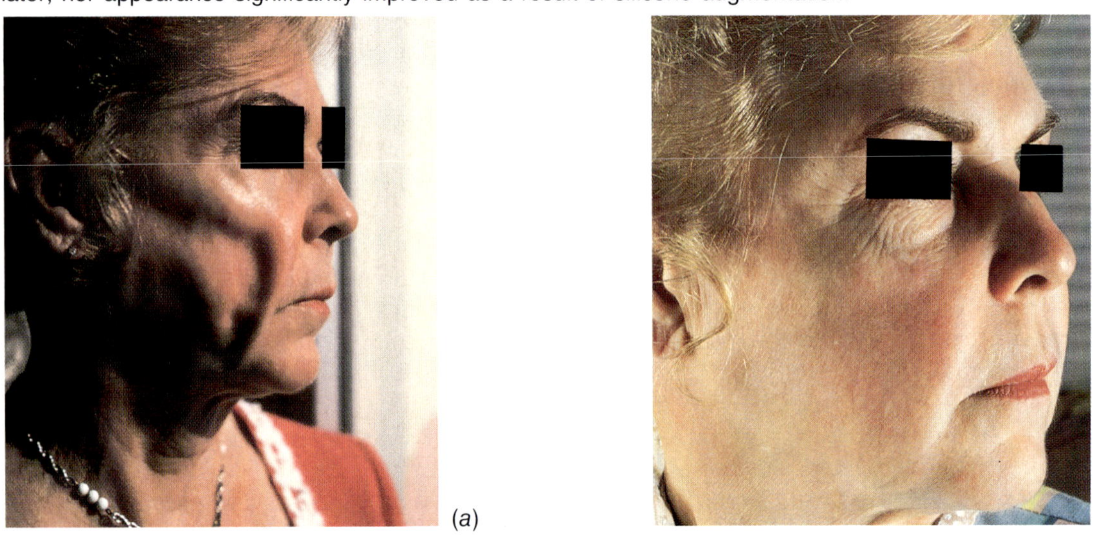

(*a*) (*b*)

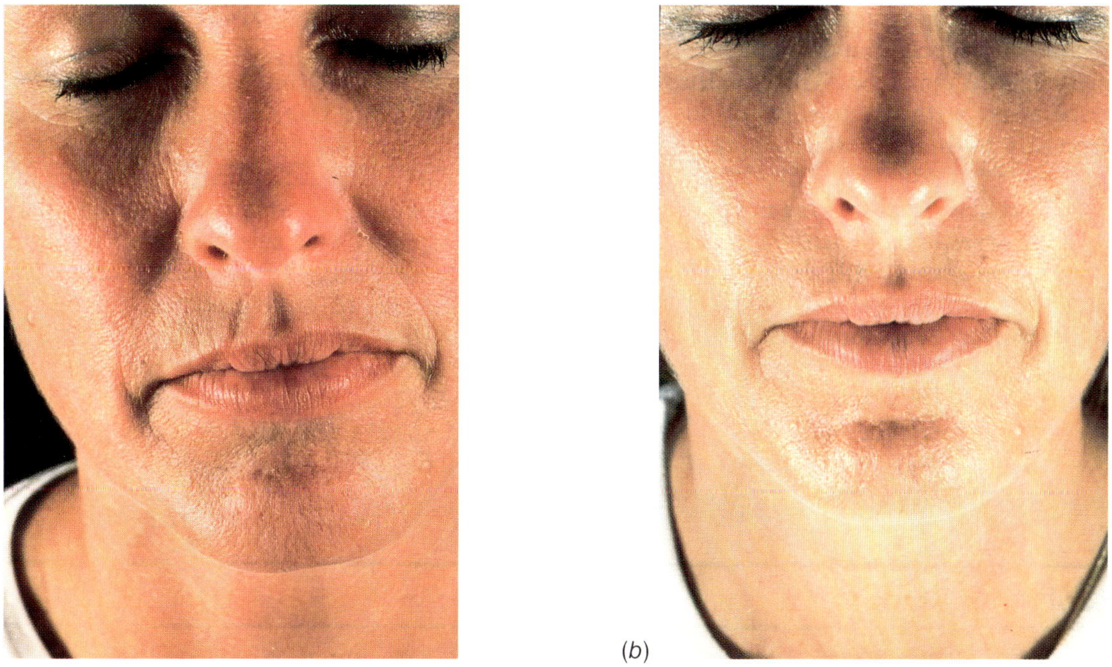

(*a*) (*b*)

FIGURE 2
(*a*) After a dog bite, this patient underwent silicone injections. (*b*) Four months later, there was significant improvement.

FIGURE 3
(*a*) The deep furrows on this man's face responded to repeated injections of silicone (*b*) over an 11-month period.

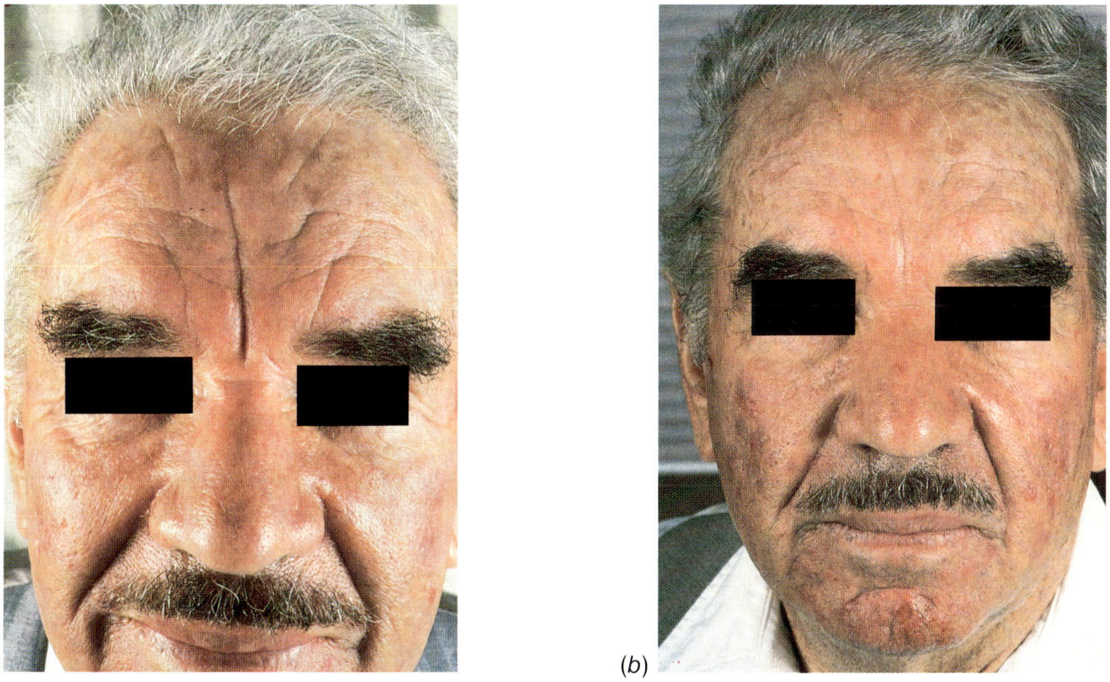

(*a*) (*b*)

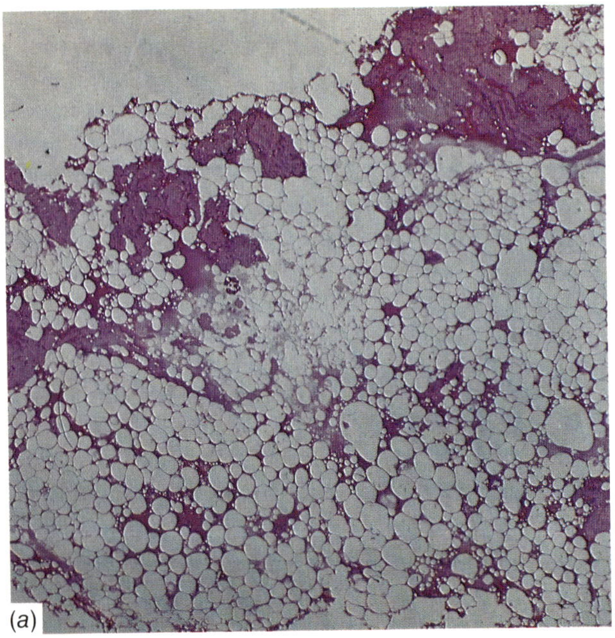

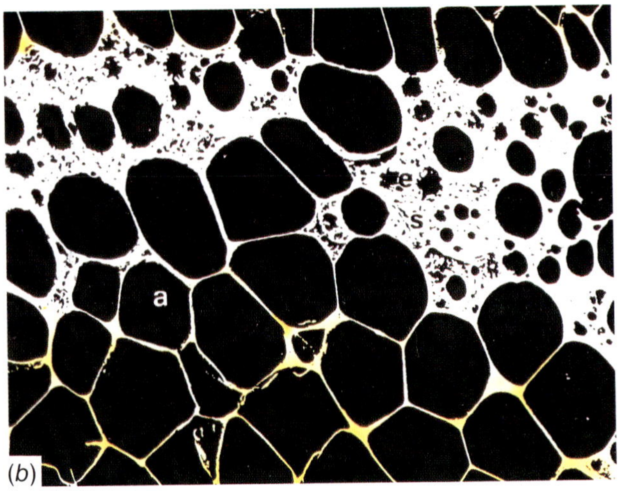

FIGURE 2
(*a*) Fat cylinder obtained with a 14-guage needle mounted on a syringe; low magnification. (*b*) Histology of a fat sliver under high magnification, showing the undamaged cells.

and have tension and pressure wrinkles; others age interiorly (tissue involution) and have sag and shrinkage wrinkles. With exterior aging, face-lift and reduction lipoplasty are necessary. With interior aging, one should replace the tissue loss with fat, the first injectable contour builder. Tissue involution involves hypotrophy not only of fat but also of muscle, bone, etc. Fat is the only tissue which can be replaced with an injectable technique.

Because fat tissue is a semi-fluid, it is the only tissue that can be replaced with an injectable technique. As with older open techniques, this new closed procedure will not change the amount of fat which will take. In fact, it will not only eliminate unnecessary scarring but will facilitate the procedure to such an extent that the patient will not be as hesitant to undergo the procedure again when necessary.

Fat removed with a suction machine should not be used, as it is damaged by the vaporization of the tissues and is manipulated to be placed into a syringe before being reinjected with a small needle. Fat which has not been damaged through suction is damaged because it is inserted with a small needle. Moreover, contact with the air may disturb the sterility of the fat.

New techniques of fat transfer have brought about advances in many areas of aesthetic surgery, such as the *face fill*, which we initiated in 1985. A face fill involves the implantation of autologous adipose tissue for cosmetic purposes such as rejuvenation and embellishment and for nonpathological indications that should be treated without hypercorrection. The adipose tissue is harvested and implanted using a closed technique. See Fig. 2. The instrument used for the harvest is a needle, a cannula, or a trocar of variable diameter and length mounted on a disposable syringe.

TECHNIQUE FOR FACE FILLS

We do face fills using two procedures. We start by using a 14-gauge needle mounted on a 2-ml insulin syringe, as in Fig. 3. The fat is extracted after infiltration with lidocaine 1% and adrenaline 1:200,000. To avoid unnecessary trauma to the fragile adipose tissue, we feel that it is better to avoid local anesthesia, which may cause hydrolical trauma from the injection and chemical trauma from the lidocaine and adrenaline. The fat should be harvested under general, twilight or block anesthesia, or cryoanesthesia. The total amount needed for each procedure is taken at the same time. The areas to be injected are marked after discussion with the patient. It is possible to inject several spots in the area of the head: glabella, temples,

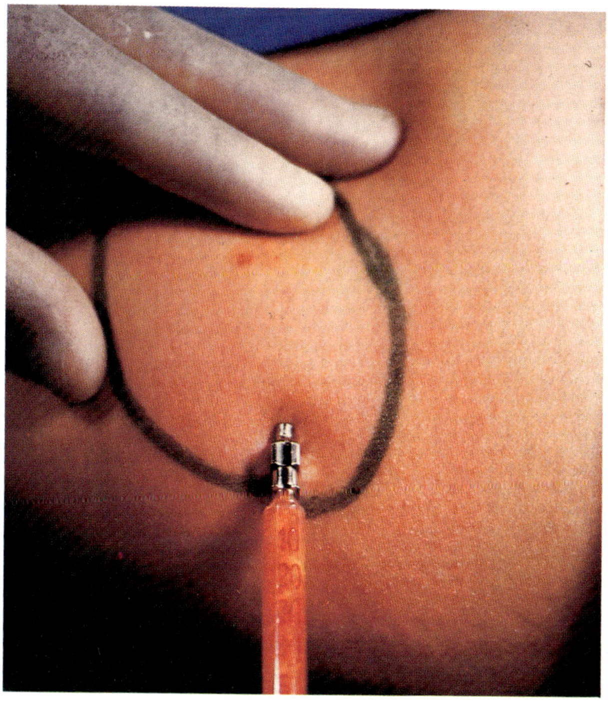

FIGURE 3
Fat slivers are easily obtained with a 14-gauge needle mounted on a 2-ml insulin syringe.

cheekbone, cheeks, nasolabial folds, upper and lower lips (red and white), chin, parotid gland area, or angles of the jaw. See, for example, Figs. 4 and 5. An estimate of the amount of fat needed is made beforehand. For each place we inject 2 to 6 ml of fat slivers obtained with a 14-gauge needle. The site where the injection is to be performed is anesthetized locally, or conventional blocks of the sensory nerves of the face are performed (intraorbital, supraorbital, mental nerve). We prefer a block or no injection at all or, when necessary, twilight or general anesthesia as shown in Fig. 6. The face is then refrigerated with ice cubes.

To reinject the fat slivers, we use the same 14-gauge needle used for extraction. A retrograde injection is performed, generally using one approach. The fat has to be distributed evenly, using a fan-shaped movement. When the retrograde injection is done, the same fan-shaped motion should be used. After the injection, the tissues are gently remodeled with the fingers. Nasolabial folds are remodeled by placing one finger in the vestibule. We immobilize the cheekbone area and the chin for 48 h.

The operation does not last more than 1 h and is

FIGURE 4
Injection in the cheekbone area: cheek and nasolabial fold. Injection of 22 ml.

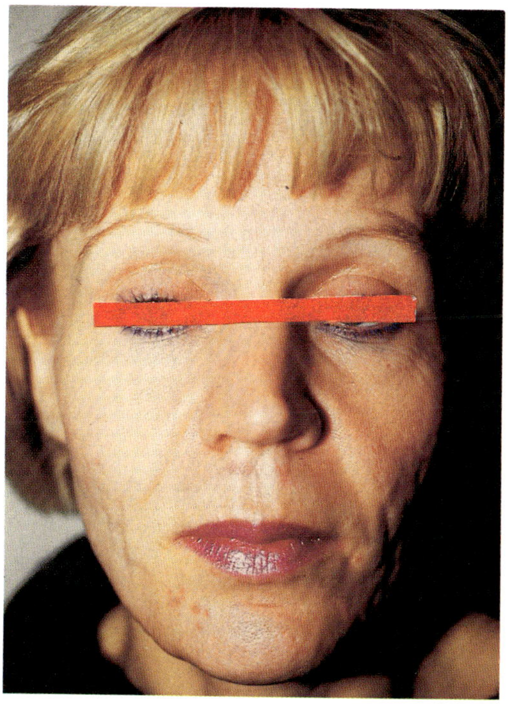

FIGURE 5
The same patient 12 months later.

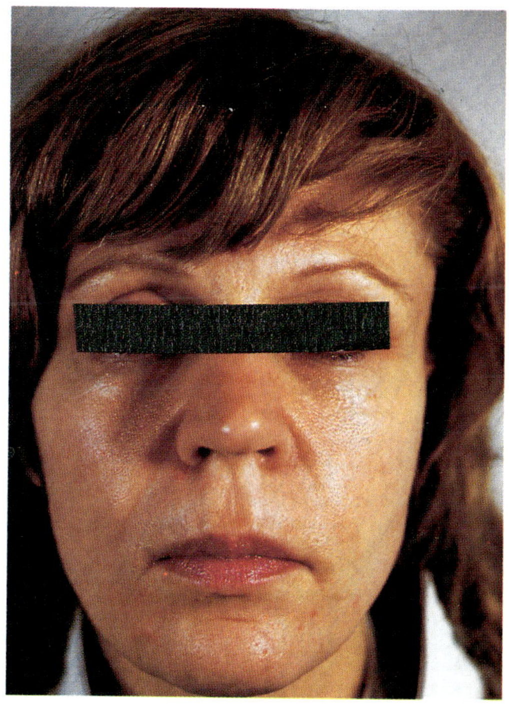

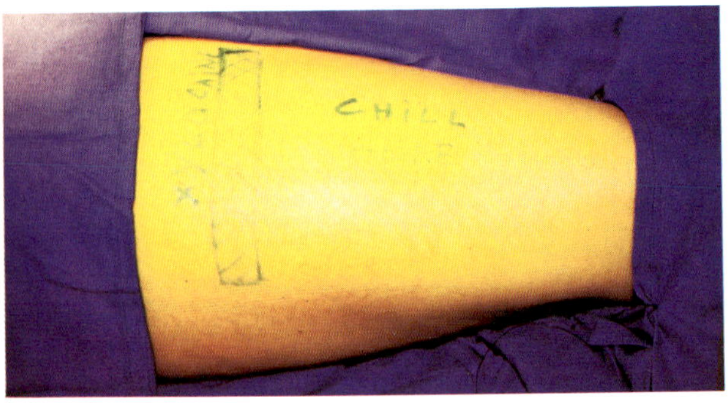

FIGURE 6
A block on the anterior thigh associated with external cryoanesthesia allows the use of a dry technique.

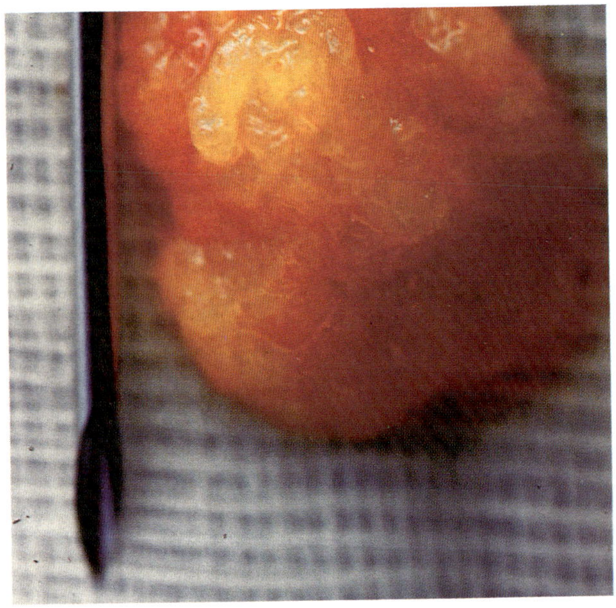

FIGURE 7
The specimen of fat obtained with a 14-gauge needle is three-dimensional.

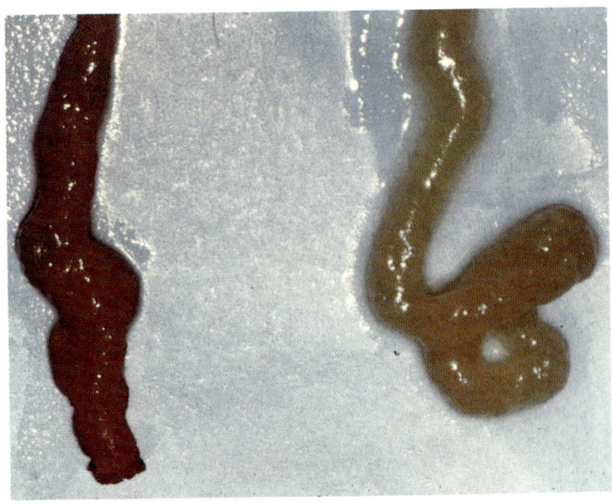

FIGURE 8
Fat slivers under low magnification.

done on an outpatient basis. To perform a successful fill, the following strictures must be observed.

Extraction should be done in an area of low vascularity, such as the limbs and trunk. Reinjection should be done in a highly vascular area, such as the face.

A small amount (2 to 6 ml) should be injected in each area, and several areas can be treated at the same time.

Reinjection in the same area can be repeated after 3 months if necessary. Reinjection may be done with or without pretunneling, using a small blunt cannula.

Reinjection should be linear, fan-shaped, or crisscross. A pocket should never be created before reinjection, only a mesh undermining.

The 14-gauge needle allows the extraction of a three-dimensional specimen of fat (as shown in Figs. 7 and 8), which is made of cylinders of adipose tissue and contains many undamaged adipose lobules, their vessels, and septa. If the periphery of the cylinder is damaged, the center will contain undamaged globules. It takes 20 s to obtain 2 ml of adipose tissue with an insulin syringe and a 14-gauge needle.

Advantages

The advantages of syringe lipoextraction and injection are evident: It is a very simple technique. Almost everyone has a rich tissue fat bank. The correction can be easily done in an area that has been overtreated if necessary. This procedure avoids solid implants and can be done in association with conventional procedures. Because only part of the fat will take, several injections have to be given in the same place.

Disadvantage

After the face fill, the patient has edema lasting 4 to 8 days. The risks of edema increase with the number of injections given; sometimes bruising is present.

With the thousands of injections we have done in the past 4 years, we have seen no complications such as infection, cysts, liquification, or distortion of the skin. The only incidents have involved hard lumps felt below the skin, and the lumps disappeared after several weeks. In some cases the graft disappeared; this happened in mature patients who had lost most of their reserves of fat in the face. We have noticed that the injected fat gravitates, but this may be prevented by immobilization. We often achieve permanent results after a year, when the area has been injected three or four times.

MODIFICATIONS FOR OTHER USES

This procedure is also used for embellishment of the hands. In this case, we inject 10 ml of fat harvested with a 14-gauge needle after a block with an anesthetic solution of lidocaine 1% with adrenaline 1/200 mg has been done on the wrist and the patient makes a fist. Then, with slight pressure, the fat diffuses in the entire dorsum of the hand. This procedure has given the best long-term results because the bones act as a splint and prevent shrinkage of the graft.

When large amounts of fat are needed, as in breast augmentation and enlargement of the calves after poliomyelitis, we harvest the fat with a 60-ml syringe on which is mounted a cannula with a blunt opening and a solid tip. The specimen obtained with such large cannulas are either cylinders of fat or pearl-shaped fragments, both of which are suitable for grafting. See Figs. 9 through 11.

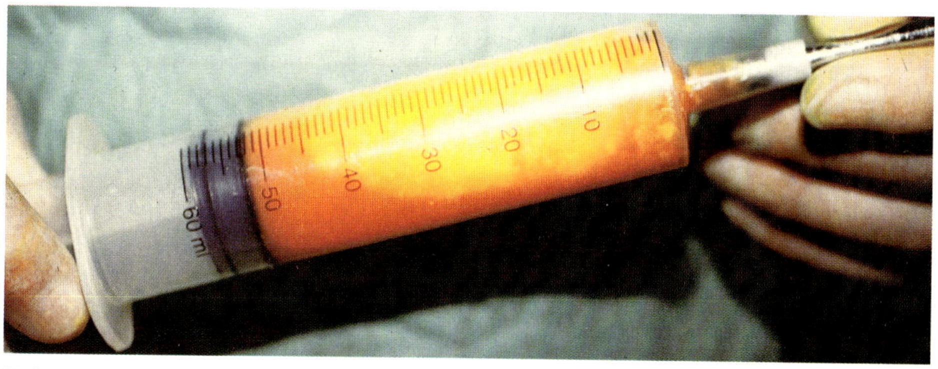

FIGURE 9
When a large amount of fat is needed, a 6-mm cannula with a solid tip mounted on a 60-ml syringe is used. In this case, a dry technique is necessary.

FIGURE 10
The specimen obtained with a 6-mm cannula mounted on a 60-ml syringe is three-dimensional. Large fat slivers are obtained with this procedure.

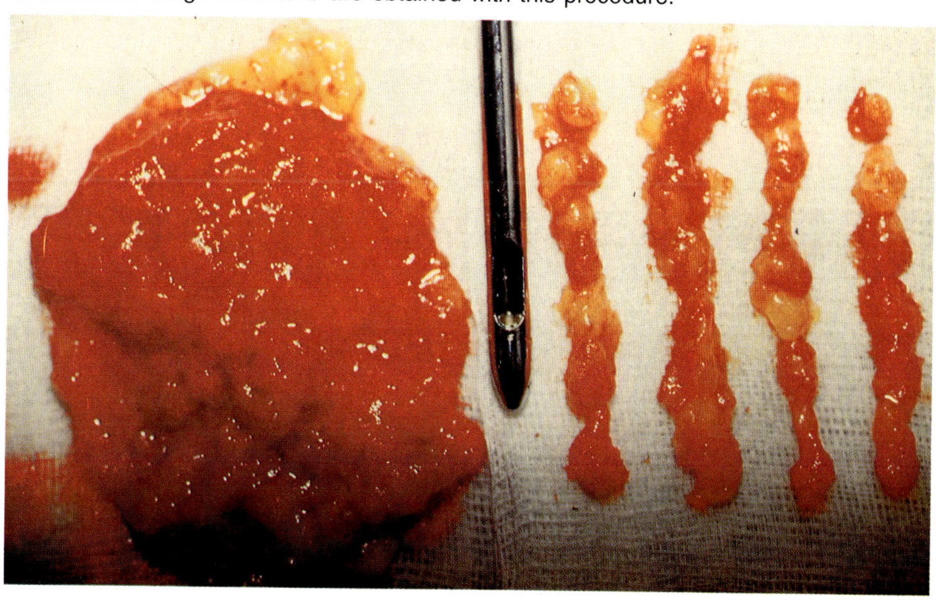

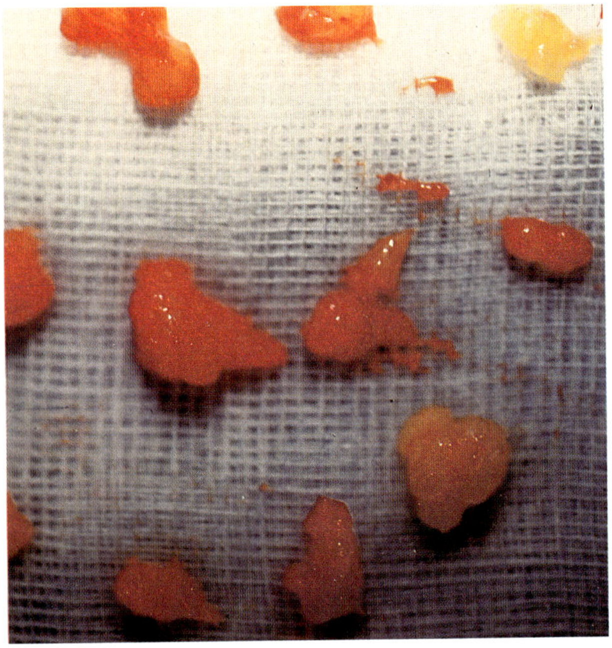

FIGURE 11
The 6-mm cannula also removes pearl-shaped fragments of fat.

We always harvest these large amounts of fat under general anesthesia, and the reinjection is done after a mesh undermining has been created in the area to be grafted (retromammary space, depression after overtreated liposculpturing in the saddlebag area, etc.). Before reinjection, the area is injected with chilled saline at 2°C with adrenaline (1 mg of adrenaline in 1 liter of chilled saline). This avoids unnecessary bleeding and keeps open the channels created by the dissection. We have injected amounts ranging from 150 to 300 ml of fat behind the mammary gland.

More recently, our group has modified the fat transferring technique by washing the fat before reinjecting it. The fat is first harvested with a 14-gauge needle mounted on a 10-ml syringe. Two milliliters of normal saline is placed in the syringe before the harvest; 5 ml of fat is then taken, followed by an additional 3 ml of normal saline. The 10-ml mixture is placed plunger down on a test tube holder; in a few seconds, the fatty component floats to the upper part of the syringe and the blood and normal saline stay on the bottom. The blood and saline are then evacuated by pushing on the plunger, and an additional 5 ml is aspirated. This maneuver is repeated several times to obtain clean yellow fat.

The syringe, filled with only the 5 ml of fat, is again placed on the test tube holder, this time with the plunger down. After several minutes the fluid fraction of the fat ascends and is put into another syringe with a transfer needle. See Fig. 12. This oily fraction, roughly 0.5 ml, is eliminated because it can be detrimental to the take of the graft.

Originally we started by injecting 2 ml in each area, but we now inject up to 6 to 8 ml in such places as the cheekbone area. In addition, we now inject into the deep fat pad area, or corpus adiposum buccae, as shown in Fig. 13. We believe that this deep pocket is the real foundation of the face and should be augmented. For this procedure we use the transcutaneous or intraoral route.

The latest modification of the face fill (subcutaneous or deep) has been to reinject not only the fat slivers harvested with a 14-gauge needle but also the tissue specimen obtained with a 19-, 20-, or even 21-gauge needle. The 19-gauge needle is the one most commonly used. We call the specimen obtained with such a needle *autologous collagen,*

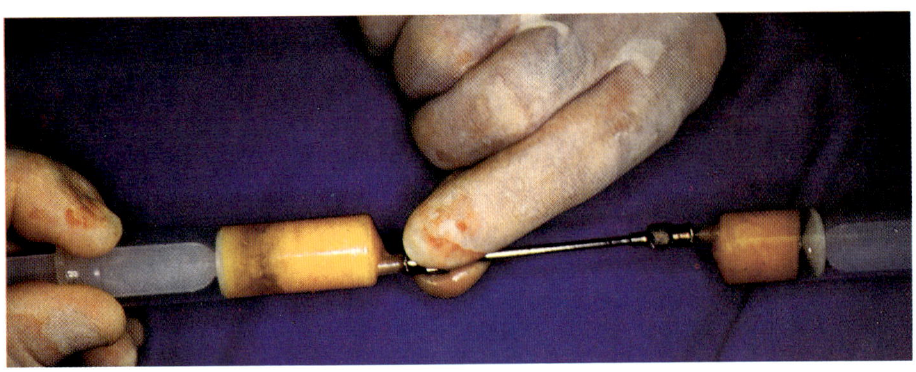

FIGURE 12
A transfer needle is useful in evacuating the oily fraction into another syringe, avoiding external manipulation.

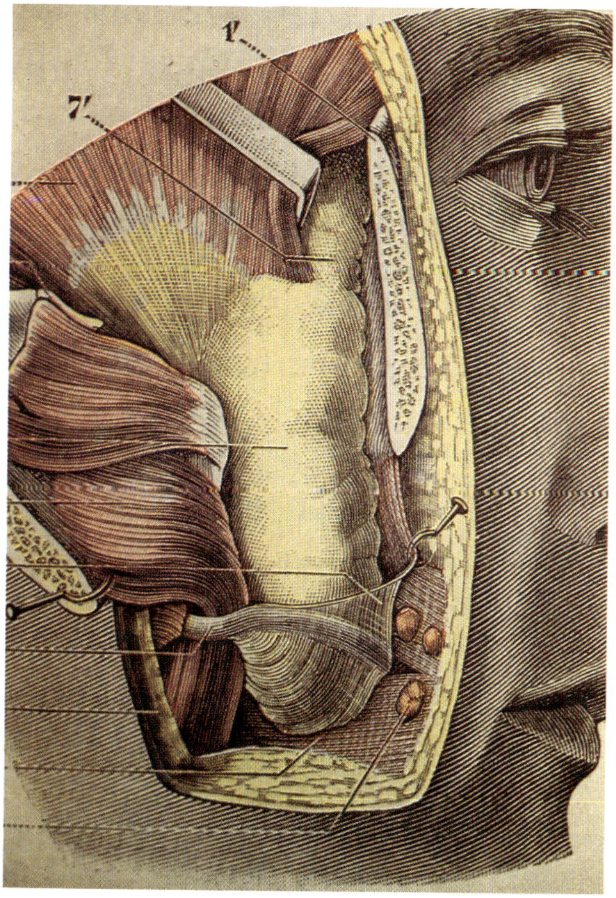

FIGURE 13
The corpus adiposum buccae is an important structure that serves as the foundation of the face.

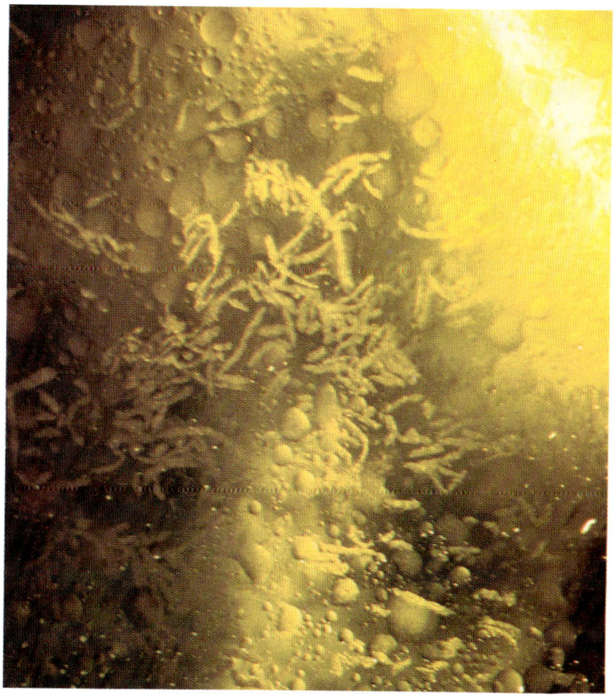

FIGURE 14
Collagen fragments collected with a 19-gauge needle.

FIGURE 15
About 50 percent of the specimen collected with a 19-gauge needle consists of fluid fat.

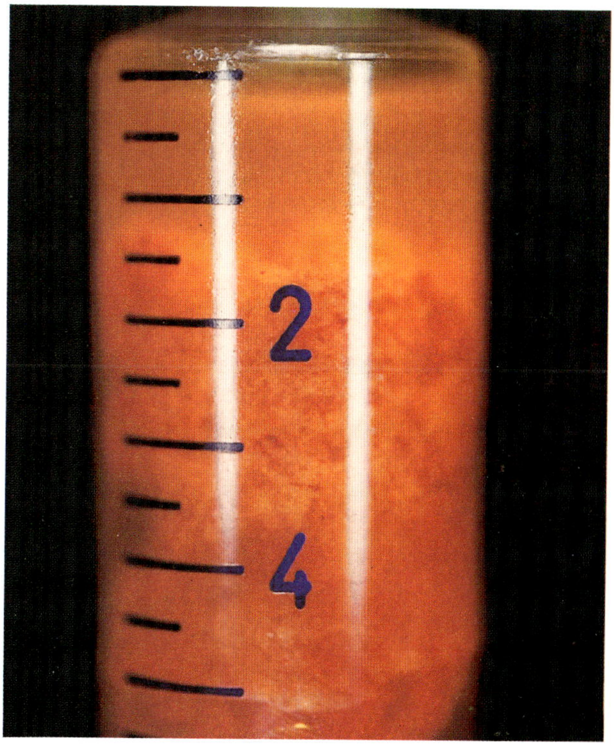

as it is made of fragments of the supporting structure of the adipose tissue: the septi. These septi give the adipose tissue its solidity, rigidity, and resistance. See Fig. 14.

After this specimen of autologous collagen is harvested with a 10-ml syringe, we employ the same cleansing procedure that is used for fat slivers harvested with a 14-gauge needle. The only difference is that the fluid fraction constitutes about 50 percent of the fatty specimen. See Fig. 15.

We use the same amount of autologous collagen as we use of fat slivers. We believe that this form of implant may last longer. We have used a 48-month observation period of autoinjection in the glabella without noticing a need for any modification of the implantation. Such an implantation is not a graft requiring revascularization by inoculation. Autologous collagen such as bovine collagen can be used

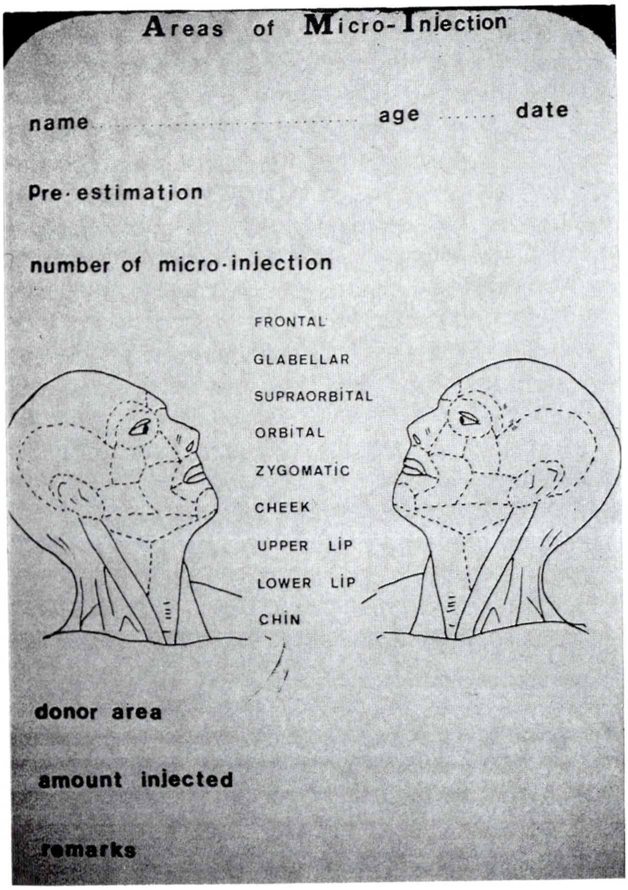

FIGURE 16
The amounts of fat injected are recorded on these schemas.

FIGURE 17
A glabellar furrow before treatment.

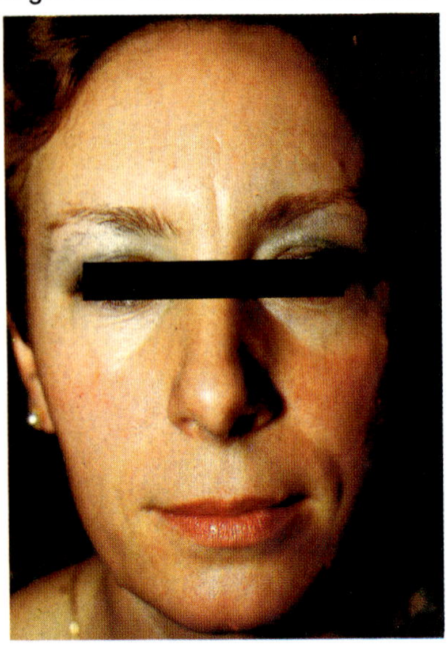

as a dermal filler. It can either be injected into the skin with the same needle used for extraction or placed into a Derma-Jet (0.1 ml is injected at a time with the latter). Aside from the longer-lasting results, the patient has less swelling and very little bruising, if any. The tissues are very easily remodeled. These autologous collagen microimplants are also injected in the pocket where the corpus adiposum buccae is located (suctorial fat pad of Bichat).

CONCLUSIONS

Fat transfer offers unique possibilities for improving areas previously thought uncorrectable or changed with much difficulty. It has comparatively few complications. Because the procedure is so new, more details and improved techniques should be forthcoming.[4]

FIGURE 18
The same glabellar furrow 2 years later, after 5 ml of fat slivers was injected.

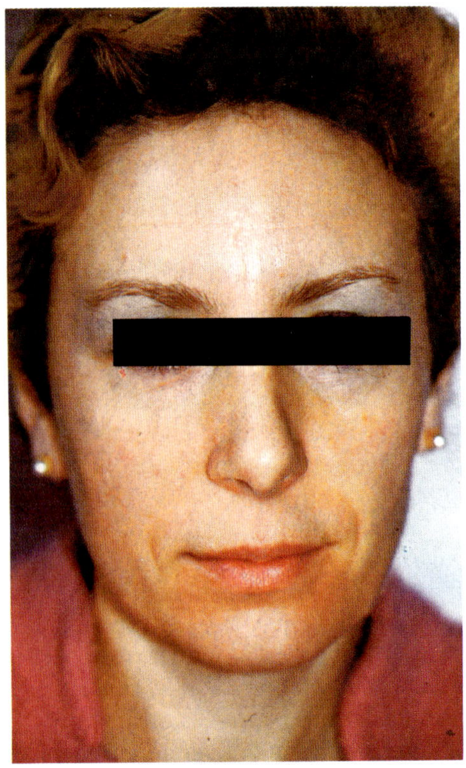

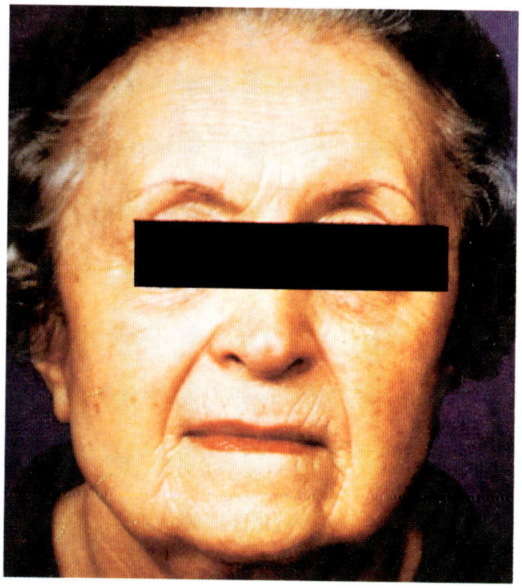

FIGURE 19
Before injection of the whole face (50 ml).

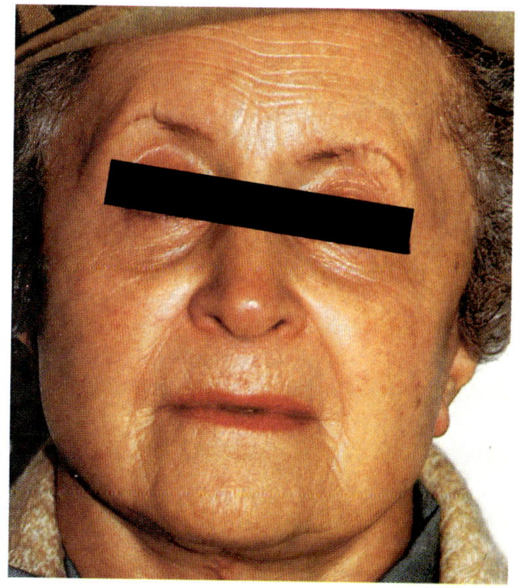

FIGURE 20
The results 30 months later. A skin resection in the neck has also been performed.

REFERENCES

1. Bailin AK, Pratt LA. Physiological consequences of human skin aging. Cutis. 1989;43:431–436.
2. Fisher A, Fisher GM. Bulletin of the International Academy of Cosmetic Surgery. Published by Tip STEI. First Surgical Treatment for Modeling Body's Cellulite with Three 5mm incisions, vol. 2. Rome, Italy, September 1976:35–36.
3. Fournier P, Otteni F. Le Traitement des Lipodystrophies localisées par Aspiration. Chirurgie Esthétique 1981–1982. Direction Scientifique: J. Faivre. Paris: 1981:59–78.
4. Fournier P, Otteni F. Honeycombed lipectomy or liposuction-dissection in body sculpturing (L.S.D. technique): The dry procedure. Presented at the annual meeting of the American Society of Plastic Reconstructive Surgery, Honolulu, October 1982.
5. Fournier P, Otteni F. Lipodissection in body sculpturing: The dry procedure. Plast Reconstr Surg. 1983; 72:598–609.
6. Fournier P, Illouz YG. Collapsing surgery and body sculpturing, in Renault P, Daniel RK (eds) Aesthetic Plastic Surgery. Boston: Little Brown, 1984:
7. Fournier P. Body Sculpturing through Syringe Liposuction and Autologous Fat Re-Injection. Del Mar, CA: Samuel Rolf, 1987.
8. Fournier PF. Microlipoextraction et microlipoinjection. Rev Chir Esthet Lang Frac. 1985;10:36–40.
9. Glogau RG. Microlipoinjection. Arch Dermatol. 1988; 124:1340–1343.
10. Illouz YG: Une nouvelle technique pour les lipodystrophies localisées. Rev Chir Esth Franc. 1980;19:15–18.
11. Newman J, Ftaiha Z. The biographical history of fat transplant surgery. Am J Cosmetic Surg. 1987;4:85–88.
12. Fournier PF. Liposculpture, ma technique. Paris: Editions Arnette, 1989.
13. Gurney CE. Experimental study of the behavior of free fat transplant. Surgery. 1938;3:680.
14. Peer LA. Loss of weight and volume in human fat graft. Plast Reconstr Surg. 1950;5:217.
15. Gillis H, Millard R. The Principles and Art of Plastic Surgery. Boston: Little, Brown, 1938:1–52.

CHAPTER 29

Expanders

WILLIAM P. COLEMAN III
GUSTAVO COLON

Although Planas in the 1940s and Neumann in 1957 experimented with subcutaneous balloons which were inflated to achieve expansion of the skin for reconstructive purposes,[1,2] the modern age of tissue expanders began with the work of Radovan.[3] Over a decade ago, he devised a silicone expander inflated by means of a subcutaneous port. His work involved the breast tissues, where he was able to demonstrate sufficient expansion to allow the use of a permanent implant for breast reconstruction.

Although this work was reported in 1976, it was not until the early 1980s that widespread use of tissue expanders began. In 1982, Austad and Rose[4] reported the use of a self-inflating tissue expander which was based on a permeable envelope with a high solute load inside. This expander depended on osmosis across the envelope to slowly expand the device without the need for injections. There has been a rapid increase in the use of tissue expanders in the 1980s for breast reconstruction, burn alopecia, defects that result from tumor removal, and elimination of large scars, tattoos, and benign tumors[5–7] (Figs. 1 through 4).

The concept of tissue expanders is based on the viscoelastic properties of the skin. As evidenced by the abdominal skin in pregnancy and the decorative stretching of the skin of the lips by African tribes, skin has a surprising tolerance for stretching. Slow stretching of the skin using a subcutaneous expander allows the design of flaps which would not otherwise be useful for closing massive defects. Expanders are available in a number of designs and shapes or can be customized for special applications (Fig. 5). These Silastic balloons are expanded by injecting saline into a nearby port on a weekly or biweekly basis. Once the skin is sufficiently expanded, the devices can be removed and the stretched skin can be employed for its intended surgical purpose.

LABORATORY STUDIES

Research on guinea pigs has shown that the expander is rapidly enveloped by a thick capsule.[8] Although the dermis and subcutaneous tissue are thinned upon expansion, the capsule continues to thicken for the first 2 to 3 months of expansion. Two years after the cessation of expansion, the dermis and subcutaneous tissue are the same thickness that they were prior to expansion and the fibrous capsule disappears.[9] Research has shown that the microcirculation of the expanded tissue is

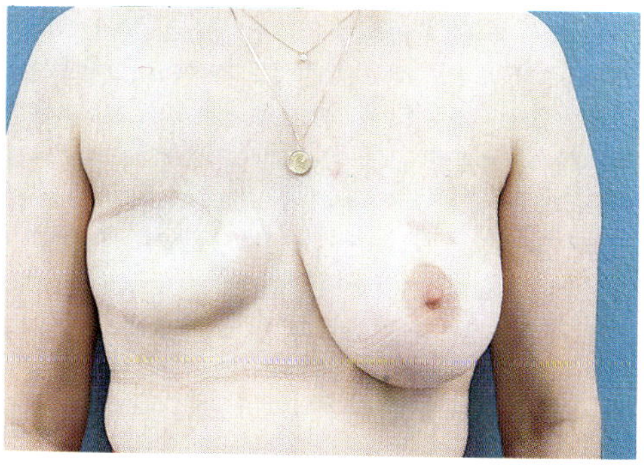

FIGURE 1
Postoperative right mastectomy and preoperative left mastectomy.

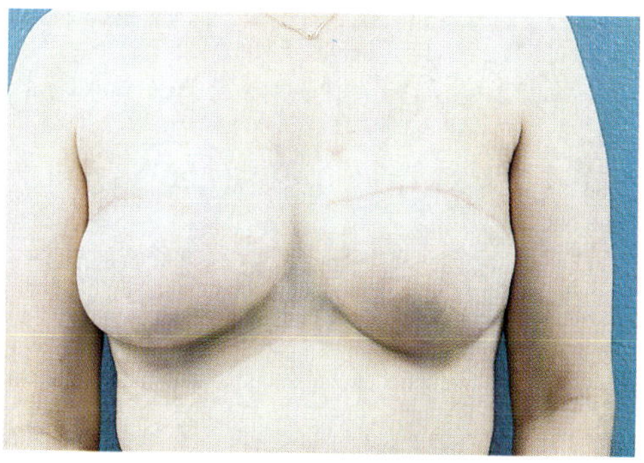

FIGURE 2
After the mastectomies shown in Fig. 1, reconstruction was achieved by the placement of permanent expanders.

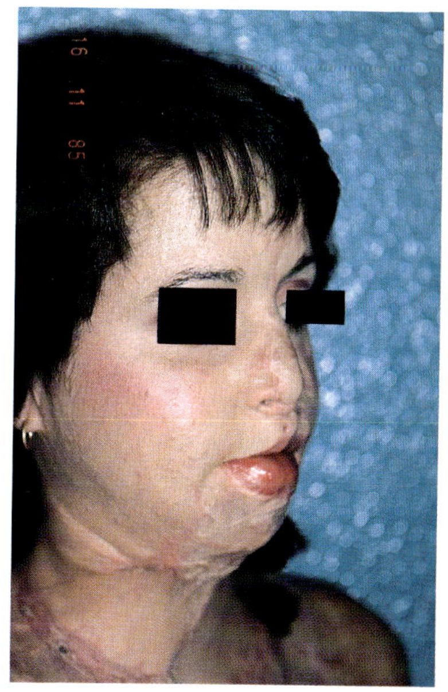

FIGURE 4
The patient in Fig. 3 after expansion. Cheek tissue advancement completed the reconstruction.

FIGURE 3
Expander in place for reconstruction of a contracted burn scar of the neck.

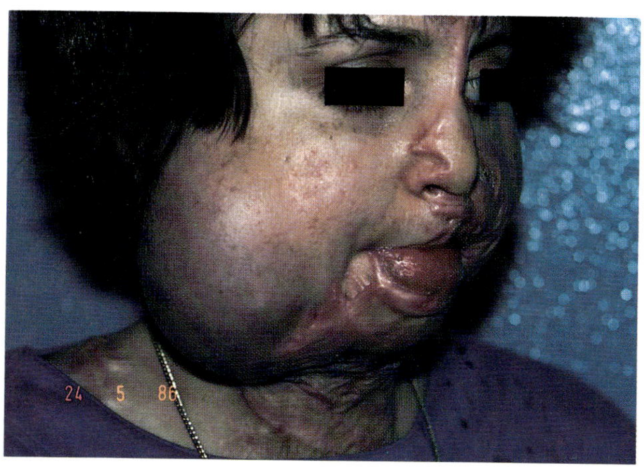

FIGURE 5
Typical tissue expander.

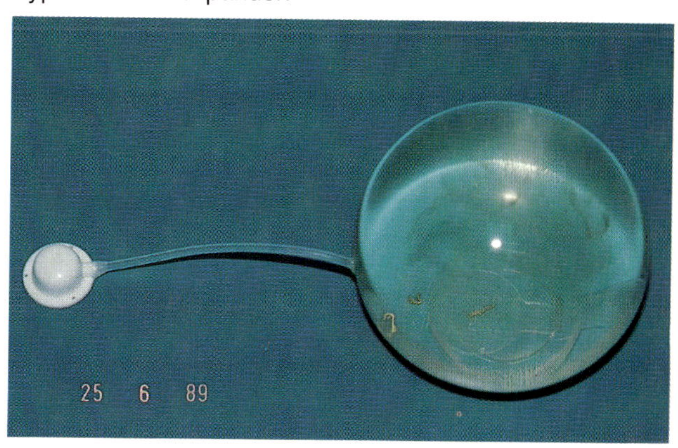

greatly enhanced.[7] This accounts for experiments which have shown that flaps constructed from expanded tissue survive better than do nonexpanded and delayed flaps.[10]

COMPLICATIONS

The major complications of tissue expansion include dehiscence of the incision, erosion of the expander envelope, implant failure, infection, and ischemia.[7] Minor complications include pain on expansion, seroma, and dogears. These complications can be minimized with proper technique but can still occur and jeopardize the success of the expansion. Proper placement of the incision and the location of the expander are important to minimize exposure. Some authors recommend the use of prophylactic antibiotics prior to implant placement to decrease the potential for infection.[6,11]

VARIATIONS ON PORT DESIGN

Most tissue expanders rely on a subcutaneous port for filling the device. This injection port is entered percutaneously with a needle. The location of the port is determined by palpating a raised ring on the surface of the expander or attached to the expander by a remote tube. Because in some situations it is difficult to palpate the port and puncture of the tube or expander is possible, various other designs have been proposed. One employs a rare-earth magnet at the base of the injection port which can be located by the use of a special "Magna-Finder."[12] Recently the use of external reservoirs has been increasing.[1] This allows the expander to be filled with much less effort by the surgeon and less pain on the part of the patient. Although this approach has been criticized for its potential for infection,[13] initial studies have shown that there is not an increased rate of infection using this approach.[14]

FILLING TECHNIQUES

The more rapidly the expander is filled, the sooner the appropriate skin expansion can be achieved; however, extremely rapid filling is painful for the patient and can decrease the circulation of the overlying skin and induce ischemia. Some surgeons recommend measuring intraluminal pressure during tissue expansion to reduce the incidence of these complications.[6,11] Monitoring the discomfort of the patient and observing the capillary flow of the overlying skin provide clinical parameters.[15] Others have recommended an "overfilling" technique in which the expanders are temporarily overexpanded to a point where the dermal capillary flow over the expander is zero.[16] The expander is then slowly deflated until the dermal circulation resumes. This approach has been hypothesized to allow accelerated tissue expansion, decreasing the number of filling sessions required.

RECOMMENDED TECHNIQUE

Placement of the incision for expander insertion must minimize scar complexity to avoid devascularizing tissue. These incisions are best placed adjacent to the defect (Fig. 6). The incision then becomes the leading edge of the advancing expanded tissue.

The expander should be placed in a generous pocket, using the largest size expander that fits. If

FIGURE 6
The expander is placed adjacent to the defect to allow subsequent advancement of skin anteriorly.

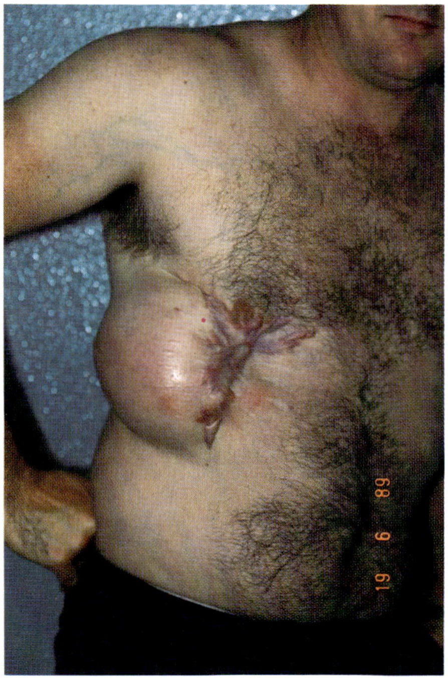

an external tube is employed, it should be brought out through the skin far away from the initial incision. If a tubed port is employed, it should also be placed well away from the body of the expander.

Tubed ports should be secured with sutures. The large incision should be closed with nonabsorbable sutures in several layers.

Prophylactic antibiotic coverage should be considered.

Filling the device begins 1 week after implantation of the expander, as follows.

1. Saline is added through the port until the patient notices tightness or severe pain.
2. The circulation of the overlying skin should be evaluated for excessive blanching or studied with a Doppler flowmeter until the dermal capillary flow is zero.
3. The expander pressure should be increased by additional injections until reaching approximately 100 mmHg for about 10 min and then reduced to around 25 to 30 mmHg.
4. Expansion continues weekly until sufficient skin stretching is achieved to generously cover the defect. This may take several months.

The expander is removed through an incision adjacent to the defect. The stretched skin can then be advanced directly if possible into the surgical defect. Simple advancement is preferred to complex flap designs to maximize the blood supply of the expanded flap. Dogears are best left unrepaired to avoid flap compromise (they often flatten out spontaneously).

SPECIAL CONSIDERATIONS

Open wounds below the knee have been shown to be a poor choice for tissue expansion. Expansion in these patients has produced a high rate of infection, dehiscence, and expander exposure.[11]

External port reservoir tissue expanders should not be employed for breast reconstruction when a permanent implant is to be inserted.[1] Prostheses which are exposed to bacterial contamination often become colonized.

Intraoperative expansion is useful when smaller amounts of tissue gain are needed. Immediate tissue expansion is most useful for reconstruction after tumor removal, but it has also been recommended to facilitate tissue movement during face lifts.[17] Reusable expanders are available for this purpose although recently disposable urinary catheters with 30cc balloons have become popular as small tissue expanders.

CONCLUSION

Tissue expansion offers an option for reconstruction of large defects when ordinary flap manipulation and serial surgery are not feasible. Tissue expansion allows movement of greater amounts of tissue than can be achieved with other methods. In spite of the inconvenience of numerous filling visits and the potential for complications, this procedure has found an important place in reconstructive surgery.

REFERENCES

1. Jackson IT, Sharpe DT, Polley J, et al. Use of external reservoirs in soft tissue expansion. Plast Reconstr Surg. 1987; 80:266–271.
2. Neumann CG. The expansion of an area of skin by progressive distention of a subcutaneous balloon. Plast Reconstr Surg. 1957;19:124–127.
3. Radovan C. Reconstruction of the breast after radical mastectomy using temporary expander. Plast Surg Forum. 1978;1:41–47.
4. Austad ED, Rose GL. A self inflating tissue expander. Plast Reconstr Surg. 1982;70:588–592.
5. Buhrer DP, Huang TT, Yee HW, et al. Treatment of burn alopecia with tissue expanders in children. Plast Reconstr Surg. 1988;81:512–515.
6. Manders EK, Graham WP III. Alopecia reduction by scalp expansion. J Dermatol Surg Oncol. 1984;10:967–969.
7. Manders EK, Schenden MJ, Furrey JP, et al. Soft tissue expansion: Concepts and complications. Plast Reconstr Surg. 1984;74:493–507.
8. Austad ED, Pasyk KA, McClatchey KD, et al. Histopathologic evaluation of guinea pig skin and soft tissue after controlled tissue expansion. Plast Reconstr Surg. 1982;70:704–710.
9. Pasyk KA, Argenta LC, Hassett C. Quantitative analysis of the thickness of human skin and subcutaneous tissue following controlled expansion with a silicone implant. Plast Reconstr Surg. 1988;81:516–523.
10. Cherry GW, Austad ED, Pasyk KA. Increased survival and

vascularity of random pattern skin flaps elevated in controlled expanded skin. Plast Reconstr Surg. 1983;72:680–688.
11. Manders EK, Oaks TE, Au VK, et al. Soft tissue expansion in the lower extremities. Plast Reconstr Surg. 1988; 81:208–217.
12. Elliot MP, Dubrul W. Magna-site tissue expander: An innovation for injection site location. Plast Reconstr Surg. 1988;81:605–607.
13. Argenta LC. Use of external reservoirs in tissue expansion. Plast Reconstr Surg. 1987;80:272–273.
14. Jackson IT. Use of external reservoirs in tissue expansion, letter. Plast Reconstr Surg. 1988;81:640–641.
15. Miller SH. Soft tissue expansion in the lower extremities. Plast Reconstr Surg. 1988;81:218–219.
16. Pietila JP, Nordstrom RE, Virkkunen PJ, et al. Accelerated tissue expansion with the "overfilling" technique. Plast Reconstr Surg. 1988;81:204–207.
17. Man D. Stretching and tissue expansion for rhytidectomy: An improved approach. Plast Reconstr Surg. 1989;84:561–569.

CHAPTER

30

Liposuction

PIERRE F. FOURNIER

Two decades ago, the only way to eliminate excess fat was open surgery which left unsightly scars, defeating the main purpose of aesthetic surgery. Another inconvenience involved the difficulties of a major operation, including hospitalization, blood transfusion, and extended convalescence. Giorgio Fischer, a cosmetic surgeon in Rome, invented the technique of liposculpturing in 1974, eliminating both scarring and major surgery. Fischer's contribution allowed a transition from open to closed surgery in body contouring. Fischer and his father demonstrated that liposculpturing is safe, without complications such as pulmonary and fat embolisms, risks which some physicians feared would be a part of the new procedure.[1]

The Fischers were selling specially designed equipment to perform the operation. In 1977, Y. G. Illouz, a cosmetic surgeon in Paris, showed that the same operation could be performed using the suction abortion equipment invented by Karman, an American gynecologist. Illouz's discovery made possible the widespread use of this technique among the members of the French Society of Aesthetic Surgery.[2] The technique soon gained momentum in France. Later, Americans came to France to study the procedure. They took their knowledge back to the United States and founded several groups that worked to improve and spread the technique.

After Illouz's simplification of the Fischer technique, a breakthrough occurred in 1985 with the development of *syringe liposculpturing*, because syringes could be employed to extract fat without the use of complicated machines. This new technique of manual liposculpturing popularized the procedure even more than Illouz's contribution because of its immediate availability, ease, and reliability. There have also been improved results due to a symmetrical and even removal because the syringe can be used as a precise unit of measurement. Liposculpturing thus evolved from the most complicated stage to a level which makes it available to any doctor who obtains the proper training.[3–7]

Syringe-assisted liposculpturing was the first step toward fat grafting in aesthetic surgery. In fact, fat grafting was used nearly 100 years ago, but only in reconstructive surgery. It was a major and open procedure, leaving scars where the fat was taken and where it was grafted. Hypercorrection was required because only part of the fat would take. The development of syringe-assisted reduction body contouring paved the way for incremental closed body sculpturing in aesthetic surgery.

SYRINGE-REDUCTION LIPOSCULPTURING

A syringe is as powerful as a machine because it creates a vacuum of one atmospheric condition. The definition of *vacuum* is an absence of air. It is possible to compress air to extremely high pressures, but it is not possible to obtain a vacuum higher than one atmospheric condition. This vacuum is easily obtained by pulling on the plunger of the syringe, and it is maintained for as long as the plunger is pulled firmly and continuously. Any kind of cannula or needle can be mounted on a syringe for lipoextraction, as shown in Figs. 1 through 3. To avoid dead space which can hinder the lipoextraction, a small amount of normal saline is placed in the syringe. The saline works as a buffer between the negative pressure and the tissues, in other words, as a shock absorber. This explains the diminished bleeding and shock that occur when a syringe is used. There is no way to use a shock absorber with a machine; the negative pressure transmitted from the jar to the tissues opens the damaged capillaries and injures the highly innervated fatty tissue. See Figs. 4 through 6.

Indications

Closed body contouring by syringe or machine is not indicated for obesity. It is an aesthetic procedure, and in many cases it requires the removal of only a few hundred milliliters of fat. When numerous adiposities have to be treated at the same time, no more than 2 liters should be removed by machine. With a syringe, up to 3 liters can be removed without the need for blood transfusion.

Liposculpturing is used to treat excess fat in areas such as the head and neck (jowls, double chin, etc.) and localized adiposities on the body (saddlebags, hips, abdomen, ankles, etc.). The ideal patient is of normal weight, can be young or mature, and has mild adiposity and good skin tonicity.

Equipment

The physician needs disposable plastic syringes in sizes of 5, 10, and 60 ml. Also required are long and short cannulas of 2.0, 2.5, 3.0, 3.5, 4.0, 5.0, 6.0 mm outside diameter. They can be bought commercially or can be custom-made by the surgeon by

FIGURE 1
The size of both the cannula and the syringe has to be adapted to the volume of the adiposity.

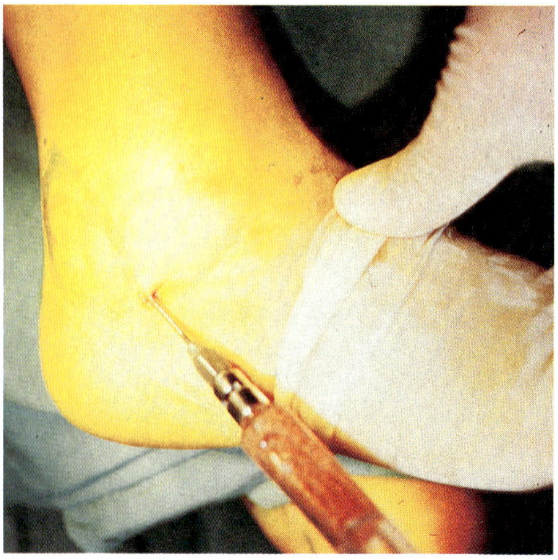

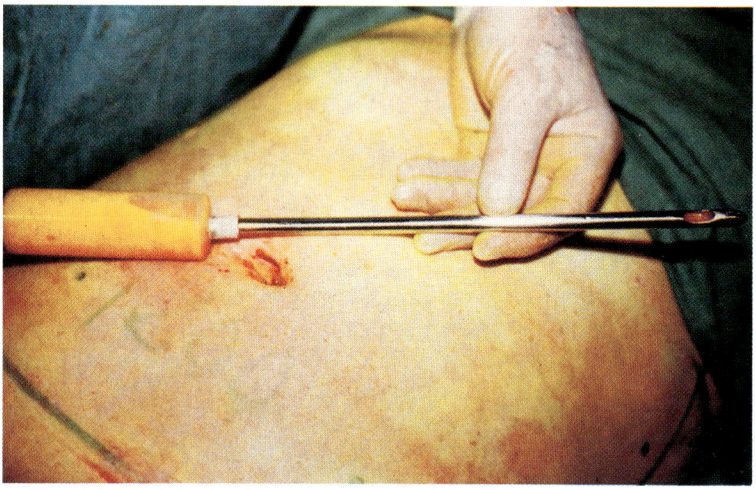

FIGURE 2
Common cannulas can be sawed and mounted on a plastic syringe.

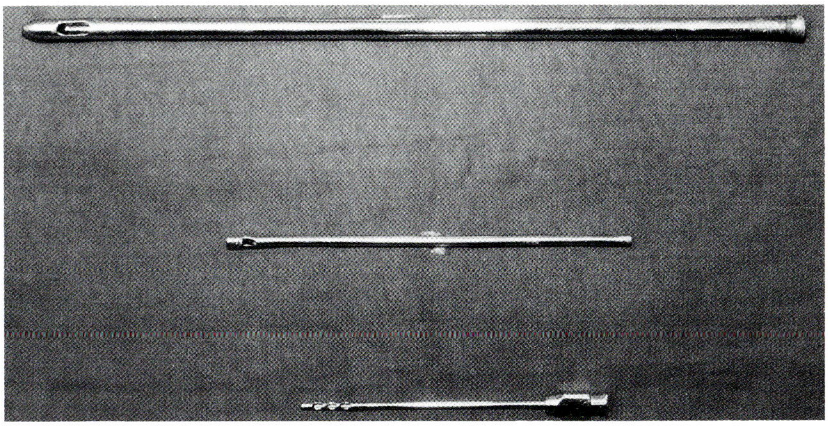

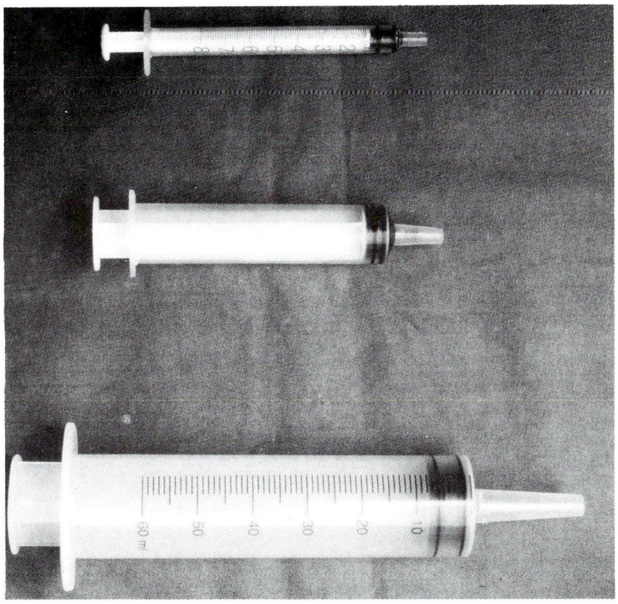

FIGURE 3
(*Left*) Any kind of reduction or incremental liposculpturing can be performed with such syringes.

cutting the handle and putting the rest of the existing cannula through the plastic syringe. Only one blunt opening with a solid tip is required.

Preoperative Procedure

As in any type of cosmetic surgery, the procedure should be done only after careful discussion with the patient about results and potential complications. All blood tests, electrocardiograms, and photographs of the patient should be done beforehand. A Polaroid study can show the patient the possibil-

FIGURE 4
It takes between 40 to 60 s to fill a 60 cc syringe when the area has been infiltrated with chilled saline at 2°C.

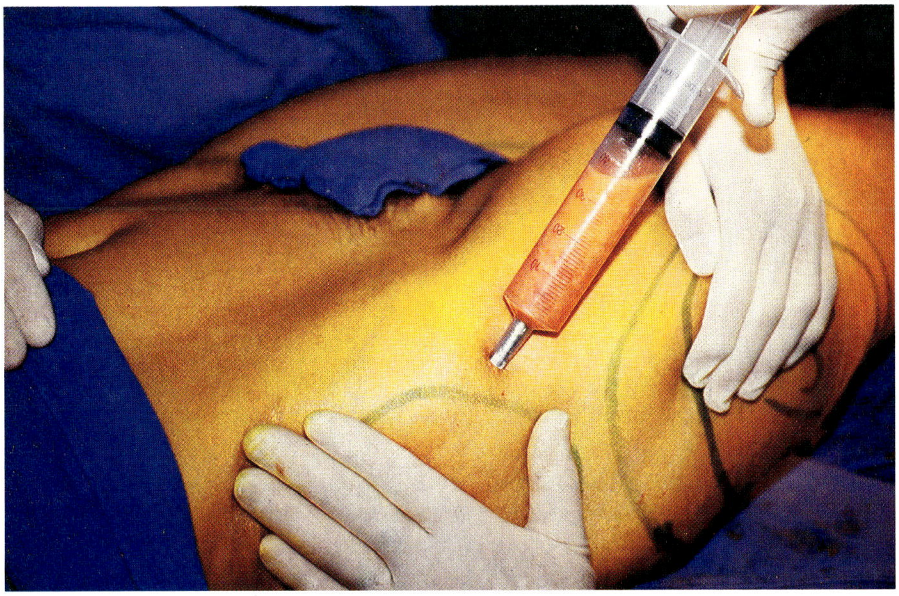

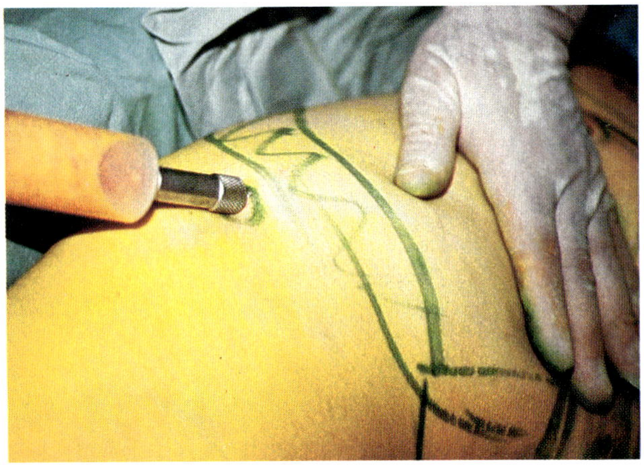

FIGURE 5
Place your hand flat on the area to be treated.

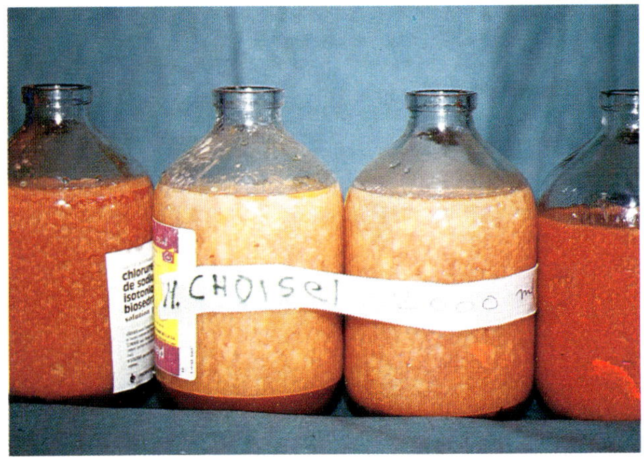

FIGURE 6
Very little blood is in the fat extracted with a syringe.

ities of the technique when one of the two pictures taken is shaded with ink.

Estimation of the Amount of Fat to Be Removed

The practitioner should know in advance approximately how much fat should be removed, knowledge that can be acquired only through experience. The practitioner must take into account the importance of the lipodysmorphism to be treated, whether the patient should be treated in one or more sessions, the tonicity of the tissue, and the age of the patient.

Marking the Patient

The adiposity is marked with a green Pentel pen or another skin marker to show where the excess fat is to be removed. The patient should be standing, as this provides the most accurate measurement. Another line is made 1 to 1.5 cm beyond the first one. The tip of the cannula will be pushed to the second marking to prevent stair step-like deformities. Beyond the adiposity, 2, 6, or 8 cm from the second marking, another marking is done to indicate the peripheral mesh undermining (PMU). Finally, the openings or incisions are marked by a point or circle to avoid permanent or transient tattooing by the ink. All the adiposities are marked before the operation, as is the site of the intended incisions or openings. The approximate amount of resection is marked in the middle of the adiposity. See Fig. 7.

Positioning the Patient

The position of the patient should be the one that is convenient for the surgeon. The choices are the supine, prone, and lateral positions. In all these positions, the arms or legs which are to be moved during the operation should be prepared. With the patient under local anesthesia, a position with the legs apart and flexed and with the feet joined (frog position) allows the patient to move or be moved if necessary; this holds true for epidural anesthesia as well. During general anesthesia, when the patient is supine, it is necessary to elevate the patient's side so that the surgeon can work on the waist, hip, or lateral chest rolls. All other areas are within easy reach: inner thighs, knees, double chin, etc. In this position it is also possible to work on the buttocks or create an infragluteal fold, although not as easily as in the prone position. By moving the patient, who has been specially prepared, it is possible to operate on almost all localized adiposities of the pelvis in the supine position.

Anesthesia

Depending on the size and surface area of the adiposity, one should use local, general, twilight, or epidural anesthesia or cryoanesthesia. To do liposculpturing under local anesthesia, the area is infiltrated as with the normal procedure. We use lidocaine 1% with adrenaline 1:200,000. Lidocaine can be used pure if only a small amount is needed or diluted to 1:2, 1:3, 1:4, or even less. It can be supplemented by external cryoanesthesia with icebags

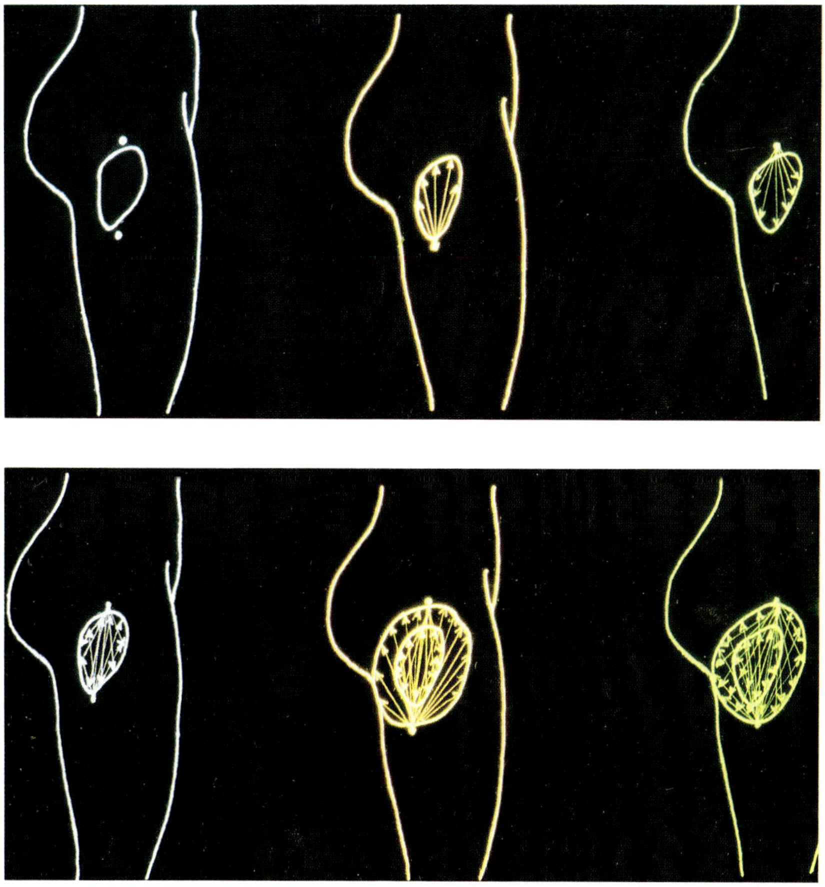

(*a*)

(*b*)

FIGURE 7
(*a*) and (*b*) Mapping out the procedures, using the following approaches: fan-shaped lesional lipectomy, criss-crossed lipectomy, peripheral mesh undermining. The result is a dermolipoplasty.

FIGURE 8
The area of the face and neck where liposculpturing is performed (real adiposities).

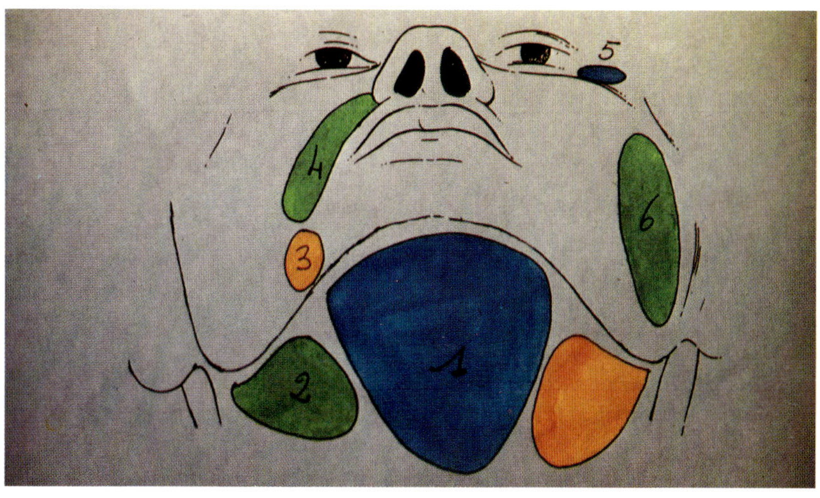

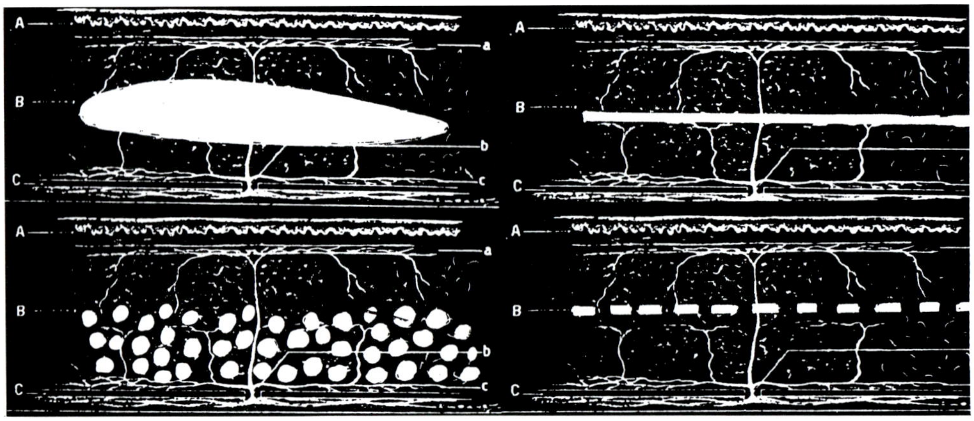

FIGURE 9
This diagram illustrates that multiple tunnels and not a single cavity have to be performed (left). On the right, a discontinuous undermining must be performed (bottom), and not a continuous one (top).

on the outside of the body. This is the *wet technique*. With the *dry technique*, the procedure is performed without injection of the fat under general anesthesia. With *cryoanesthesia*, the procedure is done after external refrigeration of the tissues. When employing general anesthesia, whatever the size of the adiposity, one should use the wet technique with chilled saline at 2°C with adrenaline (1 mg of adrenaline in 1 liter of chilled saline). The amount injected is between one-half the amount and the full amount of the fat preestimated to be extracted. This injection avoids excessive bleeding and bruising and allows the removal of more fat.

Approaches to Liposculpturing

The planned approach has to allow for easy, efficient work in the adiposity. As many approaches as necessary are performed to do crisscross work. The skin should not be incised; rather it should be punctured in the right skin tension line. In the past few years we have used an awl or ice pick to make an opening as in Fig. 10. If the awl or ice pick puncture is too small to allow the passage of the cannula, it can be easily dilated by passing first one branch and then the second branch of a hemostat and then separating the branches very gently. As there is no incision of the skin, the healing of the wound is far superior to that of a standard incision and is almost invisible. The wound must be closed in most cases with a fine nylon 5.0 suture or an inverted stitch of resorbable material.

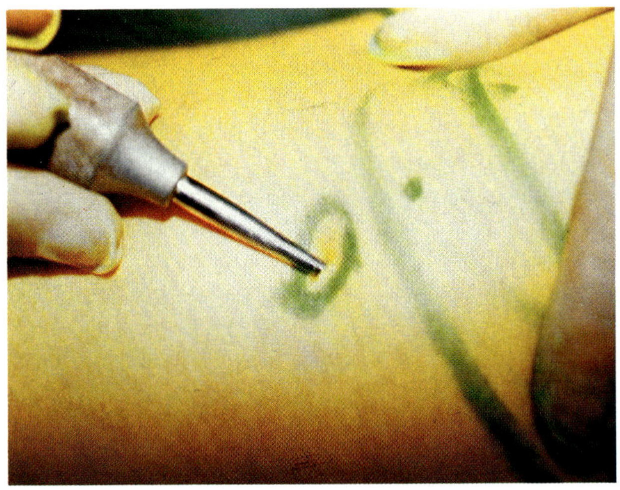

FIGURE 10
Using the ice pick.

TECHNIQUE

The following example describes work done on a hip with a 6-mm cannula and a 50-ml syringe. At the previously marked sites, incisions or openings are made (we prefer a puncture). If the opening is not large enough, it should be dilated with a hemostat. When the opening is sufficiently dilated, both limbs of the hemostat are passed through to prepare the way for the cannula. Pretunneling is not absolutely necessary but is helpful if the fat is hard. The cannula is directed into the area to be liposculptured in several fan-shaped motions. Before starting the liposculpturing, one should fill the syringe with 5 or 10 ml of chilled saline to eliminate all dead space in the cannula. The cannula is then passed through the opening while the left hand folds the skin. After insertion of the cannula, the left hand must remain flat throughout the operation.

The plunger is then withdrawn and kept withdrawn by the surgeon's right hand. The maneuver can be made easier with the use of a "stop." The cannula is moved in a fan-shaped motion approximately 5 to 10 times in the same direction. (We do not recommend that it stay in the same tunnel.) The opening of the cannula faces down during this maneuver. After 50 ml of fat is collected in the barrel, the syringe is emptied into a basin on the table. The procedure is repeated until the preestimated amount of fat is removed.

When half the preestimated amount of fat is removed from the localized adiposity, the cannula is inserted into another opening at a right angle or opposite to the first one and tunnels are made to perform crisscross work. The left hand (kept flat) still guides and follows the work of the right hand. The work of the respective hands can be summarized as follows:

Left Hand	Right Hand
Immobilize	Drill
Grasp	Extract
Lift	Dissect
Harden	Fill the syringe
Guide	Empty the syringe
Localize	Pull on the plunger
Palpate	Measure
Watch	
Pinch test	

This is the opposite of normal surgery, in which the right hand dominates. In liposculpturing, the left hand is the "brain hand" and the right hand is merely a piston.

One may in some circumstances use a smaller cannula (No. 4) to do the crisscrossing at a different level. At intervals, the left hand pinches the skin (pinch test) between the index finger and thumb to evaluate the diminution of the fold thickness. The surgeon can compare the thickness of the fold in the treated area with that of the fold made with the other hand in the nontreated paired area or on the normal neighboring tissues. The surgeon usually monitors the modification of the contour of the area treated to avoid overcorrection and also checks the volume of fat removed against the preestimate. A 1-cm uniform thickness of fat should be left covering the area, as determined by the pinch test made with the left hand. If the fat in the syringe shows too much blood, the surgeon must stop suctioning in that area and work in another part of the adiposity. If the patient complains of pain under local anesthesia, the surgeon should inject more of the anesthetic solution.

The skin must be grasped to make sure the cannula is in the right plane. The left hand should be flat and should exert some pressure on the tissues to eliminate the contained blood and stabilize the tissues. When the lipectomy has been completed, the surgeon performs a PMU, using the same openings. No suction is done during this procedure. The cannula is pushed in a fan-shaped motion until it reaches the marked line of the mesh undermining. This mesh is also done in a crisscross fashion through the area already lipectomized. The PMU allows the excess skin covering the crisscrossed lipectomy adiposity to fit better in its new bed, as less resistance is encountered in the neighboring tissues. The PMU has to be proportional to the amount of fat removed and to the quality of the skin.

When one area is completely treated, the surgeon will do similar work on the paired adiposity unless another lipoplastic surgeon has done similar work at the same time in the paired adiposity. The other adiposities are treated similarly thereafter.

Technical Considerations

The quantity of fat which has been removed constitutes the visible resection. During the procedure the to and fro movements of the cannula devitalize a certain amount of adipose tissue, which will be resorbed later by the body. This is the invisible, or biological, resection. There is adipose tissue extraction, but there is also adipose tissue destruction. The volume of fat reduction is obtained in two different ways: *mechanical disruption* and *suction friction scraping*.

The *visible resection* is achieved by the scraping motions of the cannula, which also removes part of the fat that has been mechanically disrupted. The *invisible resection* is made up of most of the devitalized fat obtained by the friction of the cannula and some of the fat that has been mechanically disrupted. Irrigation of the tissues with normal saline always removes small fragments of fat. After a certain period of time this procedure will create scar tissue, which will be followed by contraction, as in any operation on or below the skin.

This consideration is intended to enhance the performance of a thorough and even lipectomy. The PMU in the whole treated area should obtain a homogeneous contraction of the scar tissue as a result of the operating procedure. The shrinking procedure involves the skin, the fat, and the fibrous tissue. The skin is affected by the primary contraction of the muscular fibers (immediate, active process). The adipose tissue is modified by the contraction of the fibrous tissue (passive contraction, delayed). Thus, a liposculpturing procedure has an immediate effect on the contour as a result of the visible resection and a delayed effect on the volume as a result of the biological resection. The skin aspect is also modified by the primary contraction of the elastic muscle fibers immediately and by the secondary contraction of the underlying fibrous scar tissue afterward.

Precautions

As in a rhinoplasty, during a liposculpturing procedure, the most important concept to remember is not what is removed but what is left and how it is left. If too much blood is in the aspirate, one should stop working in that area and move onto another part of the adiposity or work on another adiposity. Under no circumstances should windshield wiper movements be done, as they will cut adipose columns which contain vessels, nerves, and lymphatics. When lumps are felt under the skin, a smaller cannula should be employed.

The Remodeling Dressing

When the operation is over, the incisions or punctures of the skin are closed and covered with a Steristrip. For closure of the skin, a fine nylon stitch (No. 5) is used; one or two stitches is usually enough. The suture is a transcutaneous one. The stitches are removed, together with the dressing, in about a week, depending on the healing process. If the surgeon wants to remove the stitches sooner, he or she should create a "window" in the Elastoplast dressing, which has to remain for a full week. It is also possible to do an inverted stitch on the deep dermis with a resorbable fine suture, and this will simplify the aftercare. The markings are carefully erased with ether, and this cleaning enhances the adhesion of the Elastoplast.

The width of the Elastoplast tape varies according to the surface of the adiposity treated: 3 to 5 cm in width for minor adiposities and 10 to 15 or 20 cm in width for average or major adiposities. The skin as well as the Elastoplast should not make "waves," and the positioning of the skin on the deep tissues should be done accurately. Whenever possible, the dressing should be crisscrossed (knees, abdomen). In any case, it should be a circular dressing, especially around a limb. The dressing is most important in three areas: the lateral thighs (saddlebags), the abdomen, and the back.

Fluid Balance

Blood loss should be compensated. Losses under 500 ml do not require fluid replacement. When there is over 500 ml of loss, twice the amount that has been removed should be given intravenously during the operation by the anesthesiologist or surgeon (half crystalloids, half colloids). When more than 2 liters have been removed, blood replacement may be required. Syringe liposculpturing allows a greater extent of removal without blood transfusion, as there is less blood loss.

Complications

Syringe liposculpturing has a very low rate of complications. There are the usual complications due to anesthesia, both local and general. The complications caused by the procedure are not surgical; hematoma and infection are very rarely seen. Aesthetic complications such as residual adiposity, crater depression, and checkerboard deformity may appear. They occur most often when the patient is in inexperienced hands. The surgeon should know how to treat these complications.

CONCLUSIONS

Liposuction, or body sculpturing, is an exciting modality that can improve the appearance of many patients. Used judiciously, the adverse reaction can be kept to a minimum. The results are extremely gratifying, for both patient and physician, as shown in Figs. 11 through 15.

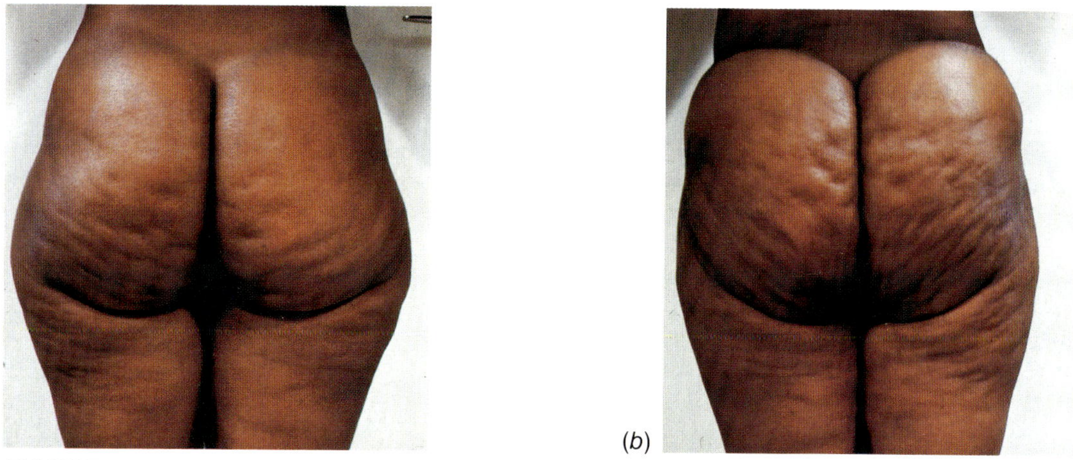

FIGURE 11
(*a*) The morphology of a patient in a relaxed position. (static morphology). (*b*) The morphology of the same patient when flexing the buttocks (dynamic morphology). This maneuver demonstrates that the patient has pseudo-saddle bags.

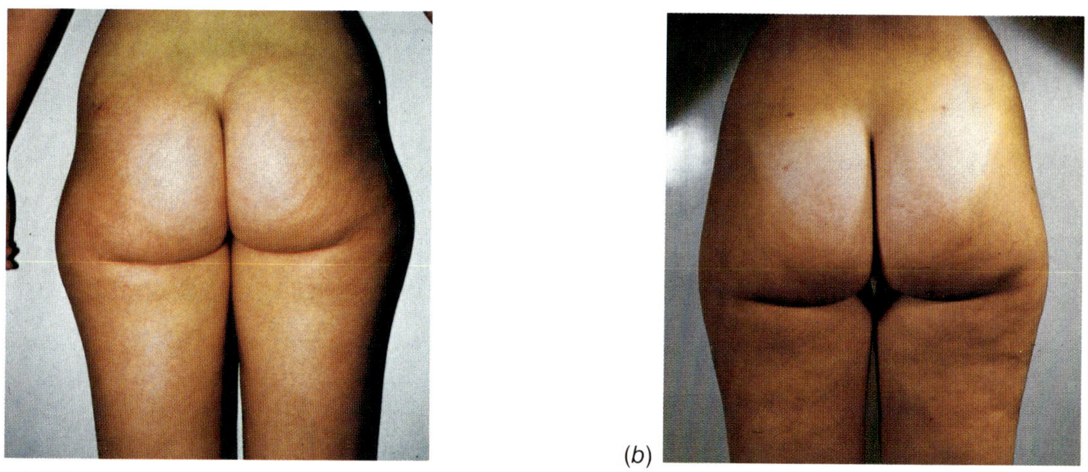

FIGURE 12
(*a*) Saddlebags before; (*b*) 6 months later.

FIGURE 13
(*a*) Hips before; (*b*) after 150 cc were removed, 6 months later.

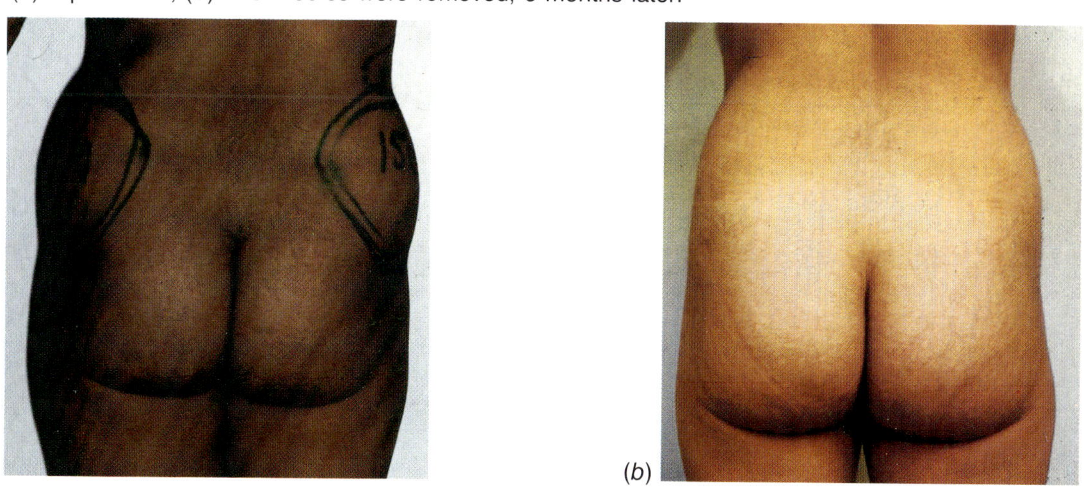

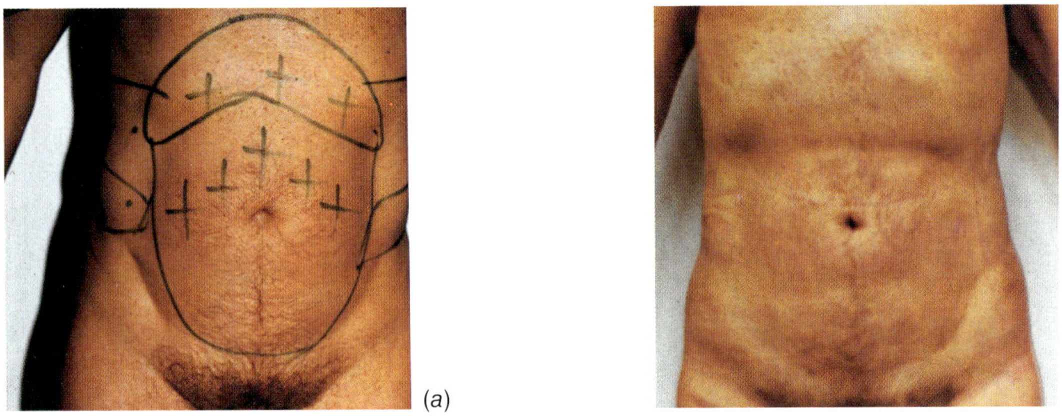

(a) (b)

FIGURE 14
(*a*) Abdomen and waist before; (*b*) after 400 cc were removed.

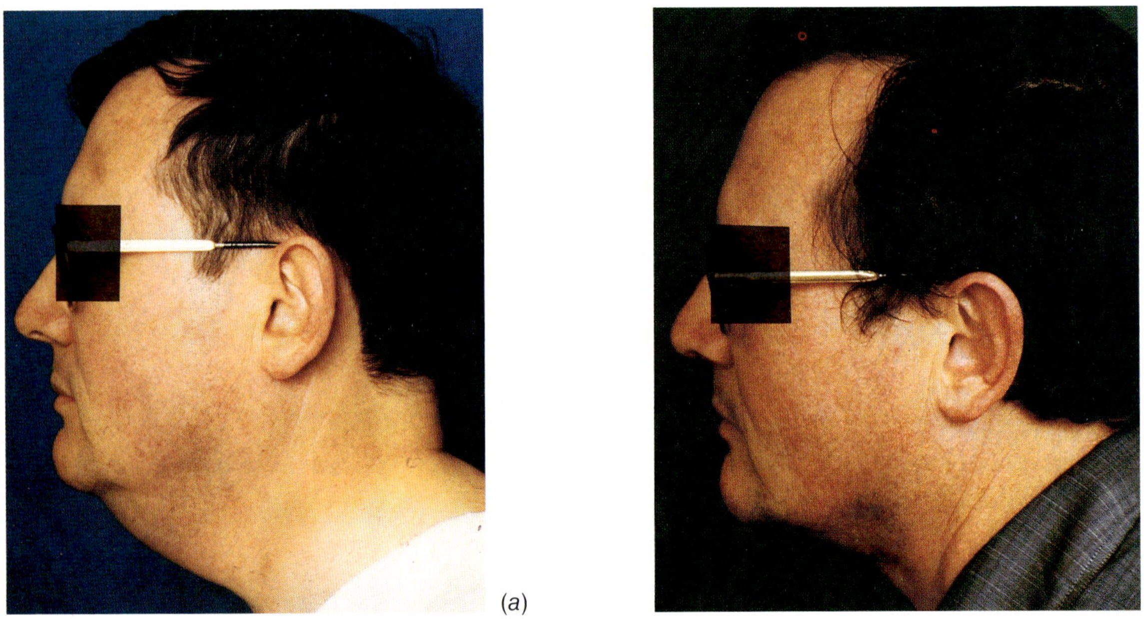

(a) (b)

FIGURE 15
(*a*) Liposculpturing of the neck and jowls before; (*b*) 6 months later.

REFERENCES

1. Illouz YG. Body contouring by lipolysis: A 5-year experience with over 3000 cases. Plast Reconstr Surg. 1983;72:591–597.
2. Fournier P, Otteni R. Lipodissection in body sculpturing: The dry procedure. Plast Reconstr Surg. 1983;72:598–609.
3. Newman J, Dolsky RL. Lipo-suction surgery: History and development. J Dermatol Surg Oncol. 1984;10:467–469.
4. Fournier PF. Liposculpture: ma technique. Paris: Arnette editeur, 1989.
5. Grazer FM. Suction-assisted lipectomy, suction lipectomy, liplysis, and lipexeresis. Plast Reconstr Surg. 1983;72:620–623.

Index